Reoperative Urology

Reoperative Urology

EDITED BY

Marc S. Cohen, M.D.

Associate Professor of Surgery, Division of Urology,
University of Florida College of Medicine;
Attending Urologist, Shands Teaching Hospital and
Veterans Affairs Medical Center, Gainesville, Florida

Martin I. Resnick, M.D.

Lester Persky Professor and Chairman,
Department of Urology,
Case Western Reserve University School of Medicine;
Director, Department of Urology,
University Hospitals of Cleveland, Cleveland

Little, Brown and Company

BOSTON   NEW YORK   TORONTO   LONDON

Library of Congress Cataloging-in-Publication Data

Reoperative urology/edited by Marc S. Cohen, Martin I. Resnick.
    p. cm.
    Includes bibliographical references and index.
    ISBN 0-316-74061-6
    1. Genitourinary organs—Reoperation. I. Cohen, Marc S.
II. Resnick, Martin I.
    [DNLM: 1. Urologic Diseases—surgery. 2. Urogenital Diseases—
surgery, 3. Reoperation—methods. WJ 168 R424 1994]
RD671,R45 1994
S 17.4'601—dc20
DNLM/DLC
for Library of Congress   94-26648
                                       CIP

Printed in the United States of America

MV-NY

Editorial: Nancy E. Chorpenning, Kristin Odmark
Production Editor: Cathleen Cote
Copyeditor: Jim Madru
Indexer: Michael Loo
Production Services: Textbook Writers Associates
Designer: Marty Tenney
Cover Designer: Linda Dana Willis

To Kris, Miriam, Michael, and Stephen
To Vicki, Andy, Missy, and Jeff
To our patients, parents, and publisher

*Their boundless courage in the uncharted
realms of life has provided us all with
insight and illumination.*

Contents

Contributing Authors

Mark C. Adams, M.D.

Assistant Professor of Urology, Indiana University School of Medicine; Attending Urologist, James Whitcomb Riley Hospital for Children, Indianapolis
28. Complications of Ureterosigmoidostomy

Lynn Banowsky, M.D.

Clinical Professor of Surgery, Division of Urology, University of Texas Medical School at San Antonio; Director, Renal Transplant Program, San Antonio Regional Hospital, San Antonio
2. Vascular Complications of Renal Transplantation

Arnold M. Belker, M.D.

Clinical Professor of Surgery, Division of Urology, University of Louisville School of Medicine, Louisville, Kentucky
21. The Failed Vasovasostomy/Vasoepididymostomy

Mitchell C. Benson, M.D.

Associate Professor of Urology, Columbia University College of Physicians and Surgeons; Director, Urologic Oncology, Columbia-Presbyterian Medical Center, New York
27. Complications of Continent Urinary Diversion

Anthony A. Caldamone, M.D.

Professor of Surgery, Division of Urology, Brown University School of Medicine; Director, Pediatric Urology, Rhode Island Hospital, Providence, Rhode Island
5. Failed Pyeloplasty

Culley C. Carson III, M.D.

Professor and Chief of Urology, University of North Carolina at Chapel Hill School of Medicine, Chapel Hill, North Carolina
7. Ureteral Calculi

Christopher Chapple, M.D.

Honorary Senior Lecturer, University of Sheffield Medical School; Consultant Urological Surgeon, Department of Urology, The Royal Hallamshire Hospital, Sheffield, England
14. Urethral Stricture

Marc S. Cohen, M.D.

Associate Professor of Surgery, Division of Urology, University of Florida College of Medicine; Attending Urologist, Shands Teaching Hospital and Veterans Affairs Medical Center, Gainesville, Florida
9. Extrinsic Ureteral Obstruction (Including Retroperitoneal Fibrosis)

Thomas W. Coleman, M.D.

Clinical Associate Professor of Urology, University of South Alabama School of Medicine, Mobile, Alabama
26. Complications Associated with Ileal and Colon Conduits

Charles J. Devine, Jr., M.D.

Professor of Urology, Eastern Virginia Medical School; Director, Devine Center for Genitourinary Reconstruction, Sentara Norfolk General Hospital, Norfolk, Virginia
19. Peyronie's Disease

John P. Donohue, M.D.

Professor of Urology, Indiana University School of Medicine; Chairman, Department of Urology, Indiana University Hospital, Indianapolis
23. Residual Lymphadenopathy after Surgery, Chemotherapy, or Radiation Therapy

Michael J. Droller, M.D.

Professor of Urology, Mount Sinai School of Medicine of the City University of New York; Chairman, Department of Urology, The Mount Sinai Medical Center, New York
11. Bladder Cancer

John W. Duckett, Jr., M.D.

Professor of Urology, University of Pennsylvania School of Medicine; Director, Pediatric Urology, Children's Hospital of Philadelphia, Philadelphia
16. Failed Hypospadias Repair

Jack S. Elder, M.D.

Professor of Urology and Pediatrics, Case Western Reserve University School of Medicine; Director, Pediatric Urology, Rainbow Babies and Children's Hospital, Cleveland
22. The Failed Orchiopexy

Deborah R. Erickson, M.D.

Assistant Professor of Surgery, Pennsylvania State University College of Medicine; Attending Surgeon, Division of Urology, Milton S. Hershey Medical Center, Hershey, Pennsylvania
15. Stress Incontinence

David Esrig, M.D.

Assistant Professor of Surgery, Section of Urology, Yale University School of Medicine, New Haven, Connecticut
8. Ureteral Strictures

Richard S. Foster, M.D.

Associate Professor of Urology, Indiana University School of Medicine; Attending Surgeon, Urology Department, Indiana University Hospital, Indianapolis
23. Residual Lymphadenopathy after Surgery, Chemotherapy, or Radiation Therapy

Jackson E. Fowler, Jr., M.D.

Professor and Chairman of Urology, University of Mississippi School of Medicine; Attending Surgeon, Division of Urology, University of Mississippi Medical Center, Jackson, Mississippi
1. Renal Cancer

Edmond T. Gonzales, Jr., M.D.

Professor of Urology, Baylor College of Medicine; Head, Department of Surgery and Chief, Urology Service, Texas Children's Hospital, Houston
29. Vesicostomy, Ureterostomy, and Pyelostomy

C. William Hinnant, Jr., M.D.

Attending Physician, Department of Urology, Anderson Area Medical Center, Anderson, South Carolina
3. Nonvascular Complications of Renal Transplantation

Jeffry L. Huffman, M.D.

Associate Professor of Urology, University of Southern California School of Medicine, Los Angeles
8. Ureteral Strictures

Charles Lee Jackson, M.D.

Chairman, Department of Urology, The Cleveland Clinic, Fort Lauderdale, Florida
4. Renovascular Complications Unrelated to Renal Transplantation

Gerald H. Jordan, M.D.

Professor of Urology, Eastern Virginia Medical School; Attending Surgeon, Sentara Norfolk General Hospital, Norfolk, Virginia
19. Peyronie's Disease

Evan J. Kass. M.D.

Chief, Division of Pediatric Urology, William Beaumont Hospital, Royal Oak, Michigan
10. Recurrent Vesicoureteral Reflux

Aaron E. Katz, M.D.

Assistant Professor of Urology, Columbia University College of Physicians and Surgeons; Assistant Urologist, Columbia-Presbyterian Medical Center, New York
27. Complications of Continent Urinary Diversion

Michael A. Keating, M.D.

Assistant Professor of Urology, Indiana University School of Medicine; Attending Pediatric Urologist, James Whitcomb Riley Hospital for Children, Indianapolis
16. Failed Hypospadias Repair

Lowell R. King, M.D.

Professor of Surgery and Pediatrics, Duke University School of Medicine; Head, Section of Pediatric Urology, Duke University Medical Center, Durham, North Carolina
12. Exstrophy of the Bladder

R. Lawrence Kroovand, M.D.

Professor of Surgery, Division of Pediatric Urology, Bowman Gray School of Medicine of Wake Forest University; Head, Section on Pediatric, Adolescent, and Reconstructive Urology, North Carolina Baptist Hospital, Winston-Salem, North Carolina
17. Complications of Neonatal Circumcision

Elroy D. Kursh, M.D.

Professor of Urology, Case Western Reserve University School of Medicine; Attending Urologist, University Hospitals of Cleveland, Cleveland
13. Vesicovaginal Fistulas

Russell K. Lawson, M.D.

Professor and Chairman of Urology, Medical College of Wisconsin; Attending Urologist, Froedtert Memorial Lutheran Hospital, Milwaukee
24. Prostatectomy for Benign Disease

Ronald W. Lewis, M.D.

Professor of Urology, Mayo Medical School; Consultant in Urology, Mayo Clinic, Rochester, Minnesota
20. Failure of the Penile Prosthesis

John A. Libertino, M.D.

Assistant Clinical Professor of Surgery, Harvard Medical School, Boston; Chairman of Surgery and Chairman of Urology, Lahey Clinic, Burlington, Massachusetts
26. Complications Associated with Ileal and Colon Conduits

William R. Morgan, M.D.

Staff Urologist, Urology Center, Richmond, Virginia
20. Failure of the Penile Prosthesis

Andrew C. Novick, M.D.

Chairman, Department of Urology, The Cleveland Clinic Hospital, Cleveland
4. Renovascular Complications Unrelated to Renal Transplantation

Carl A. Olsson, M.D.

Professor and Chairman of Urology, Columbia University College of Physicians and Surgeons; Attending Urologist, Columbia-Presbyterian Medical Center, New York
27. Complications of Continent Urinary Diversion

Louis L. Pisters, M.D.

Faculty Associate, Department of Urology, The University of Texas M. D. Anderson Cancer Center, Houston
9. Extrinsic Ureteral Obstruction (Including Retroperitoneal Fibrosis)

J. Edson Pontes, M.D.

Professor and Chairman of Urology, Wayne State University School of Medicine, Detroit
25. Radical Prostatectomy

Shlomo Raz, M.D.

Professor of Urology, Department of Surgery, University of California, Los Angeles, UCLA School of Medicine, Los Angeles
15. Stress Incontinence

Martin I. Resnick, M.D.

Lester Persky Professor and Chairman, Department of Urology, Case Western Reserve University School of Medicine; Director, Department of Urology, University Hospitals of Cleveland, Cleveland
6. Stone Surgery

Alan B. Retik, M.D.

Professor of Surgery, Division of Urology, Harvard Medical School; Chief, Division of Urology, Children's Hospital, Boston
28. Complications of Ureterosigmoidostomy

Arthur I. Sagalowsky, M.D.

Professor of Urology, University of Texas Southwestern Medical Center at Dallas, Dallas
3. Nonvascular Complications of Renal Transplantation

Steven M. Schlossberg, M.D.

Associate Professor, Departments of Urology and Anatomy, Eastern Virginia Medical School, Norfolk, Virginia
19. Peyronie's Disease

Ernest M. Sussman, M.D.

Clinical Fellow, Division of Urology, University of California, Los Angeles, UCLA School of Medicine, Los Angeles
15. Stress Incontinence

Samuel T. Thompson, M.D.

Methodist Hospital Advanced Fertility Institute, Indianapolis
6. Stone Surgery

Richard Turner-Warwick, C.B.C., F.R.C.P., F.R.C.S., F.R.C.O.G.

Professor of Reconstructive Surgery, Emeritus Surgeon, The Middlesex Hospital, London
14. Urethral Stricture

Chester C. Winter, M.D.

Professor Emeritus of Urology, Ohio State University College of Medicine, Columbus, Ohio
18. Priapism

August Zabbo, M.D.

Assistant Professor of Surgery, Division of Urology, Brown University School of Medicine; Chief of Urology, Rhode Island Hospital, Providence, Rhode Island
5. Failed Pyeloplasty

Preface

Library shelves teem with textbooks describing the pathophysiology of urologic disease processes and techniques for surgical intervention. What we have found to be lacking is information regarding those situations in which previous intervention has produced less than optimal results and reoperation is felt to be necessary. This book was initiated to address this deficiency. We hope it will benefit urology trainees as well as attending urologists with years of experience who must confront and manage unexpected complications of urologic surgery.

Reoperative procedures can be difficult for all concerned. For patients and their families, it is a time when feelings of hope of improvement after prior surgery may be replaced with fear, frustration, and anger. Similar feelings may be experienced by the surgical team. Experience dictates that reoperative surgery is rarely easier or as clear cut as the "first time in."

We believe that a textbook dealing specifically with reoperative techniques is therefore appropriate. This book is not intended to be a comprehensive textbook of urology or an atlas of operative technique; we have chosen rather to focus on management strategies for selected problems in urologic surgery that can necessitate reoperation. In preparing this text, we were fortunate to enlist authors with experience and expertise in a wide range of reoperative techniques. To these expert individuals we are most grateful. We have encouraged each author to provide his or her own unique approach to a variety of reoperative scenarios. If the reader is able to identify a technique or approach that makes a particular reoperative procedure less stressful for either the surgeon or the patient, and achieves a successful outcome for both, then our intent in preparing this text will be fulfilled.

M.S.C.
M.I.R.

Reoperative Urology

Notice

The indications and dosages of all drugs in this book have been recommended in the medical literature and conform to the practices of the general medical community. The medications described do not necessarily have specific approval by the Food and Drug Administration for use in the diseases and dosages for which they are recommended. The package insert for each drug should be consulted for use and dosage as approved by the FDA. Because standards for usage change, it is advisable to keep abreast of revised recommendations, particularly those concerning new drugs.

Renal Cancer

JACKSON E. FOWLER, JR.

Renal cell carcinomas affect about 24,000 men and women in the United States each year. In a majority of cases the tumors are not associated with distant metastases at the time of diagnosis and are managed by radical nephrectomy. This procedure, which involves removal of the entire kidney, upper ureter, ipsilateral adrenal gland and surrounding perinephric fat, and Gerota's fascia, is curative in about 50 percent of patients. Parameters that predispose to treatment failure include regional lymph node metastases, tumor infiltration beyond the renal capsule, and tumor extension into the inferior vena cava. Postoperative radiation therapy or chemotherapy does not improve the survival of patients with these unfavorable tumor characteristics. In addition, biologic response modifiers which have some activity against metastatic renal cancer, such as interleukin 2 (IL-2) and LAK cells, IL-2 alone, or γ-interferon, have not as yet proved useful in the adjuvant setting.

Persistent cancer after a radical nephrectomy is most often manifested by lung or bone metastases within 1 to 2 years of surgery. The metastases are usually multiple and preclude operative intervention as primary treatment. In about 10 percent of cases, however, the persistent disease is localized to the renal fossa, and excision of the mass, or a "reoperation," is a reasonable therapeutic option.

A partial nephrectomy is an alternative surgical treatment for renal cell carcinomas that are located in the periphery or polar regions of the kidney. About 5 percent of patients who are managed with this operative technique, however, will develop a local recurrence, and about 20 percent will develop distant metastases with or without coexisting local recurrences. Incomplete exci-

sion of the recognized lesion, nonapparent multifocality of the tumor within the kidney, regional lymph node metastases, and subclinical distant metastases are responsible for these treatment failures. The indications for "reoperations" due to persistent disease are the same as those following a radical nephrectomy. However, since local recurrences are usually contiguous with the remnant kidney that in most cases was spared because of severe dysfunction, absence, or tumor involvement of the contralateral kidney, and because the size of local recurrences at the time of diagnosis is often small, excision of recurrent disease alone and excision of the recurrent disease and the remnant kidney are both therapeutic options.

The adverse impact of recurrent cancer on ultimate longevity requires no discussion, and the advisability of a partial nephrectomy that may result in incomplete local tumor control has been the subject of considerable debate and commentary. Few would argue that the operation deserves careful consideration in elderly patients with bilateral tumors or a functionally solitary kidney that contains an easily resectable peripheral cancer, because the morbidity and mortality of dialysis probably outweigh the risks of recurrent disease. The procedure also may be reasonable in younger patients when the tumor is only 1 or 2 cm in diameter and a generous tumor-free margin can be achieved with absolute certainty or in young patients with von Hippel–Lindau's disease and unilateral or bilateral tumors. However, the advisability of "nephron-sparing" surgery in younger patients with a functionally solitary kidney and a tumor that is not clearly amenable to partial excision or in any patient with a normal contralateral kidney is questionable at best. In the former circumstances, transplantation is usually feasible if the patient remains free of disease for 6 to 12 months. In the latter situation, the threat of recurrent cancer is of substantially greater concern than the theoretical possibility of impaired renal function from hyperperfusion of a solitary kidney or the remote possibility of irreparable damage to the remaining kidney from traumatic injury, renovascular disease, or calculogenesis. Indeed, I have always been intrigued by urologic surgeons who favor partial nephrectomies in patients with a normal contralateral kidney but have no concern about the sequelae of a nephrectomy that is performed for the purpose of living-related kidney transplantation.

This chapter focuses on surgery for locally recurrent renal cell carcinoma after a radical or partial nephrectomy. Operative intervention also may be warranted in selected patients to remove solitary pulmonary, brain, or bony metastases that develop after excision of the primary lesion. These procedures may be of symptomatic benefit or extend longevity but are customarily performed by other surgical subspecialists.

Reoperations after a Radical Nephrectomy

Local tumor recurrences after a radical nephrectomy are characteristically advanced at the time of diagnosis. This reflects the lack of symptomatology that accompanies most retroperitoneal masses and the infrequency with which the retroperitoneum is monitored during postoperative surveillance. Most patients present with low back pain due to tumor infiltration of the posterior abdominal wall, gastrointestinal symptomatology due to bowel obstruction, and such systemic complaints as weight loss and lethargy. A hard, fixed mass is often palpable on careful examination of the abdomen.

The diagnosis is established with computed tomography (CT) or magnetic resonance imaging (MRI), and a thorough extent of disease evaluation is undertaken to rule out distant metastases that by and large contraindicate excision of the local disease. The components of this workup include a complete physical examination, bone scan, and CT of the chest and abdomen. CT of the brain is also warranted if there are symptoms or signs of cerebral metastases.

Primary renal tumors and their metastases are characteristically hypervascular, and an arteriogram is performed routinely to provide a road map of the arterial blood supply of the lesion. In some cases the mass is perfused in large part by branches of the lumbar, gonadal, and iliac arteries that can be embolized before surgery or ligated and secured before attacking the mass

during surgical exploration. In a limited experience with recurrent local cancer after a radical nephrectomy, however, a well-defined arterial supply has not been demonstrable. The arteriogram is also a sensitive tool for assessing invasion of the bowel or intraabdominal viscera because renal cell carcinomas often parasitize the vasculature of the organ that they infiltrate (Fig. 1-1). A barium examination of the small and large bowels is performed if intestinal invasion is at all suspect, and MRI or inferior vena cavography is performed if tumor invasion of the vena cava is a possibility.

Patient Preparation

Most patients with recurrent renal cancer are middle-aged or elderly, and preoperative evaluation by an internist is warranted to optimize the control of chronic cardiac, respiratory, and metabolic diseases. In addition, medical complications of the surgery or medical diseases that are exacerbated by the surgery are managed more effectively if the internist is already familiar with the patient. When a major vascular reconstruction is a contingency but the urologist's skill with this work is limited, a vascular surgeon should be consulted before the operation and should be available to assist during the procedure.

The candidate for surgical exploration is thoroughly counseled about the potential morbidity and mortality of the operation and must consent to removal of adjacent viscera. The necessity for an intestinal resection usually cannot be established before surgery, and a complete mechanical and antibiotic bowel preparation is always warranted. For the same reason, a perioperative antimicrobial regimen consisting of an aminoglycoside, ampicillin, and parenteral metronidazole is begun on the evening before the operation as prophylaxis against wound infection. Full-length hose or pneumatic compression boots are applied to reduce venostasis in the lower extremities, and minidose heparin is administered if the patient is at high risk for thromboembolic complications. Supplemental parenteral hyperalimentation is advisable if there is severe debility, and a pneumococcal vaccine is given if the mass lies adjacent to the spleen and a splenectomy may be necessary for a satisfactory resection.

Four to six units of packed red blood cells should be available to replace the often prodigious intraoperative blood loss, and arrangements should be made to have an autotransfusion device available at the time of surgery. An arterial line and a Swan-Ganz catheter are routinely used to monitor the hemodynamic response to abrupt intraoperative hemorrhage and to facilitate fluid man-

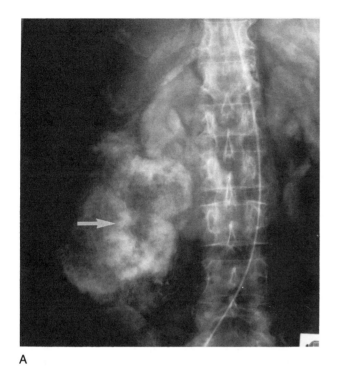
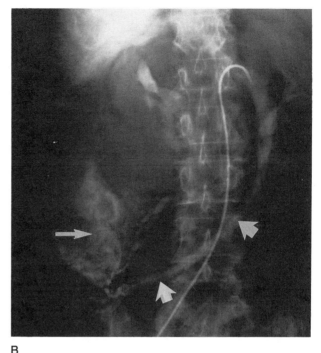

A   B

Figure 1-1. *Parasitization of mesenteric vessels by a primary right renal cell carcinoma. A. The early phase of the arteriogram shows the hypervascular tumor* (arrow). *B. The late phase shows contrast material within the tumor* (left arrow) *and in the inferior mesenteric vein* (right arrow).

agement in the early postoperative period, and a urethral catheter is introduced at the time of surgery to monitor the urinary output.

Operative Technique

The retroperitoneum is approached through a generous transperitoneal midline or thoracoabdominal incision. The latter is always advisable if the mass occupies the upper retroperitoneum. To exploit the cephalad exposure provided by the thoracoabdominal approach, the thoracic cavity is routinely entered through the eighth or ninth rib bed or intercostal space.

After entry of the abdominal cavity, the viscera are inspected and palpated to identify unsuspected metastases or invasion of the mesenteric bowel, liver, spleen, or female reproductive organs. In the absence of metastatic disease, however, the feasibility of a complete resection usually cannot be established until the anterior aspect of the mass has been exposed and an attempt is made to establish planes of dissection between the tumor and contiguous retroperitoneal structures.

Laterally placed masses that are not bulky often can be exposed satisfactorily by medial reflection of the colon. However, if extensive midline exposure is required

for the management of masses that abut the aorta or vena cava, the posterior peritoneum from the cecum to the ligament of Treitz is incised, and the cecum and ascending colon are reflected superiorly (Fig. 1-2). Adherence of the mass to the colonic mesentery should be anticipated, and the mesentery is routinely excised en bloc with the tumor if there is any evidence of invasion (Fig. 1-3). This maneuver will rarely lead to colonic ischemia if the marginal artery is preserved. In addition, cephalad exposure of tumors that extend into the upper left retroperitoneum is enhanced by dividing the peritoneum lateral and superior to the spleen and reflecting the splenic flexure, the spleen, and the tail of the pancreas medially.

The need for en bloc resection of the large bowel, the spleen, or the tail of the pancreas or invasion or encasement of the porta hepatis, superior mesenteric artery, or duodenum is generally recognized at this stage of the procedure. The latter findings usually mandate abandonment of the resection because a grossly incomplete excision has little or no therapeutic benefit and merely leads to excessive blood loss and an increased incidence of postoperative complications.

Attention is then turned to the medial and posterior aspects of the dissection. Masses that encroach on the

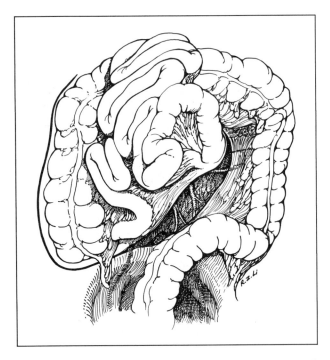

Figure 1-2. *The posterior peritoneum is incised, and the ascending colon and small bowel are reflected superiorly to expose midline masses. (Reproduced with permission from Fowler, JE, Jr. Manual of Urologic Surgery. Boston: Little, Brown, 1990.)*

great vessels are peeled from the adventitia, taking care to identify and ligate lumbar arteries and veins. If a satisfactory plane cannot be established, excision of the infrarenal aorta and replacement with a synthetic graft or ligation and resection of the infrarenal vena cava may be warranted. The latter, however, can lead to significant postoperative morbidity and should be undertaken only when the prospects of complete tumor resection are great.

Local recurrences after a radical nephrectomy arise next to the musculature of the posterior abdominal wall, and tumor infiltration should be anticipated. The posterior dissection, therefore, encompasses the superficial psoas or quadratus lumborum muscle (Fig. 1-4). This maneuver does not lead to functional impairment and is probably accompanied by less bleeding than a posterior dissection immediately adjacent to a hypervascular mass.

The retroperitoneum is liberally irrigated with sterile water after the surgical specimen is removed, and residual bleeders are secured with hemostatic clips or suture ligatures. Water lyses red blood cells and facilitates the identification of bleeding arteries and veins. When feasible, the tumor bed is covered with the colonic mesentery, and the posterior peritoneal incisions are

approximated with interrupted sutures. The small bowel is then repositioned in the abdominal cavity, and the wound is closed in the standard manner with heavy nylon or 28-gauge wire sutures. Drainage of the retroperitoneum is rarely indicated.

Complications and Results

The incidence of postoperative complications and the duration of convalescence are directly related to the age and general medical condition of the patient and to the magnitude of the operative procedure. Potential complications that are shared by all major transabdominal or retroperitoneal operations include bleeding, abscess, venous thrombosis with pulmonary embolism, cardiac events, and intestinal obstruction. Colonic ischemia due to excision of the mesentery may lead to diarrhea or crampy abdominal pain but is unusual if the marginal arteries are preserved.

Meaningful data concerning the therapeutic benefit of reoperations for local tumor recurrence after a radical nephrectomy are not available. However, because of the probability of subclinical distant metastases and of the general observation that the constraints of solid tumors usually exceed the borders of the visible lesion, the likelihood of cure is limited at best. Death within 1 to 2 years of surgery is the rule if the operation is not curative. The thoughtful surgeon will always keep these dismal realities in mind during the resection and avoid heroic attempts to excise a mass that cannot be removed in its entirety.

Reoperations after a Partial Nephrectomy

The size of recurrent local tumor after a partial nephrectomy is characteristically less than after a radical nephrectomy and in one series was reported to range from 3 to 8 cm only (Fig. 1-5). This reflects an understandable concern about the risk of recurrent disease and the routine use of ultrasonography and CT for postoperative surveillance of the remnant kidney. In addition, hematuria may be the first sign of recurrent cancer, a finding that is not seen in patients with local recurrences after a radical nephrectomy. Excision of the tumor only is not unreasonable if the lesion is amenable to local resection with generous tumor-free margins and the considerations that prompted the initial partial nephrectomy remain relevant and compelling. Sacrifice of the remaining normal renal tissue, however, is always warranted when the contralateral kidney is normal or complete

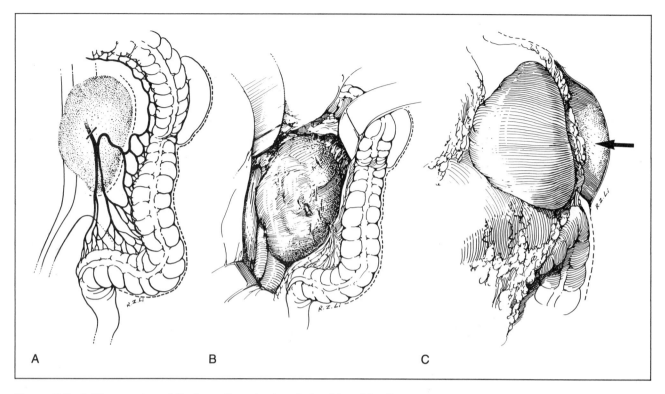

Figure 1-3. *A. The mesentery of the descending colon is excised en bloc with adherent recurrent tumor masses. B. Exposure of the left retroperitoneum is enhanced by incising the left paracolic gutter and the peritoneum superolateral to the spleen. C. This permits medial reflection of the colon, spleen, and tail of the pancreas. (Reproduced with permission from Fowler, JE, Jr. Manual of Urologic Surgery. Boston: Little, Brown, 1990.)*

excision of the recurrence is not possible without a nephrectomy.

The presence or absence of distant metastases is assessed with CT of the abdomen and chest and with a bone scan. As a general rule, distant metastases contraindicate surgical intervention unless there are solitary lesions that also can be excised. Renal angiography is advisable for diagnostic purposes and is mandatory to assess the extent of the lesion and the relationship of the cancer to the normal renal vasculature if excision of the tumor only is contemplated. MRI or inferior vena cavography is performed if tumor extension into the inferior vena cava is at all suspect.

Patient Preparation

The preparation of a patient for excision of the local recurrence and remnant kidney parallels that of a radical nephrectomy and is by and large limited to a mechanical bowel preparation and measures that will reduce the risks of thrombophlebitis. Tumor invasion of adjacent viscera or musculature is uncommon because the le-

sions are usually not extensive and are encompassed by Gerota's fascia that is draped over the kidney after the initial partial resection.

When excision of the recurrent cancer only is planned, arrangements should be made to have iced saline slush available at the time of surgery for renal cooling during the obligatory period of renal artery occlusion. Similarly, the materials and perfusate needed for ex vivo renal surgery must be available if this technique is a contingency. The patient with an absent or severely impaired contralateral kidney must accept the inevitability of dialytic treatments if the remnant kidney is to be removed and the possibility of temporary dialysis if excision of the recurrent cancer only is anticipated. It is helpful to make preparations for dialysis before the operative event.

Operative Techniques

The basic technique for removal of the recurrent tumor and remnant kidney parallels that of a primary radical nephrectomy. The kidney is approached in a trans-

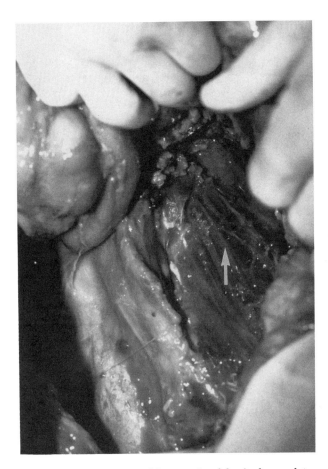

Figure 1-4. *Appearance of the posterior abdominal musculature after excision of the superficial psoas muscle* (arrow). *(Reproduced with permission from Fowler, JE, Jr. Operations for primary retroperitoneal tumors. In JE Fowler, Jr (ed), Mastery of Surgery: Urologic Surgery. Boston: Little, Brown, 1991.)*

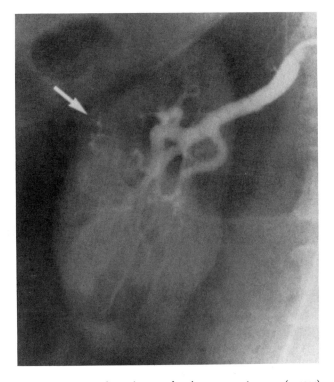

Figure 1-5. *Renal arteriogram showing recurrent cancer* (arrow) *after a partial nephrectomy for renal cell carcinoma. (Reproduced with permission from Novick, AC, and Straffon, RA. Management of locally recurrent renal cell carcinoma after partial nephrectomy. J Urol 138:607, 1987.)*

peritoneal fashion through a subcostal, midline, or thoracoabdominal incision. After careful inspection of the intraabdominal viscera, the renal vessels are exposed through an incision in the posterior peritoneum medial to the inferior mesenteric vein (Fig. 1-6). The artery and vein are then sequentially isolated and ligated to reduce the risks of brisk blood loss while manipulating the kidney and the theoretical possibility of hematogenous dissemination of malignant cells. The tumor-bearing kidney is then exposed by medial reflection of the ascending or descending colon. The plane between the colonic mesentery and the kidney may be difficult to establish due to prior surgery, but sacrifice of the mesentery because of suspected tumor invasion is rarely necessary unless the mass lesion is bulky.

I prefer to mobilize the inferior, inferomedial, and posterior aspects of the kidney before the superior and superomedial aspects. With this approach, the dissec-

tion adjacent to the adrenal gland is performed last, and control of troublesome bleeding is simplified because the specimen can be removed quickly. For the same reason, there may be some benefit to addressing the tumor-bearing portion of the kidney after the remainder of the surgical specimen has been mobilized to facilitate the control of bleeding from vessels that are parasitized by the tumor from adjacent musculature or viscera. Regardless of one's preference with respect to the sequence of the surgery, however, the plane of dissection is maintained superficial to Gerota's fascia throughout the operation.

The ureter and gonadal vessels are identified at the pelvic brim, individually ligated with nonabsorbable sutures, and transected. The ureter with surrounding fat and Gerota's fascia is then freed to the lower pole of the kidney, and a plane is established between the posterior Gerota's fascia and the quadratus lumborum and psoas muscles. The dissection is then extended to the medial border of the psoas muscle, the ureter and lower pole of the kidney are retracted laterally, and the medial fibrous and nodal tissues adjacent to the aorta or vena cava are

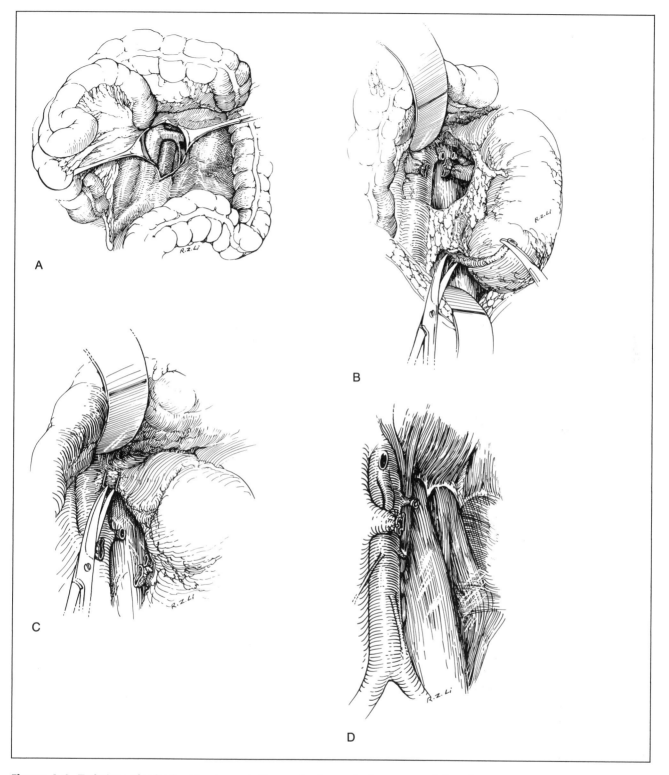

Figure 1-6. *Technique of radical nephrectomy. A. The renal artery and vein are exposed through an incision of the posterior peritoneum. B. After reflection of the colon and transection of the ureter, infero-medial fibrous tissue is divided to the level of the renal vessels. C. The adrenal vasculature is controlled with hemostatic clips and divided before the surgical specimen is removed. D. Appearance of retro-peritoneum after a left radical nephrectomy. (Reproduced with permission from Fowler, JE. Manual of Urologic Surgery. Boston: Little, Brown, 1990.)*

incised to the level of the previously transected renal vessels.

The superior aspect of Gerota's fascia above the adrenal gland is dissected from the diaphragm, taking care to avoid splenic or hepatic injury from overzealous retraction. Working medially, the adrenal arteries and veins are identified and secured with ligatures or hemostatic clips. Gerota's fascia above the renal vessels is then freed from the aorta or vena cava and the surgical specimen is removed. After the renal fossa is liberally irrigated with sterile water and residual bleeders are identified and ligated, the posterior peritoneal and paracolic incisions are closed with interrupted sutures. Drainage of the renal fossa is not necessary.

The rationale for a regional lymphadenectomy during a primary tumor nephrectomy or a secondary nephrectomy is arguable. If undertaken, however, the appropriate superior level of the dissection is the origin of the superior mesenteric artery, and the appropriate inferior level is the origin of the inferior mesenteric artery. For right-sided tumors, tissue lateral to the vena cava and between the vena cava and aorta is removed, and for left-sided tumors, tissue lateral to the aorta and between the aorta and vena cava is removed.

The technique for excision of a local recurrence only parallels that of a standard partial nephrectomy. However, since preservation of the remnant kidney can be justified only if the contralateral kidney is nonfunctional or absent, extreme care must be taken to avoid ischemic injury throughout the operation. The risks of acute tubular necrosis are greater with ex vivo surgery than with in situ surgery, and the latter is always recommended unless technically impossible. In addition, obliteration of normal tissue planes due to the previous surgery should be anticipated, and it is preferable to approach the kidney through a transperitoneal incision. This facilitates isolation of the renal vessels and reduces the risks of injury to the normal renal parenchyma.

The renal artery is exposed using the techniques described for a secondary nephrectomy and secured with a vessel loop. The colon is then reflected medially, and the kidney and encompassing Gerota's fascia are isolated in their entirety. A plastic sheet is then draped around the renal pedicle to hold the iced slush. I prefer to use a Lahey intestinal bag that is open on the bottom and secured around the renal pedicle by tightening the straps on the top. Gerota's fascia is incised adjacent to the palpable interface of the tumor and normal renal parenchyma so that fat and fascia overlying the lesion can be removed en bloc with the tumor. Whenever possible, the line of excision is made along the antici-

pated margins of the segmental arterial supply to the kidney. Delineation of the superior or inferior renal segments can be achieved by isolation and temporary occlusion of the corresponding segmental artery.

The renal artery is occluded with a noncrushing bulldog clamp, and the plastic drape is filled with iced saline slush. Cooling of the kidney in this manner reduces metabolic requirements, and acute tubular necrosis is uncommon despite $1/2$ to 1 hour of total ischemia. After excision of the tumor with sharp dissection, the surgical specimen is assessed with frozen-section examination to determine the adequacy of the surgical margins. Transected calyces are then oversewn with a continuous fine absorbable suture (Fig. 1-7), and the arterial clamp is released to permit identification and ligation of residual bleeders. The denuded renal parenchyma is covered with vascularized omentum or a patch of peritoneum. Nephrostomy drainage is prudent if there is concern about the integrity of the closure of the collecting system.

Figure 1-7. *Secondary partial nephrectomy for recurrent cancer. After the tumor is excised, the collecting system is closed with a fine continuous absorbable suture, and residual bleeding vessels are ligated. The denuded renal parenchyma is covered with a patch of peritoneum or vascularized omentum. (Reproduced with permission from Fowler, JE.* Manual of Urologic Surgery. *Boston: Little, Brown, 1990.)*

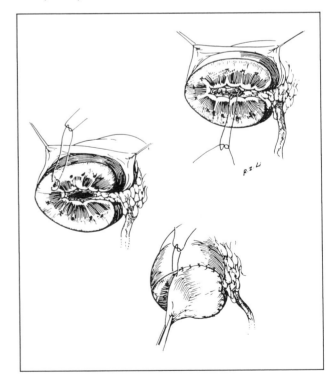

Complications and Results

There is no evidence that the operative morbidity of a secondary partial or total nephrectomy for local recurrences is substantially greater than that of a primary operation of equivalent magnitude. However, subsequent disease-free survival is usually complicated by the side effects of dialytic therapy or renal transplantation if an anticipated or unexpected sequela of the surgery is severe renal insufficiency.

The groups at the Cleveland Clinic and at the Mayo Clinic have reported on the efficacy of partial nephrectomy for renal cell carcinoma and the fate of patients with recurrent local tumor only. In the Cleveland Clinic series, 23 of 100 patients had recurrent cancer. The treatment failures were manifested by a local recurrence alone in 5 patients, a local recurrence and distant metastases in 4 patients, and distant metastases only in 14 patients. The 5 recurrences that were confined to the renal remnant were detected 3 to 6 years (mean 4.6 years) after the initial surgery. Each of the patients with a local recurrence only underwent a secondary operation with apparent complete excision of the residual tumor. Two of 3 patients who were treated with a repeat partial nephrectomy developed subsequent recurrences but were alive at the time of the report, and 1 was free of disease 6 months after surgery. Of 2 patients managed with a nephrectomy, 1 was free of disease 3 years after surgery and is awaiting a transplant, and 1 died 3 months after surgery due to the complications of renal insufficiency.

Five of 104 patients in the Mayo Clinic series developed a local recurrence only that was identified 3 to 183 months (mean 57 months) after surgery. Each was managed by resection of the recurrence only. Three of the patients died of metastatic disease 3 to 30 months after the secondary operation, 1 was alive 15 months after surgery but had a pulmonary metastasis, and 1 died of other causes.

References

deKernion, JB, Ramming, KP, and Smith, RB. The natural history of metastatic renal cell carcinoma: A computer analysis. J Urol 120:148, 1978.

Finney, R. An evaluation of postoperative radiotherapy in hypernephroma treatment: A clinical trial. Cancer 32:1332, 1973.

Finney, R. The value of radiotherapy in the treatment of hypernephroma: A clinical trial. Br J Urol 45:258, 1973.

Marshall, FF, and Walsh, PC. In situ management of renal tumors: Renal cell carcinoma and transitional cell carcinoma. J Urol 131:1045, 1984.

Morgan, WR, and Zincke, H. Progression and survival after renal-conserving surgery for renal cell carcinoma: Experience in 104 patients and extended followup. J Urol 144:852, 1990.

Mukamel, E, Konichezky, M, Engelstein, D, and Servadio, C. Incidental small renal tumors accompanying clinically overt renal cell carcinoma. J Urol 140:22, 1988.

Novick, AC, Streem, S, Montie, JE, et al. Conservative surgery for renal cell carcinoma: A single-center experience with 100 patients. J Urol 141:835, 1989.

Phillips, E, and Messing, EM. Local recurrence in a subset of patients with aggressive renal cell carcinoma. Presented at the North Central Section Meeting of the American Urological Association, 1990.

Rafla, S. Renal cell carcinoma: Natural history and results of treatment. Cancer 25:26, 1970.

Smith, RB, deKernion, JB, Ehrlich, RM, et al. Bilateral renal cell carcinoma and renal cell carcinoma in the solitary kidney. J Urol 132:450, 1984.

Topley, M, Novick, AC, and Montie, JE. Long-term results following partial nephrectomy for localized renal adenocarcinoma. J Urol 131:1050, 1984.

van der Werf-Messing, B. Carcinoma of the kidney. Cancer 5:1056, 1973.

Wickham, JE. Conservative renal surgery for adenocarcinoma: The place of bench surgery. Br J Urol 47:25, 1975.

Vascular Complications of Renal Transplantation

LYNN BANOWSKY

In vascular surgery, the first operation is always technically less difficult than secondary operations. All phases of the secondary operation (opening, dissection of the blood vessels, anastomoses, and wound closure) are more difficult. This is especially true of repeat operations for vascular complications in renal transplantation. Since the renal allograft is almost always in the retroperitoneal space, it is encased in scar tissue. The dissection necessary to mobilize the transplanted kidney and identify its vital components is both tedious and difficult. An error in dissection can result in an inadvertent injury to the artery, vein, or ureter that is always time consuming to repair and can produce either immediate or delayed loss of the allograft.

Repeat operations for vascular complications following renal transplantation are confined almost exclusively to the repair of renal artery stenosis. Successful repair of renal artery stenosis in a transplanted kidney requires careful preoperative assessment and planning. During the operation itself, the surgeon must display patience, precision, and at times creativity. The stakes for the patient are high. Successful repair of the vascular lesion results in a return of the blood pressure to normal and continued function of the renal allograft. An unsuccessful repair most often causes arterial thrombosis and an immediate return to chronic hemodialysis.

Several surgical principles are applicable to any repeat operation and are especially helpful in the repair of renal arterial stenosis in a transplanted kidney. A careful review of the original operative note is mandatory. This not only informs the surgeon of the type of arterial anastomosis but also may alert him or her to any unusual anatomy in either the kidney or the recipient that could pose an intraoperative problem. Surprises in the operating room are usually unpleasant.

If possible, it is preferable to avoid the old incision. An incision that is above, below, or on either side of the old incision allows one to open through relatively normal tissue. Dissection can then be initiated where a plane can be easily established before the bed of scar tissue is entered. Avoiding the old incision also allows for recognition of anatomic landmarks that may be difficult to identify through the previous operative site. It is always prudent to go from the known to the unknown rather than starting in the unknown.

There are several helpful techniques for dissecting and mobilizing any tubular structure (artery, vein, ureter). Begin the dissection from an area where the structure is relatively normal and easily identified. This permits one to establish a plane before entering the scar tissue. The safest plane in which to dissect a blood vessel is directly on top of the vessel. Sharp dissection is necessary and preferable most of the time. The surgeon and first assistant should provide traction and countertraction on the vessel using forceps so that small snips with the scissors will release the artery or vein from its investing scar tissue. The crux of any repeat operation is the safe dissection of the structure to be repaired; when this is done well, the repair itself is relatively simple. This chapter will attempt to use these basic principles to illustrate their applicability in the repair of renal artery stenosis in a transplanted kidney.

General Information

Renal artery stenosis in renal transplant recipients occurs with a reported frequency of 2 to 23 percent. There are three types of postoperative stenoses. Suture-line stenosis is the result of a faulty anastomosis or of damage to the intima of the renal artery at the time of nephrectomy or during the process of renal profusion and hypothermic storage. A tubular type of stenosis occurs away from the suture line in some end-to-side arterial anastomoses. The etiology of this type of stenosis is obscure, but turbulent flow secondary to the end-to-side anastomosis is a probable contributing factor. The third type of stenosis occurs away from the suture line and typically is in multiple sites in the segmental renal arteries. Histologically, these lesions are characterized by intimal proliferation. The etiology of these multiple sites of arterial obstruction is most often vascular injury caused by rejection. Cyclosporin A also may be an etiologic agent in some cases. Only the third type of stenosis is usually not amenable to surgical correction.

The diagnosis of renal artery stenosis should be considered in the following clinical settings: (1) uncontrollable hypertension, (2) hypertension that requires the use of three to four potent hypertensive drugs to effect control, and (3) hypertension, controlled or not, that is associated with an unexpected rise in the serum creatinine level. The diagnosis can only be made accurately by renal arteriography. All screening tests, including renal scans, etc., are sufficiently inaccurate that the decision to perform a renal angiogram should be made on the basis of the patient's course and clinical history. To minimize possible renal injury from the contrast material, the patient should be adequately hydrated prior to the examination and receive 12.5 gm of intravenous mannitol 30 minutes before the contrast material is to be injected. In the future, color Doppler studies may be an ideal screening procedure, and should they become accurate enough, they may very well supplant renal angiography as the diagnostic procedure of choice.

Selection of the Type of Procedure

The initial choice of the type of procedure is deciding between an open operation and a percutaneous angioplasty. For some types of stenoses, percutaneous angioplasty is preferred, but for many lesions, this procedure is associated with an inordinately high rate of intimal dissection and thrombosis. Should intimal dissection and thrombosis occur, it is extremely difficult to salvage the renal allograft. For any tight suture-line or tubular stenosis, my choice is for open operative repair. Over the last 7 years, eight renal artery stenoses have been corrected surgically with the loss of no renal allografts.

Once an open operative procedure has been decided on, a number of surgical techniques exist to accomplish revascularization of the renal allograft. Resection of the stenotic area and reanastomosis of the artery, arteriotomy, and saphenous vein patch have all been reported as means of repairing renal artery stenosis. While the surgeon's experience and training undoubtedly have a heavy influence on the type of open operation selected, it is my feeling that the bypass graft is not only the most consistently successful type of repair but also the most versatile.

There are several types of grafts that may be selected for an arterial bypass. Saphenous vein, hypogastric artery, and some type of Dacron synthetic graft are the most common types of material used. For all operations autogenous tissue such as the saphenous vein or the hypogastric artery are preferable to any synthetic graft. Autogenous tissue not only has higher reported rates of patency but also is less likely to become infected. The synthetic grafts also are a problem in that it is difficult to find reliable grafts of less than 5 to 6 mm in size. This frequently is a great deal larger than the renal artery to be repaired and creates an excessive size discrepancy between the bypass graft and the renal artery. This discrepancy in size results in turbulent flow and can lead to thrombosis. The only advantage of the synthetic grafts is that they are always available, and some patients may not have a usable saphenous vein or hypogastric artery.

Autogenous saphenous vein is the bypass graft of choice because of unusually high patency rates and a low risk of infection. The saphenous vein is easily accessible through a small incision in the thigh, and a sufficient length can be obtained to do a single anastomosis or to create multiple sidearms when there are multiple sites of stenoses involving both the main renal artery and some of the segmental branches (Fig. 2-1). The hypogastric artery is also an excellent vessel to use, and if it is harvested with its branches, it avoids the creation of sidearms to repair multiple-branch lesions. The disadvantage of the hypogastric artery is that it is frequently unusable because of significant atherosclerotic disease either at its origin or down into the area of the bifurcation. It also requires a major incision on the opposite side to harvest the contralateral hypogastric artery. In addition to being a more complicated recovery of the vessel, it disturbs the opposite iliac fossa should that area ever be needed for a second transplant.

Surgical Technique

Patient Preparation

It should be noted that prior to interruption of the renal circulation the patient has been adequately hydrated,

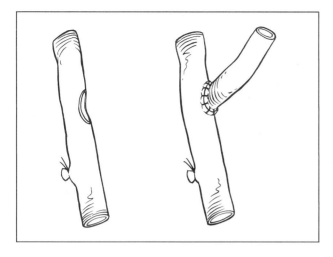

Figure 2-1. *Should there be more than one arterial lesion to be repaired, sidearms may be created off the saphenous vein. A small venotomy is made, and an appropriate length and diameter of saphenous vein are removed and sutured with interrupted 6-0 silk sutures into the side of the previously created venotomy. This allows great flexibility in repairing lesions that involve not only the main renal artery but also its branches.*

has been given 12½ gm of intravenous mannitol and 2500 to 5000 units of aqueous heparin. Following removal of the vascular clamps, if it is necessary, the patient is reversed with a third to half the original dose of heparin with protamine sulfate.

Harvesting the Saphenous Vein

The saphenous vein runs a course from proximal to distal from the medial aspect of the knee diagonally and superiorly toward the femoral vein (Fig. 2-2). There are numerous valves present in this portion of the vein. An awareness of their presence is necessary to establish correct flow in the bypass graft. A skin incision is made over the course of the saphenous vein to allow for the recovery of a sufficient length so that a number of repairs are possible. It should be remembered that it is always desirable to have an excess of vein rather than too little. After the skin and subcutaneous tissue have been divided, two Gilpy retractors are used to maintain exposure. The saphenous vein is found and freed from its surrounding adventitia (Fig. 2-3). Several branches of the vein will be encountered, and these should be suture ligated. Suture ligation is preferable because the vein will be under arterial pressure, and pulsation could cause a simple free-hand tie to roll off. Prior to harvesting the vein, a sterile marking pen should be used to draw a line down the anterior surface of the vein so that kinking or torsion can be avoided during the vascular

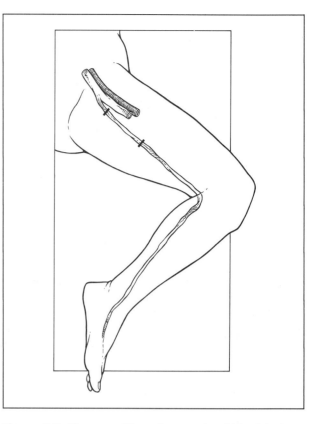

Figure 2-2. *The course of the saphenous vein, which originates on the medial aspect of the lower extremity and runs a course up to the femoral vein. A small incision in the upper thigh is usually sufficient to recover a sufficient length of the vein for most repairs of renal artery stenosis. This segment is usually long enough to allow the creation of multiple sidearms should that be necessary.*

repair. Zero silk suture is used to ligate the proximal and distal ends of the saphenous vein prior to its division. After removal, a Titus needle is inserted into the proximal portion of the vein, and a small bulldog clamp is placed across the distal end of the vein in order to distend the vein with heparinized saline (Fig. 2-4). This allows the surgeon to determine if there are any points of leakage or adventitial obstruction along the course of the vein. Once the integrity of the saphenous vein has been established, it should be stored in a pan of cold heparinized saline. The Titus needle should be left attached until the anastomosis is begun so that there will be no confusion about the correct direction of flow.

Incision

In order to avoid the intense scar tissue surrounding the renal allograft, a lower abdominal transperitoneal midline incision is preferred (Fig. 2-5). This incision not only avoids the scar tissue in the fascial and muscular

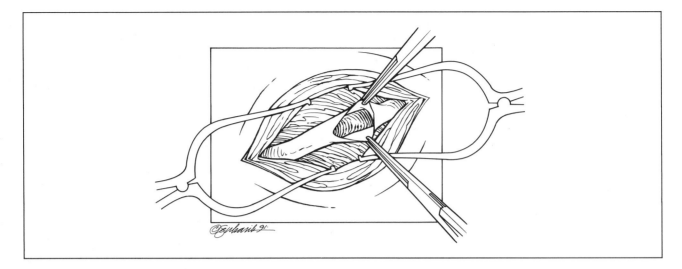

Figure 2-3. *Two small Gelpi retractors are helpful in holding the subcutaneous tissue open during dissection of the saphenous vein. Any small side branches that are identified should be suture ligated with 4-0 or 5-0 vascular silk. The Gelpi retractors allow the saphenous vein to be harvested easily by one surgeon.*

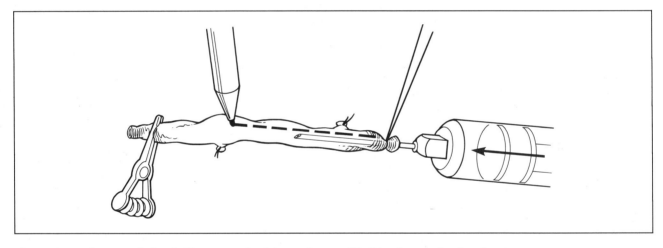

Figure 2-4. *After removal of a suitable segment of saphenous vein, a small bulldog clamp is placed on the distal end of the vein graft so that it is totally occluded. A Titus needle attached to a syringe filled with heparinized saline is inserted into the proximal end of the vein and is fixed with a 4-0 silk suture tie. The vein is then hydrodistended so that any leaks may be found and corrected prior to the actual revascularization procedure. With the vein distended, a blue sterile marking pen is used to draw a line down the center of the vein so that torsion or twisting of the vein can be avoided during the revascularization operation. In this illustration, two small branches have been fixed with suture ligatures.*

layers but also allows easy visualization through the peritoneal cavity of the renal allograft and the external iliac artery.

Dissection

After the peritoneal cavity has been opened, the patient is placed in the Trendelenburg position, and the small and large intestines are retracted cephalad with a moist laparotomy pad. Some type of self-retaining retractor,

e.g., Balfour, Smith ring, Wilkinson, is preferred to maintain exposure.

Whether the original vascular anastomosis was performed end-to-side with the renal artery to the external iliac artery or end-to-end between the renal artery and the hypogastric artery, the first step is to control the common and/or external iliac artery both proximally and distally. The more difficult repair of an end-to-side anastomosis will be used to illustrate the repair of the renal artery stenosis. The posterior peritoneum is in-

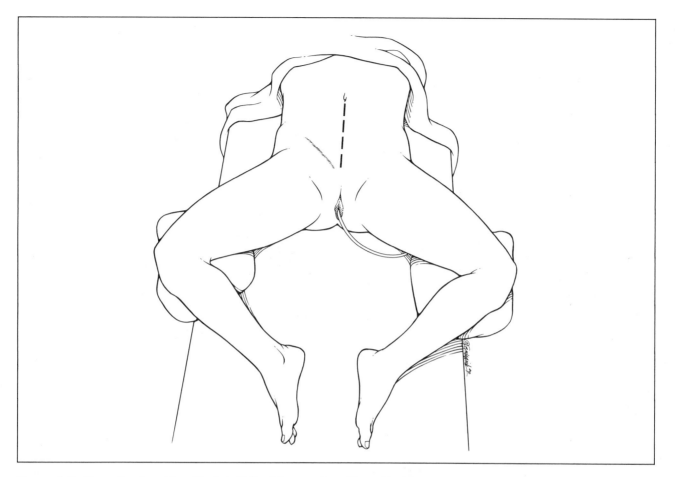

Figure 2-5. *The patient is positioned in the middle of the operative table, and both legs are placed in a frogleg position to facilitate the recovery of saphenous vein from either thigh. An indwelling Foley catheter is used to monitor urine output. A lower abdominal transperitoneal midline incision is made to avoid the scar tissue from the previous incision, which is shown in the right lower quadrant.*

cised first over the common or proximal external iliac artery (Fig. 2-6). The peritoneum is sharply dissected from the anterior, medial, and lateral surfaces of the artery in that order. A right-angle clamp is used to complete the dissection of the posterior aspect of the artery. Upon completion of the dissection, a vascular loop is passed twice around the artery. The same type of dissection is done to gain control of the distal external iliac artery. Control of the iliac arterial system is mandatory for safe dissection of the renal iliac arterial anastomosis.

Dissection is begun on the proximal external iliac artery using Metzenbaum scissors and some type of vascular forceps (Fig. 2-6, *inset*). This dissection is most easily and safely done by using a combination of traction and countertraction. The surgeon and the first assistant use vascular forceps to lift and stretch the adventitia and scar tissue surrounding the artery. Metzenbaum scissors are used to alternately cut and spread this tissue.

This type of dissection is used to mobilize the external iliac artery until the site of the previous arterial anastomosis is found. For the subsequent vascular repair to be performed successfully, the renal artery must be dissected for a sufficient length so that the anastomoses can be done without tension and control of the distal renal artery can be accomplished to prevent back-bleeding. Sufficient exposure of the artery also guarantees that the entire area of obstruction will be bypassed. It is desirable to only mobilize the external iliac artery, the iliac renal arterial anastomosis, and the renal artery itself. In some instances, this is not possible, and complete mobilization of the renal allograft, the renal artery, the renal vein, and the iliac arterial system is necessary. Great care must be taken to avoid injury of the vital structures surrounding the renal artery. The renal vein and ureter are in close proximity, and their injury can produce severe consequences. Again, a review of the previous

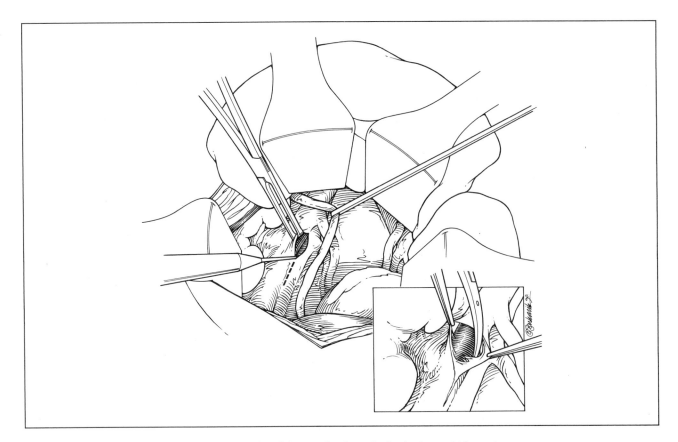

Figure 2-6. *The peritoneal cavity has been opened, and exposure has been obtained using moist laparotomy pads and the Smith ring retractor. The common and external iliac arteries are easily seen through the posterior peritoneum. The ureter is retracted out of this area, and an incision is made in the posterior peritoneum over the common and external iliac arteries. (Inset) Using sharp and blunt dissection with the Metzenbaum scissors, the anterior surface of the artery is freed first. Attention is then turned to the medial and lateral aspects of the artery. It is only after a sufficient length and mobilization of these three sides of the artery that attention should be turned to freeing the artery in its posterior plane. Most branches of the arteries and veins in this area originate posteriorly.*

operative note can be of great help in giving the surgeon some idea of where these important structures are most likely to be found. When the renal arterial dissection has been completed, it is secured with a vascular loop (Fig. 2-7).

The Vascular Anastomosis

The proximal anastomosis between the saphenous vein and the external iliac artery is performed first. A number of vascular clamps can be used to control the iliac artery. My preference is for the pediatric renal artery clamp. This instrument is not only atraumatic but also can be applied so that it is out of the surgeon's way. Bulldog clamps or Debakey clamps are also quite satisfactory. A no. 11 blade is used to make the initial arteriotomy in the anterior arterial wall. Once the artery is opened, an

aortic punch is used to create a smooth elliptical arteriotomy that will allow for laminar rather than tubular flow (Fig. 2-8). A 6-0 double-arm Prolene vascular suture is placed from inside out through the apex of the spatulated proximal saphenous vein. The other end of the suture is then picked up, and the needle is again passed inside out through the arteriotomy in the iliac artery (Fig. 2-9). Each suture is then tied with seven knots. The sutures are then run from either end toward the middle of the arteriotomy, where they are tied to each other. The same procedure is repeated on the opposite side. Great care must be taken to adequately visualize the placement of each suture so that the intima is securely tacked down. Upon completion of this portion of the anastomosis, a small bulldog clamp is placed on the most proximal portion of the saphenous vein graft, and the controlling clamps are removed from the iliac ar-

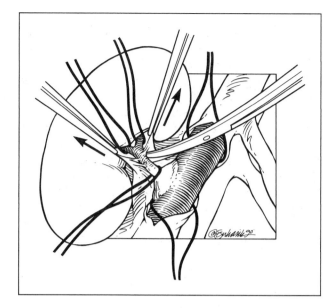

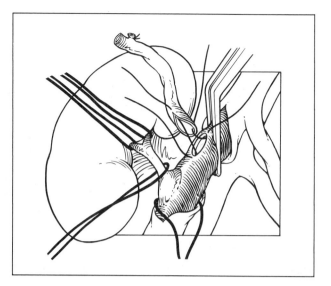

Figure 2-7. *Dissection of the iliac and renal arteries is most safely and quickly accomplished by the surgeon and the first assistant using a combination of traction and countertraction on the scar tissue that encases the vessel. When this scar tissue is placed under tension, small snips with the Metzenbaum scissors followed by spreading will easily release the artery from its encasing scar tissue. In this illustration, this technique is being used to free up the renal artery. Control has already been obtained of the proximal and distal iliac artery, and dissection is now being carried out in the distal portion of the main renal artery and its branches.*

Figure 2-8. *Once control of the iliac artery has been obtained and the renal artery has been completely dissected, a small arteriotomy is made in the proximal external iliac artery using a no. 11 blade. The lumen of the artery is then flushed with heparinized saline, and an aortic punch, usually in sizes 4 to 4.4 mm, is used to create a smooth elliptical opening in the iliac artery. This minimizes turbulent flow.*

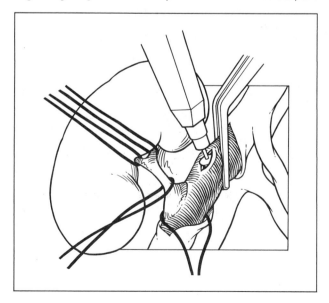

Figure 2-9. *The saphenous vein graft is spatulated and two 6-0 double-arm Prolene sutures are then placed through both the apex and the base of the saphenous vein graft and through either end of the iliac arteriotomy. These sutures are then tied securely, and the vein graft is fixed to the iliac artery. The proximal anastomosis can then be done by running either end of the 6-0 double-arm Prolene from each end of the arteriotomy to the middle, and there they are tied. This same process is repeated on the opposite wall.*

tery. This allows one to check the patency of the anastomosis and repair any leaks in the suture line. The saphenous vein graft is then passed over to the renal artery and measured so that the vein graft can be trimmed to a satisfactory length to avoid either excessive tension or excessive length, which would predispose to torsion or kinking of the artery. A piece of umbilical tape is quite satisfactory to accomplish this measurement. There is frequently a size discrepancy between the renal artery and the saphenous vein graft, with the renal artery being the smaller of the two structures. Should this be the case, the renal artery is spatulated prior to initiating the anastomosis. Since the anastomosis involves a significantly smaller vessel than the proximal anastomosis between proximal saphenous vein and external iliac artery, it is performed most often with interrupted 6-0 double-arm silk suture. Sutures are placed at the apex and base of the saphenous vein graft and affixed to the spatulated renal artery (Fig. 2-10). Interrupted sutures are then placed from either end toward the middle, with care being taken so that each suture is placed under direct vision to avoid kinking of the renal artery. The distal renal artery has been controlled previously with a very small atraumatic bulldog clamp. Following completion of the first side of the anastomosis, the vessel is then flipped,

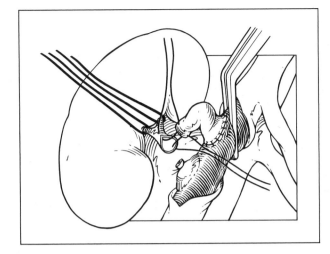

Figure 2-10. *There is usually a size discrepancy between the renal artery and the distal end of the saphenous vein graft. This size discrepancy can be minimized by spatulating the renal artery. Since this anastomosis is much smaller than the proximal anastomosis between the saphenous vein and the external iliac artery, interrupted 6-0 silk double-arm sutures are preferred because they are less constricting than a running anastomosis with Prolene. The first two sutures are placed from the apex of the renal artery through the comparable segment on the saphenous vein and then through the base of the renal artery through its comparable segment of the saphenous vein. These two sutures are then tied, and the anastomosis is completed on either side using interrupted 6-0 silk sutures. The interrupted placement of the sutures also allows one to visualize each suture as it is placed so that one is certain that the intima has been securely tacked down on both sides.*

Figure 2-11. *The completed iliac renal bypass graft. One should note that the saphenous vein describes a gentle curve and there is no torsion or kinking of the vein graft.*

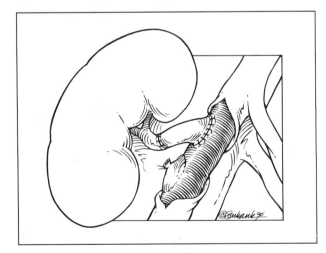

and the posterior side of the anastomosis is performed in the same way using interrupted 6-0 silk sutures beginning from either end and suturing toward the middle. Following completion of this anastomosis, the distal bulldog clamp on the renal artery is removed so that back-bleeding can occur and small leaks may be seen and repaired while the system is under low pressure. Following the repair of any leaks, the proximal clamp is removed, and the anastomosis once again is checked for patency and hemostasis (Fig. 2-11). If the anastomosis is satisfactory, the wound is irrigated with approximately 1 liter of normal saline and then closed in two layers using interrupted 0 neurolon or interrupted no. 28 wire. The subcutaneous tissue is closed with 3-0 plain catgut, and the skin is most often closed with a staple gun.

Postoperative Care

Normalization of blood pressure even under ideal circumstances may take 24 to 48 hours. If the blood pressure is excessively high immediately following surgery (diastolic $\geq$ 120 mm Hg), control is most safely established with a nitroprusside drip. Many patients will still require one or two antihypertensive drugs for maintenance.

Adequate volume replacement and the avoidance of hypovolemia are the goals of postoperative fluid management. Monitoring of the central venous pressure can be a very helpful guide. Acute renal failure with oliguria is uncommon. Any anuria that does not respond promptly to furosemide or mannitol should be investigated aggressively with a technetium-99m renal flow scan. If there is no flow, the patient should be taken back to the operating room immediately for exploration of the artery.

Bibliography

Banowsky, LHW. Surgical complications of renal transplantation. In JF Glenn (ed), Urologic Surgery, 2nd Ed. New York: Hoeber, 1974, pp 252–266.

Belzer FO. Technical complications after renal transplantation. In PJ Morris (ed), Kidney Transplantation: Principles and Practice. New York: Grune & Stratton, 1971, pp 267–284.

Clements, R, Evans, C, and Salaman, JR. Percutaneous transluminal angioplasty of renal transplant artery stenosis. Clin Radiol 38:235, 1987.

Nonvascular Complications of Renal Transplantation

ARTHUR I. SAGALOWSKY
C. WILLIAM HINNANT, JR.

Renal transplantation is the preferred management of end-stage renal disease in suitable patients. During the past 45 years, the surgical procedure has become standardized, and great progress has been made in obtaining safe and effective immunosuppression. Current 1-year graft and patient survival for primary cadaveric renal allograft recipients is approximately 85 and 95 percent, respectively. Results remain slightly higher for recipients of living, related donor kidneys. Nevertheless, management of transplant recipients remains challenging. Reoperation for acute complications of the transplant procedure or late complications due to chronic immunosuppression or the natural history of the patient's primary disease process (e.g., diabetes mellitus) is not uncommon.

This chapter will focus on reoperation for nonvascular complications of renal transplantation. In a narrow sense, all the complications directly related to the transplant procedure may be categorized as either vascular, urologic, or wound problems, as listed in Table 3-1. However, such an approach avoids the many indirectly related problems that may present either early or late after transplantation. Therefore, in order to place chronologic and numeric perspective on these events, we have reviewed all nonrenovascular reoperations performed on renal transplant recipients at our institution between January of 1985, and September of 1990 (Table 3-2). During this period, 451 renal transplants were performed in 363 adult and 88 pediatric recipients. Reoperation for renovascular problems is discussed in another chapter in this book. Several points must be emphasized to interpret the data in Table 3-2 correctly. Some of the operations were performed on patients who received an allograft earlier than 1985. Thus the numbers do not reflect an incidence for a given procedure or complication but do reflect relative frequency. Second, a given complication may have required more than one initial or delayed procedure. Thus the subcategories cannot necessarily be added to obtain totals.

Currently, the great majority of transplant patients remain on corticosteroids indefinitely. Prior to undergoing anesthesia, these patients should receive stress doses of steroids. Although the frequency of acute steroid insufficiency without such coverage is said to be rare, it is unpredictable and is potentially life-threatening. Patients tolerate the chronic anemia of renal failure from a cardiovascular standpoint. Transfusion prior to induction of anesthesia may be reserved for patients with active bleeding or those who are in a chronic debilitated state. We believe that broad-spectrum perioperative antibiotic coverage minimizes wound infections in transplant recipients. Patients receive Aztreonam and ampicillin preoperatively and for 24 hours postoperatively.

Exploration of the Allograft

Bleeding

Reexploration of the allograft during the first week postoperatively almost invariably is due to bleeding. The crucial step is recognition of the problem and proper timing of reexploration. Most patients accumulate a small hematoma in the iliac fossa after transplantation. Excessive pain out of proportion to the surgery, tachycardia, or peripheral vasoconstriction may be early signs of significant bleeding. Later, the findings of a tense,

Table 3-1 *Categories of Surgical Complications after Renal Transplantation*

Vascular:
  Arterial, venous, or both
    Anastomotic bleeding
    Stenosis
    Thrombosis
Urologic:
  Ureter
    Leak
    Obstruction
  Bladder leak
Wound:
  Hematoma
  Infection
  Lymphocele

Source: Adapted from Sagalowsky, AI, and Dawidson, I. Surgical complications of renal transplantation. In H Jacobson, GE Striker, and S. Klahr (eds), The Principles and Practice of Nephrology. Philadelphia: B.C. Decker, 1991, pp 843–846.

Table 3-2 *Reoperations on Renal Allograft Recipients, 1985–1990, UT Southwestern*

Category	Perioperative 0–7 Days	Early, 8–90 Days	Late, >90 Days
Expl. Tx			
Evac. hematoma	7	5	
Anast. bleed, arterial	4		
Hilar bleed	2		
Tx. rupture		1	
Open biopsy		2	6
Iliac arteriorrhaphy			1
Tx. neph	2	26	58
Urol., open			
Ureteral leak	2	6	2
Excise + nephrost		5	
Excise + reimplant	2	1	
Second-degree pyeloureterost + native neph			4
Native neph.			8
Nephrost		1	2
UVj obst., reimplant		1	1
UPJ obst., pyeloplasty			1
Bladder leak	1	2	
Suprapubic cystost.	1	2	2
Vesicost. closure			1
Penectomy			2
Penile prosthesis			5
Urol., endoscopic			
Cysto	4	3	43
Cysto alone	1		8
Cysto + RGPG		1	10
Cysto + ureteral stent			7
Cysto + double J stent			17
Cysto + clot evac	3	2	
Cysto + VIU			1
Perc. nephrost.		2	4
Wound			
Lymphocele		16	5
Perc.		9	5
Open, internalized		3	1
Open, external		4	1
Infection		2	4
Incisional hernia			4

Table 3-2 *(Continued)*

Category	Perioperative 0–7 Days	Early, 8–90 Days	Late, >90 Days
Expl. lap			
UGI bleed	1	1	
SBO	1	2	1
S.B. perf.	1		
Colon bleed		2	
Colon perf., colost.			2
Coloves. fistula, colost.			1
Colost. closure			1
Cholecystect.			2
Pancreatitis		1	2
Retroperit. absce			2
Urinary ascites			2
Rad. cystect., ileal conduit			1
Augment. cystoplast.			4
Skin abscess, I & D			
Labial			2
Perirectal			5
Axillary			1
Leg			5
Scrotal			2
Amputations			
Upper, digit			1
Lower			
Digit, ray		1	5
B-K			5
A-K			1
Other			
Hip prosthesis			12
Parathyroidect			2
Subtotal			1
Total			1
Cardiac			
CABG			1
Valve			1
Vena caval filter			2
C-section			1

bulging wound, hemodynamic instability, and a falling hematocrit make the diagnosis obvious. In our experience, patients do not continue to make urine in the face of ongoing bleeding. Blood clots also can accumulate in the collecting system (Fig. 3-1).

The wound must be reopened with care, and the peritoneum must be mobilized off the renal surface without creating capsular tears or parenchymal fracture. In the absence of massive hemorrhage, the hematoma should be evacuated carefully as the next step. Then a systematic search for the potential important sources of bleeding should be made. This includes viewing the arterial and venous anastomoses, the renal hilum, and the parenchymal surface. An early arterial anastomotic bleed occurred in 0.9 percent of our patients and was reparable in each instance. The potential causes are technical error, a severely atherosclerotic recipient ves-

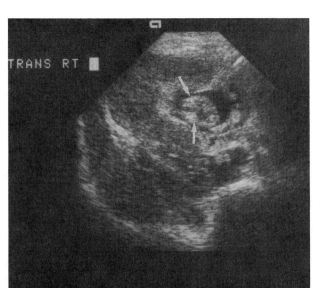
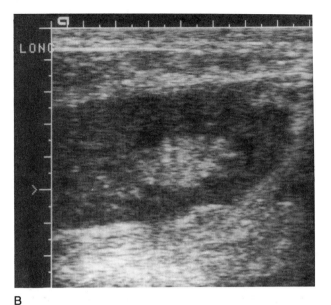

A　　　　　　　　　　　　　　　　　　　　B

Figure 3-1. *A. Hematoma* (arrows) *within the collecting system of a transplanted kidney. B. Magnification demonstrating hypoechoic blood clot within the collecting system. Hematoma was noted through days after transplantation.*

sel, or sudden hypertension. Venous anastomotic bleeding is very rare and was not seen in our experience.

Small renal hilar vessels that are severed during organ procurement are another potential source of postoperative hemorrhage. However, in the majority of instances, no source of the hematoma is found, as was the case in 7 of our 13 perioperative explorations for bleeding. Late arterial bleeding suggests anastomotic infection and pseudoaneurysm formation. Nephrectomy and resection of the anastomosis are the safest policy.

Allograft rupture can be categorized under the general problem of bleeding. Patients describe sudden and severe pain directly over the allograft, followed by signs of hemorrhage. Acute rejection is the most common cause of allograft rupture due to intense parenchymal swelling. Nephrectomy usually is required in these patients.

Transplant Nephrectomy

Transplant nephrectomy is the most common reason for reexploration of a renal transplant, and our experience, shown in Table 3-2, is representative. Renal artery thrombosis is the usual cause of perioperative nephrectomy. Hyperacute humoral rejection is rarely seen with modern histocompatibility techniques. Acute rejection that is unresponsive to maximal immunosuppression is the most common reason for nephrectomy in the first

3 months following transplantation; so-called chronic rejection is the predominant cause thereafter.

Transplant nephrectomy is not required in every instance of a failed allograft. Indeed, the frequency is in part a reflection of the bias of the particular transplant team. Once a patient reaches "end-stage" rejection and is back on maintenance dialysis, the ongoing risks of immunosuppression are not justified. Cyclosporine and/or azathioprine are discontinued abruptly, and steroids are tapered over several weeks before being stopped. Very few patients who lose graft function from rejection in the first few months are able to have the allograft left in place. Fever and painful swelling of the allograft are the rule. Patients who ultimately lose a graft to chronic rejection after years of successful function may tolerate withdrawal of immunosuppressants asymptomatically. If the patient begins to have vague malaise, low-grade fever, and intermittent subjective allograft pain, often with hematuria, in the absence of any other source of infection or illness, then transplant nephrectomy is performed. Invariably all the symptoms and findings resolve following transplant nephrectomy in this setting.

In the perioperative period, transplant nephrectomy is straightforward. The fresh extraperitoneal wound is reentered, and the renal vessels and ureter are secured and divided. The renal vein anastomosis is a low-pressure system that may be left intact. The renal vein should be suture ligated near the iliac vein. This will minimize the risk for clot formation and pulmonary embolism from the venous stump. Ideally, the high-pressure arterial anastomosis should be entirely resected. For end-to-end anastomosis to the hypogastric artery, this is a simple matter. In patients with an end-to-side anastomosis to the external or common iliac artery, removal of the anastomosis may require an autogenous vein patch arteriorrhaphy to avoid significant narrowing in the closure. The ureter is avulsed from the neocystostomy site, and the bladder wall is oversewn with absorbable suture. A bladder catheter is left in place for 24 to 48 hours in patients with output from the native kidneys.

Transplant nephrectomy beyond the perioperative period is another matter entirely. The kidney is immobilized by a dense rind of scar with the peritoneum adherent anteriorly and the iliac vessels posteriorly. One approach is to open the peritoneum along the length of the original incision and approach the iliac vessels through the posterior parietal peritoneum. This requires extensive dissection and may be associated with postoperative paralytic ileus. We prefer to dissect extraperitoneally along the lines of the prior incision onto the surface of the renal capsule. The kidney is then mobilized either by extracapsular or subcapsular dissection. This approach close to the renal surface and hilum is more expeditious and is preferred by most transplant surgeons. However, the safety and efficiency depend more on the surgeon's experience and knowledge of where the renal vessels and ureter should be than on wide exposure, as in most other surgeries. If the kidney has been fully mobilized, a Satinsky vascular clamp can be placed quickly across the renal pedicle in case of sudden bleeding. However, this is not desirable electively because it risks tangential injury to the iliac vessels and is not a substitute for attempting to identify the renal vessels. The renal arterial and venous branches are each ligated and divided as they are encountered close to the surface of the kidney. The ureter is divided only as far distally as is prudent. After the kidney has been removed, each vascular branch is checked for hemostasis. We do not recommend removal of the arterial anastomosis in chronic cases because the risk of injuring the iliac vessels is high. Often a closed suction drain is left in place until after the first dialysis without significant drainage.

Urologic Procedures

Major urologic procedures on the transplant obviously are also a form of transplant exploration but are listed separately for clarity.

Open

The main transplant-related urologic complications requiring reoperation can be divided into urinary leak and obstruction. Urinary leak is by far the more urgent problem. Urine in a wound is a strong chemical irritant and predisposes to infection and disruption of the vascular anastomoses. Early diagnosis and elimination of further leakage are essential in minimizing morbidity and mortality. The clinical findings of urine leak are fullness over the wound, oliguria, weight gain, and increased serum creatinine and chloride. Patients often describe pain radiating into the groin during voiding from urine dissecting through the external inguinal ring into the labia or scrotum.

Demonstration of a fluid mass on ultrasonography is the best test for a suspected urine leak (Fig. 3-2). The diagnosis of leak is confirmed if the creatinine content of aspirated fluid is higher than that of serum. Next, the source of the leak must be determined. Bladder leak may occur from the cystotomy suture line or from the ureteral-bladder mucosal anastomosis in patients with intravesical and extravesical ureteral reimplants, respectively. Cystography usually will demonstrate cystotomy leakage but may fail to demonstrate extravasation from the reimplant site itself. Although Foley catheter drainage alone may suffice for a small bladder leak, larger leaks are better handled by direct open repair and placement of a suprapubic catheter and/or ureteral stent if the bladder repair is fragile.

Upper urinary tract leakage may occur from ureteral necrosis or a calyceal fistula secondary to ischemia from loss of periureteral or renal hilar blood supply during organ procurement. Retrograde pyelography to confirm ureteral leak or to allow placement of a ureteral stent is difficult with a fresh ureteral reimplant. Placement of a percutaneous nephrostomy will allow contrast studies to localize the leak site and will provide proximal urinary diversion and stabilization of the patient. If the ureter appears healthy and the leak is only at the reimplant site, antegrade placement of a ureteral stent may provide definitive treatment. However, if ureteral necrosis is suspected, open repair is necessary.

A disrupted or leaking ureteral reimplant with an otherwise healthy ureter may be repaired by redoing a ureteral neocystostomy over a stent. If the distal ureter is necrotic, attempting to repeat the implant is risky even if the length appears adequate. In these patients, we prefer to resect the ureter nearly to the renal pelvis, which is closed after a nephrostomy and drain are placed. A delayed reconstruction of the urinary tract by

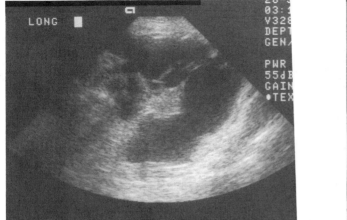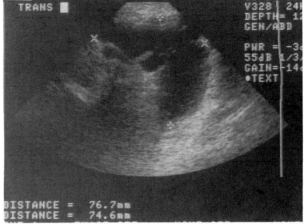

Figure 3-2. *Longitudinal (A) and transverse (B) ultrasound scans demonstrating large urinoma associated with renal transplantation. Urinoma was noted 6 days after renal transplantation.*

ureteropyelostomy of the native ureter to the transplanted renal pelvis is performed in 4 to 6 months.

Over the last 5 years, we have seen early urinary leak in only 2.4 percent of patients (11/451) (Table 3-2). As might be anticipated, the two ureteral leaks in the first postoperative week were simple partial anastomotic disruptions that were repaired by debridement and a repeat reimplantation. Five of six ureteral leaks identified during the second to third postoperative weeks were due to extensive ureteral necrosis. Four of these patients were treated successfully with debridement and a nephrostomy followed by secondary repair as described above.

Ureterovesical junction obstruction is quite uncommon after renal transplantation. Transient perioperative obstruction by clots or swelling is self-limited. True early technical obstruction was not seen in our experience. Later ureteral obstruction, as was seen in two of our patients, is due to fibrosis. Symptoms are rare, and findings are a subtle rise in serum creatinine and mild obstruction on renal scan or ultrasound. Retrograde or antegrade placement of a ureteral stent with or without balloon dilation often corrects the problem and avoids a difficult open repeat ureteroneocystostomy.

Other uncommon secondary urologic problems requiring major open surgery, such as bladder cancer, colovesical fistulas, contracted noncompliant bladder, ureteropelvic junction obstruction, and penile gangrene, as reflected in Table 3-2, each may be treated exactly as in nontransplant patients. Although the surgical morbidity might be anticipated to be higher in transplant recipients, no complications in fact were seen in these patients in our series.

Endoscopic

Cystoscopy is a common procedure following renal transplantation. The perioperative indications are almost always for clot evacuation. Late indications may be for hematuria of variable degree and to define or exclude and/or treat obstruction. Percutaneous nephrostomy is invaluable in defining true obstruction in late cases of mild hydronephrosis and chronic renal deterioration. The large number of cystoscopies for insertion of a double-J stent in our experience represent interval catheter changes in two patients with distal ureteral obstruction. Surgical correction was deferred because of marginal renal function or poor general health in these patients.

Wound

Lymphocele

Persistent leak from lymphatics that are disrupted during exposure of the iliac vessels at the time of transplantation may be troublesome. Some authors advocate dissecting only the shortest possible length along the iliac vessels to minimize this problem. The best prevention, however, is meticulous ligation before dividing the lymphatics. Although ultrasonography reveals lymphoceles in many transplant recipients, clinically significant lymphoceles are present in only approximately 5 percent of patients. The overall incidence of lymphoceles in our experience was 4.7 percent (21/451). Of these, 76 percent (16/21) occurred early, as expected, and 24 percent (5/21) occurred later. The reasons for late appearance of a lymphocele are unclear. The signs and symptoms of a clinically significant lymphocele are due either to extrinsic obstruction of the ureter producing elevated serum creatinine with or without hydronephrosis or compression of the iliac vein producing edema of the involved lower extremity. The size of the lymphocele may not correlate with the degree of functional impairment. The diagnosis is confirmed by ultrasound-guided aspiration and chemical analysis compared with the values of serum creatinine, or potassium. Complete percutaneous aspiration is the initial treatment. If fluid reaccumulates, repeated aspirations, percutaneous tube drainage, and open surgical repair are options. Tube drainage tends to be protracted over 4 to 6 weeks but usually is successful if exit-site infection is avoided. Internal surgical drainage into the peritoneum is effective for large collections and avoids external drains. Surgical exploration and external drainage by means of a closed suction catheter are successful for smaller collections. The success of each of these treatments ultimately depends on collapse of the cavity and sclerosis of the lymphatics.

Other

Wound infection is a potentially serious complication in the immunosuppressed patient. Current use of perioperative antibiotics and the avoidance of external drains whenever possible have reduced this problem to a minimum. Wound infections occurred in only 1.3 percent (6/451) of our patients since 1985. Only two of these infections occurred in the early postoperative period.

Incisional hernias are infrequent following renal transplantation.

Exploratory Laparotomy

Data on the frequency of major intraabdominal events requiring exploratory surgery in contemporary series utilizing modern immunosuppression are few. Therefore, we have reviewed our total experience since 1985. Only two patients required surgery for upper gastrointestinal bleeding secondary to peptic ulcer disease. In the one perioperative case, the ulcer was very large and clearly was present prior to transplantation, even though the patient denied symptoms. Despite a prolonged and stormy course, both the patient and the allograft were saved. One perioperative small bowel obstruction and perforation occurred from iatrogenic injury during wound closure. This patient ultimately died of peritonitis despite early cessation of all immunosuppression and prompt surgical repair.

The two colon bleeds that occurred during the second and third postoperative months were due to cytomegalovirus in highly immunosuppressed patients following antirejection therapy. The three late colon perforations, one with a colovesical fistula, were secondary to perforated diverticula. Patient survival was 80 percent (4/5) following emergency surgery for colonic problems.

Late retroperitoneal abscesses were seen in two patients and carried a 50 percent mortality rate. In one patient the abscess appeared to originate from the native kidney. Acute cholecystitis, severe pancreatitis mimicking an acute abdomen, and gross urinary ascites following removal of a percutaneous nephrostomy were the remaining causes for exploratory laparotomy. A successful outcome was obtained in each. The other urologically related cases (bladder cancer, augmentation cystoplasty) were discussed earlier.

Other

Skin Abscesses

There were 15 patients who required formal drainage in the operating room. Numerous smaller abscesses that were drained in the outpatient clinic are not listed.

Amputation

Partial, serial, or complete loss of limbs is a major chronic morbidity in renal transplant recipients. Most of the patients in our series suffering this complication had renal failure secondary to diabetes mellitus and have the progressive vascular ravages of that disease.

Miscellaneous

For completeness, the remaining surgical procedures performed in our patients are listed under "Other" in Table 3-2. The relatively low number of patients requiring hip prostheses is mainly a result of improved immunosuppression requiring lower doses of corticosteroids in the cyclosporine era. Occasionally, secondary hyperparathyroidism persists following successful renal transplantation and requires subtotal or total parathyroidectomy.

Summary

Renal transplantation has become a highly successful form of management that offers patients with end-stage renal disease an improved lifestyle. The surgical technique is fairly standardized, and the early surgical complication rates are low. We have presented a detailed review of reoperations in our last 451 renal transplant recipients. In contrast to earlier reviews, which emphasized how frequent complications were and how difficult they were to deal with, we have shown that early and late events are relatively few. There can be no doubt that renal transplant recipients face additional surgical risks due to immunosuppression and cardiovascular disease. However, major surgery is possible following transplantation when necessary. Prompt diagnosis, keen clinical judgment, and attention to detail are essential for a satisfactory outcome.

Bibliography

Sagalowsky, AI, and Dawidson, I. Surgical complications of renal transplantation. In HR Jacobson, GE Striker, and S Klahr (eds), The Principles and Practice of Nephrology. Philadelphia: B. C. Decker, 1991, pp 843–846.

Sagalowsky, AI, Helderman, JH, and Peters, PC. Renal transplantation. In JY Gillenwater, JT Grayhack, SS Howards, and JW Duckett (eds), Adult and Pediatric Urology. Year Book Medical Publishers, Chicago, 1987, pp 715–751.

Renovascular Complications Unrelated to Renal Transplantation

CHARLES LEE JACKSON
ANDREW C. NOVICK

Renal revascularization is an effective treatment for hypertension and renal insufficiency secondary to renal artery stenosis. Approximately 90 percent of patients undergoing primary renal revascularization will benefit with improved postoperative renal function and blood pressure control. Approximately 10 percent, however, will demonstrate recurrent hypertension or further deterioration in renal function within a few months to several years following primary renal revascularization. Recurrent vascular disease may be caused by secondary stenosis of the previously repaired renal artery, new stenosis of the unoperated contralateral renal artery, or progressive parenchymal nephrosclerosis. Regular long-term postoperative follow-up will help identify those patients with recurrent disease. Their identification is followed by careful evaluation to determine the specific cause of recurrence and to guide treatment. Treatment options include primary revascularization of contralateral disease, angioplasty or secondary revascularization of recurrent ipsilateral disease, and nephrectomy for parenchymal disease. The following discussion will focus on the preoperative evaluation, operative considerations, and postoperative management of recurrent stenosis of the previously repaired renal artery.

Evaluation and Treatment Options

Routine postoperative evaluation after renovascular surgery should include blood pressure measurement, serum creatinine, and nuclear renography at 6- to 12-month intervals. The blood pressure and serum creatinine level are sensitive indicators of recurrent disease, and any new or persistent elevation in blood pressure or deterioration in renal function should prompt further radiographic investigation. Suspected recurrent renal artery disease must be confirmed angiographically (Fig. 4-1). Intraarterial digital subtraction angiography will identify and characterize recurrent ipsilateral stenosis or new contralateral disease with a minimum of contrast material. Lateral aortic views to demonstrate the celiac trunk and pelvic views should be obtained at the time of angiography to guide subsequent treatment decisions.

Hemodynamically significant stenosis in the unoperated contralateral renal artery without evidence of stenosis in the renovascular graft should be evaluated and managed as any other primary unilateral renal artery stenosis. Angiographic evidence of significantly recurrent stenosis or occlusion of the previously operated renal artery may be managed with percutaneous transluminal angioplasty, secondary revascularization, or nephrectomy. Treatment selection depends on the extent of the recurrent stenosis and renal salvageability.

With a totally occluded renal artery, renal salvageability is suggested by a renal length of greater than or equal to 9 cm, reconstitution of intrarenal vessels by collateral vessels, and evidence of renal function on a nuclear scan. An intraoperative renal biopsy demonstrating histologic evidence of viable glomeruli without extensive hyalinization or sclerosis further supports renal viability and attempted secondary revascularization. Advanced nephrosclerosis without evidence of renal salvageability, however, should be managed by nephrectomy.

Percutaneous renal angioplasty may be attempted for short, well-defined focal stenosis of a previously repaired renal artery. This approach may avoid a technically difficult secondary revascularization, but there are

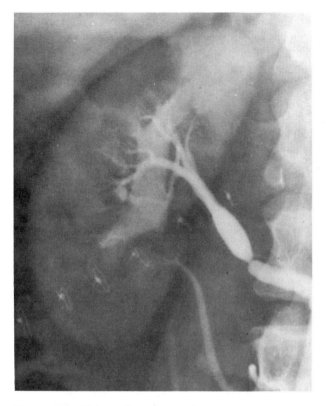

Figure 4-1. *Right renal arteriogram shows stenosis at distal anastomosis of aortorenal bypass graft to renal artery.*

little data to describe long-term results with this approach for recurrent renal artery disease. Angioplasty is not recommended for diffuse vascular graft stenoses due to intramural ischemia of the venous graft or complete vascular graft occlusion. These lesions are best managed by secondary reoperative renal revascularization.

Operative Considerations

Secondary renal revascularization is a difficult and challenging procedure. The operative field is often obliterated by dense retroperitoneal fibrosis that encases the diseased renovascular graft and obscures its identification. Successful secondary revascularization depends on an operative approach that avoids anatomy distorted by previous surgical dissection and on careful identification and dissection of the renovascular graft. Intraoperative Doppler ultrasound may be helpful in locating the diseased renovascular graft with a diminished pulse and to identify its relationship to contiguous structures such as the renal vein and ureter. Intraoperative aortography is rarely required but may, on occasion, supplement preoperative studies and guide dissection.

Great care and time are required to establish a plane between the vascular graft and the surrounding fibrous scar. Fine Metzenbaum scissors, an endarterectomy knife, and a finely tipped right-angle Moynihan should be applied as required to slowly and tediously separate the vascular graft from the surrounding scar without tearing the graft or injuring contiguous structures. Dissection into the renal hilum for a distal anastomotic stricture is especially difficult and may risk renal injury and loss. This dissection may be best performed extracorporeally with optical magnification and surface cooling of the kidney in iced saline. Bench dissection and repair with subsequent autotransplantation are also recommended for recurrent stenotic disease extending into the renal arterial branches.

Dissection for proximal anastomotic stenoses or for total arterial graft occlusion may be simplified by avoiding areas of previous dissection as much as possible. This may be achieved in part by selecting an extraaortic technique for secondary revascularization. Splenorenal bypass, hepatorenal bypass, and iliorenal bypass avoid dissection on the previously operated aorta and reduce the risk of aortic injury, hemorrhage, or embolization of atheromatous debris into the peripheral circulation. They also avoid the potential risks of systemic heparinization and aortic cross-clamping.

Preoperative Preparation

Preoperative preparation should be done to avoid the same extrarenal vascular complications that attend primary renal revascularization. Operative morbidity and mortality are consequences of coronary and cerebrovascular disease. The renovascular patient should therefore be evaluated with a history, physical examination, ECG, and thallium cardiac stress test. If coronary artery disease is suspected, further evaluation with coronary angiography and left ventriculography is recommended. Patients with significant correctable coronary artery disease should be considered for myocardial revascularization or angioplasty prior to secondary renal revascularization. Doppler ultrasound evaluation of the carotids, followed by surgical correction of high-grade lesions, is also advised to protect against cerebral circulatory compromise during secondary renal arterial reconstruction. In addition, careful perioperative monitoring is required and may include admission to the intensive care unit for Swan-Ganz catheter placement. Antihypertensive medications and diuretic-induced hypovolemia often diminish renal perfusion and function in the patient with recurrent renovascular disease. Swan-Ganz catheter placement is helpful to optimize fluid balance and guide pharmacologic treatment to decrease cardiac work and increase cardiac reserve.

Operative Procedures

The patient is brought to the operating room well hydrated to limit ischemic renal injury by ensuring optimal renal perfusion prior to and following renal arterial clamping. Mannitol is infused at the beginning of the procedure and intraoperatively to further protect against ischemic renal injury. An extraaortic technique is most often selected for secondary revascularization.

Splenorenal Bypass

Splenorenal bypass is an ideal procedure for revascularizing a failed aortorenal bypass to the left kidney. Its success depends on the patency of the celiac trunk, which should be demonstrated preoperatively on a lateral aortic film. The left kidney is exposed by mobilizing the pancreas and mesentery off the anterior surface of the left kidney to expose the splenic artery and vein and the left renal artery and vein. Previous dissection to expose the left kidney for initial revascularization may complicate this dissection, and great care must be exercised to avoid pancreatic and renal vein injury. The splenic artery is identified superior to the splenic vein. It is mobilized proximally to take advantage of the greater

diameter of the proximal splenic artery and to avoid distal splenic atherosclerotic disease. The splenic artery may be completely divided in anticipation of a direct end-to-end anastomosis to the left renal artery without compromising splenic viability. The spleen will receive adequate collateral blood supply from the remaining gastroepiploic and short gastric vessels. The proximal splenic artery may then be anastomosed to the distal left renal artery with a spatulated end-to-end single anastomosis (Fig. 4-2).

Hepatorenal Bypass

Hepatorenal bypass to revascularize the right renal artery also depends on the patency of the celiac axis (Fig. 4-3). The common hepatic artery is dissected and mobilized to expose its division into the main hepatic artery and the gastroduodenal artery. Small bulldog clamps or circumferential vessel loops may be used to occlude these vessels to allow a saphenous vein interpositional graft to be placed end-to-side at the division of the common hepatic artery to create a trifurcation.

The right kidney is exposed, and the renal artery is mobilized with care to avoid injury to the duodenum, vena cava, or right renal vein. The venous interpositional graft is then anastomosed end-to-end to the spat-

Figure 4-3. *Aortogram in patient with previously inserted right aortorenal bypass graft shows severe proximal stenosis of native artery to solitary right kidney. The bypass graft is occluded and is not visualized. This patient underwent right hepatorenal bypass for secondary renal vascular reconstruction.*

Figure 4-2. *Aortogram following splenorenal bypass shows patent left renal vascular reconstruction.*

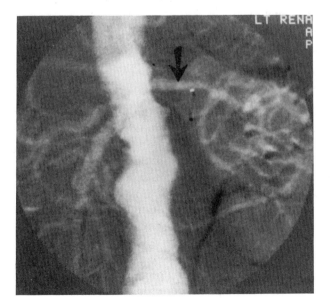

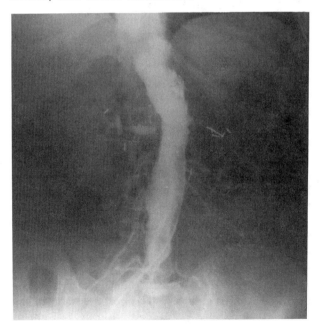

ulated distal right renal artery. An end-to-side distal anastomosis is avoided, if possible, to minimize turbulent renal arterial blood flow and potential recurrent stenosis.

An end-to-side proximal anastomosis, however, is important to avoid ischemic complications of the gallbladder. There is minimal risk of ischemic hepatic injury if the hepatic artery is completely divided due to a rich collateral hepatic arterial supply and increased oxygen extraction from the portal venous circulation, but the gallbladder may become ischemic in this setting, and its arterial flow should be preserved.

Iliorenal Bypass

When a splenorenal or hepatorenal bypass is not an acceptable alternative for secondary revascularization due to advanced disease of the celiac trunk or previous dissection, an iliorenal bypass from the common iliac arteries may be performed (Fig. 4-4). Atherosclerosis is a segmental disease and will often spare portions of the common iliac artery to allow renal revascularization. The procedure is performed by mobilizing a disease-free portion of the ipsilateral common iliac artery to allow arterial clamps to be applied (see Chap. 2). A saphenous vein or synthetic graft is then anastomosed end-to-side to the common iliac artery. The graft is brought cephalad and anastomosed end-to-end to the renal artery. This procedure is limited, however, by the possibility of subsequent compromise of the iliac vessels by progressive atherosclerotic disease, and it also requires a lengthy saphenous vein or synthetic graft.

Supraceliac Aortorenal Bypass

When the above-described techniques are not possible due to previous surgery or atherosclerotic disease of the celiac and common iliac arteries, a supraceliac aortorenal bypass may be possible. The supraceliac aorta is often spared from segmental atherosclerosis and can be used for renal revascularization.

The procedure is performed transabdominally and also frequently requires a transthoracic incision. The left lobe of the liver and stomach are mobilized and retracted to the right. The crural tissue at the aortic hiatus is divided to expose the supraceliac aorta. The aorta is partially occluded with a Satinsky clamp following mobilization of the renal artery. A reversed saphenous vein graft is anastomosed end-to-side to the supraceliac aorta and end-to-end to the spatulated renal artery (Fig. 4-5). On the left, the graft is placed behind the stomach and pancreas. Supraceliac revascularization to the right re-

nal artery is more difficult and requires the vascular graft to be tunneled behind the hepatoduodenal ligament and through the foramen of Winslow.

Postoperative Management

Postoperative management of the renovascular patient begins in the intensive care unit with careful monitoring of urine output, blood pressure, and central venous pressure. These patients are commonly hypertensive despite a patent renal arterial anastomosis due to hypervolemia, hypothermic vasoconstriction, pain, or renal ischemia.

Continuous infusion of nitroprusside is titrated to maintain the diastolic blood pressure between 90 and 100 mgHg. This ensures adequate renal perfusion to avoid graft thrombosis and to prevent elevated blood pressures, which can cause hemorrhage from a fresh vascular anastomosis. A patent anastomosis is confirmed on the first postoperative day with a technetium-99m nuclear renal scan. The uncomplicated renovascular patient will typically stabilize within 48 hours postoperatively and may then be transferred to a regular ward. Invasive monitoring catheters are removed prior to transfer, and the nitroprusside infusion is replaced by maintenance antihypertensives. Serial blood pressure measurements are continued on the ward along with routine postoperative care. Special attention is given to serum creatinine and electrolyte levels, as well as overall fluid status. The patient is generally ready for discharge within 7 to 10 days postoperatively. The patient returns 1 month postoperatively to resume a follow-up program that monitors serum creatinine, blood pressure, and renal function with nuclear renography at 6- to 12-month intervals.

Postoperative Complications

Complications following secondary renal revascularization are similar to those seen with primary renal revascularization. Since these operations are performed transabdominally, atelectasis, pneumonia, bowel obstruction, pulmonary embolus, myocardial infarction, and cerebrovascular accidents may occur. Complications specific to secondary renal revascularization include hemorrhage, renal arterial thrombosis, and injury to contiguous viscera.

Hemorrhage following renal revascularization is a consequence of a poorly performed arterial anastomosis

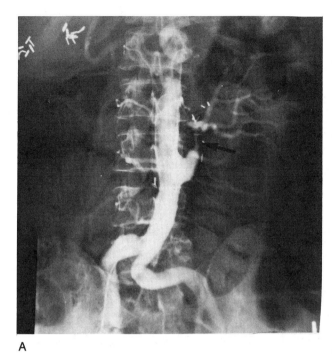

A

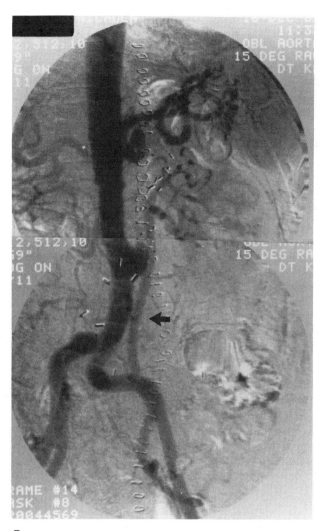

B

Figure 4-4. *A. A 64-year-old man with bilateral high-grade renal artery stenosis underwent a left aortorenal bypass and a right saphenous vein patch angioplasty in 1982. Recurrent hypertension 2 years later was evaluated with aortography and demonstrated complete occlusion of the right renal artery and recurrent stenosis of the left aortorenal bypass graft. Secondary aortorenal bypass with a distal end-to-side anastomosis to the left renal artery was performed. Recurrent hypertension and deteriorating renal function 3 years later were evaluated angiographically and demonstrated a diffuse stenosis of the left saphenous vein graft. Attempted percutaneous transluminal renal angioplasty was unsuccessful. B. Reoperative revascularization with iliorenal bypass using a synthetic graft was performed. Blood pressure and renal function were improved at 3-month follow-up.*

or inadequate surgical hemostasis. Surgical hemostasis may be especially difficult to achieve following a dissection for secondary renal revascularization due to distorted and absent anatomic planes and dense retroperitoneal fibrotic scar. Postoperative bleeding is most likely to occur from poorly secured lumbar vessels in the fibrotic retroperitoneal bed and from the vascular anastomosis, ipsilateral adrenal gland, or an unsecured branch of the saphenous vein graft. Bleeding from these sites may be promoted by poorly controlled postoperative hypertension, incomplete heparin reversal, or coagulopathy. Severe hemorrhage will require rapid central venous fluid replacement and immediate reoperation for hemostasis.

Early postoperative renal arterial thrombosis may occur secondary to hypotension, hypovolemia, or a hypercoagulable state. It also may be caused by intrarenal arteriolar nephrosclerosis associated with parenchymal

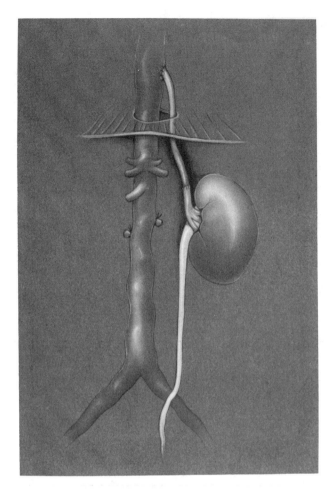

Figure 4-5. *Sketch illustrating thoracic aortorenal bypass to the left kidney with a saphenous vein graft.*

loss and loss of renal function. Kidneys demonstrating advanced nephrosclerosis following primary renal revascularization should be managed with nephrectomy.

The most common cause of renal arterial thrombosis is improper construction of the vascular anastomosis. Technical compromise of the anastomosis may be caused by traumatic injury to the vascular graft during a difficult secondary dissection, embolization of atheromatous debris, or kinking and angulation of the bypass graft. If renal arterial thrombosis following secondary revascularization is confirmed angiographically, emergency reexploration for bypass graft revision and thrombectomy should be undertaken with a view toward renal salvage. Nephrectomy may be required if the kidney is no longer viable due to irreversible ischemic injury.

Visceral complications may occur as a result of difficult secondary dissection. Mobilizing the bowel, duodenum, and pancreas from the anterior surface of the previously exposed kidney for purposes of splenorenal

or hepatorenal bypass exposes the spleen, duodenum, and pancreas to possible retraction injury, pancreatitis, pseudocyst formation, or duodenal fistula. Similarly, dissection and mobilization of the previously repaired renal artery exposes the contiguous renal vein, vena cava, and urinary collecting system to injury. These injuries can only be avoided by taking the necessary time and care during secondary dissection. Potential life-threatening aortic complications of hemorrhage or cardiac compromise from aortic clamping are avoided by using extraaortic techniques when possible for secondary renal revascularization.

Results

The results of secondary renorevascularization are similar to those achieved with primary revascularization. The criteria for measuring the results are also the same. The renovascular patient is considered cured if the postoperative blood pressure is 150/90 mm Hg without medication. If the patient is normotensive with medication, or if the diastolic blood pressure is between 90 and 100 mm Hg and at least 15 percent lower than the preoperative levels, the patient is considered improved. If the diastolic blood pressure is greater than 90 mm Hg but less than 15 percent lower than the preoperative values, or if the diastolic blood pressure is greater than 110 mm Hg, the patient is considered a treatment failure.

Applying these criteria, Stanley and colleagues demonstrated a 97 percent combined rate of improvement or cure in blood pressure following secondary renal revascularization. The associated operative mortality rate was 1.4 percent, and this event was largely limited to patients with significant extrarenal atherosclerotic disease.

The incidence of nephrectomy at reoperation has been approximately 40 percent. Nephrectomy is the reoperative procedure of choice for the nonsalvageable renin-producing kidney and will yield blood pressure control equivalent to secondary revascularization. It does not, however, preserve renal function and should be avoided, if possible, when there is evidence of renal salvageability. The relatively high incidence of nephrectomy further emphasizes the potential for renal injury and loss during secondary renal revascularization.

Summary

Secondary renal revascularization is a technically difficult surgical procedure. It is indicated for the approximately 10 percent of patients with recurrent disease following primary revascularization and produces comparable results. It is associated with a low mortality rate but a high risk of renal loss by nephrectomy and should proceed only after careful preoperative evaluation and preparation. Morbidity and mortality may be further minimized by applying extraaortic techniques for secondary revascularization and by early identification of recurrent disease by careful postoperative monitoring.

Bibliography

Ekestrom, S, Liljeqvist, L, Nordhus, O, and Tidgren, B. Persisting hypertension after renal artery construction: A follow-up study. Scand J Urol Nephrol 13:83, 1979.

Erturk, E, Novick, AC, Vidt, DG, and Cunningham, R. Secondary renorevascularization for recurrent renal artery stenosis. Cleve Clin J Med 56:427, 1989.

Fowl, RJ, Hollier, LH, Bernatz, PE, et al. Repeat revascularization versus nephrectomy in the treatment of recurrent renovascular hypertension. Surg Gynecol Obstet 162:37, 1986.

Fry, RE, and Fry, WJ. Supraceliac aortorenal bypass with saphenous vein for renovascular hypertension. Surg Gynecol Obstet 168:181, 1989.

Kaylor, WM, Novick, AC, Ziegelbaum, M, and Vidt, DG. Reversal of end stage renal failure with surgical revascularization in patients with atherosclerotic renal artery occlusion. J Urol 141:46, 1989.

Khauli, R, Novick, AC, and Ziegelbaum, M. Splenorenal bypass in the treatment of renal artery stenosis: Experience with sixty-nine cases. J Vasc Surg 2:547, 1985.

McElroy, J, and Novick, AC. Renorevascularization by end-to-end anastomosis of the hepatic and renal arteries. J Urol 134:1089, 1985.

Novick, AC. Management of intrarenal branch arterial lesions with extracaporeal microvascular reconstruction and autotransplantation. J Urol 126:150, 1981.

Novick, AC. Complications of renovascular surgery and percutaneous transluminal angioplasty. In R Marshal (ed), Urologic Complications. St. Louis: Mosby–Year Book, 1990.

Novick, AC, and Banowski, LH. Iliorenal saphenous vein bypass: Alternative for renal revascularization in patients with surgically difficult aorta. J Urol 122:243, 1979.

Stanley, JC, Whitehouse, WM, Zelenock, GB, et al. Reoperation for complications of renal artery reconstructive surgery undertaken for treatment of renovascular hypertension. J Vasc Surg 2:133, 1985.

Failed Pyeloplasty

ANTHONY A. CALDAMONE
AUGUST ZABBO

As with any surgical procedure, postoperative success depends on careful preoperative evaluation of the anatomic abnormality with thought as to the options available for surgical correction of the problem. This discussion will be divided into the following areas: preoperative planning, intraoperative factors, postoperative evaluation, and reoperative considerations. Consideration will be given to both open operative techniques and percutaneous endourologic options.

Preoperative Planning

In the evaluation of the functional status of an obstructed kidney, it is important to determine whether a pyeloplasty would be beneficial as opposed to a nephrectomy. This is a particularly difficult consideration in very young children. While one may be able to ascribe a percentage function based on a nuclear renal scan, one is unable to determine recoverability of function. Therefore, the traditional consideration of 10 percent function being borderline for salvageability does not carry the same weight in a newborn as in an adult. If one is indecisive as to whether a pyeloplasty should be performed, temporary placement of a percutaneous nephrostomy tube preoperatively may be helpful. Decompression may result in a better assessment of kidney function over several weeks' time. Additionally, an accurate creatinine clearance could be determined from the affected kidney.

The preoperative voiding cystourethrogram (VCUG) is indicated in most children with ureteropelvic junction (UPJ) obstruction, since coincidental reflux is often seen. Although it is uncommon that the reflux needs to be addressed and dealt with directly, it may have some effect on the postoperative course in potentiating leakage from a repair. Generally, it is a straightforward decision whether the reflux or the UPJ obstruction requires correction in those patients in whom both exist. The decision can be made by performing an upper tract imaging study, either an excretory urogram or a DTPA scan, with a catheter in the bladder to obviate the reflux.

The presence of a dilated ureter on the preoperative ultrasound may indicate a concomitant ureterovesical junction obstruction as well. This should be searched for diligently. Some would choose to do a retrograde pyelogram on all patients preoperatively to rule out this possibility; however, this may not be wise in the newborn and young-infant age group, particularly in boys. However, it is strongly advised in reoperative patients to best determine the extent of narrowing of the ureteropelvic junction and where normal ureteral caliber begins.

Intraoperative Factors

The first decision that must be made is related to the type of repair. This generally comes down to a decision between dismembered pyeloplasty versus some form of a V-Y on nondismembered pyeloplasty. The basic difference between the two is that the dismembered pyeloplasty would be more likely to excise the entire diseased segment if that is the cause of the obstruction, whereas the V-Y plasty would incorporate the stenotic segment into the repair. Theoretically, therefore, the V-Y plasty may have a higher postoperative obstruction rate.

The operative approach to the kidney probably has little bearing on the ultimate outcome. The approach would be more influenced by the surgeon's preference and familiarity with the anatomy than by the cause of the UPJ obstruction itself. In general, however, we have found an anterior approach to work better in those patients in whom we anticipate vessels crossing at the ureteropelvic junction (Fig. 5-1). This may provide for better visualization of the anatomic arrangement between the ureteropelvic junction and the crossing vessels.

It is quite likely that the handling of the ureter may be the single most important factor leading to postoperative success or failure. The vascularity of the ureter must be given the utmost respect. In mobilizing the ureter, it is best to leave as much tissue with the ureteral adventitia as possible. One should avoid placing a vessel loop or umbilical tape around the ureter, since traction may lead to some degree of devascularization. It is safest to handle the ureter by placing a seromuscular 5-0 stitch at its superomedial margin. This not only minimizes the traumatic handling of the ureter but also will serve as a reminder as to its orientation and, therefore, prevent twisting at the time of anastomosis.

When the diseased segment of ureteropelvic junction or proximal ureter is quite obvious, all the segment should be removed. This generally accounts for only a few millimeters to half a centimeter in older patients. The ureter should be widely spatulated along its lateral aspect. It is helpful to place stay sutures at the superomedial and inferolateral aspects of the pelvis, therefore marking the extent of the pelvic incision. Whether the pelvis should be reduced is somewhat controversial. It is likely quite helpful, however, when there is a large re-

Figure 5-1. *IVP of a 7-year-old boy with bilateral UPJ obstruction and crossing lower-pole vessels. Note contrast material just below the UPJ on the right.*

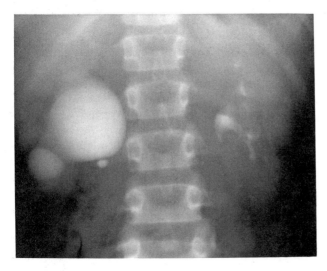

dundancy of the pelvis even after decompression of the system, to reduce the pelvis along its medial and inferior margins. This will generally result in decreased stasis and more prompt drainage.

The ureteral anastomosis is best accomplished with interrupted sutures at the apex and for a short distance on both the anterior and posterior walls, followed by running sutures for that portion of the ureteropelvic anastomosis which is well away from the apex itself. It is quite likely that this will reduce the amount of ischemia to the anastomosis, which is most critical at the apex, the most dependent portion. Whether the ureter-to-pelvis anastomosis is done first or the residual pelvis-to-pelvis anastomosis is done first probably makes very little difference. When the ureteropelvic anastomosis is done first, however, one need not guess as to the length of the pelvis-to-pelvis anastomosis that remains. It is helpful to have a small feeding tube or ureteral catheter through the ureteropelvic junction while performing the anterior wall anastomosis. If one notices an excessive amount of mobility in the kidney, which may result in postoperative angulation and kinking at the ureteropelvic junction, the kidney capsule may be sutured to the psoas muscle to prevent postoperative angulation. The detailed technique of this anastomosis was best described by Hendren.

The use of stents, splints, and nephrostomy tubes remains a controversial area, at least when dealing with the pediatric patient. In most repairs in the adult population, an internal stent is employed. The stent can be extracted under local anesthesia transurethrally, which likely influences its frequent use. In the pediatric population, however, indwelling stents are not used as routinely. Proponents of their use argue that it is likely that they will result in reduced urinary extravasation and urinoma formation. In newborns in particular, a very tight anastomosis complicated by mucosal edema may result in early postoperative obstruction. However, reviews by Homsy and associates and Persky and Tynberg have not supported a more successful outcome with the use of splints and nephrostomy tubes. In fact, both studies documented no significant difference in the postoperative outcome. The study by Persky and Tynberg in particular had a slightly higher complication rate in the stented group. It is possible that the use of stents may increase complications due to increased postoperative infection rate or increased tissue reaction from the stent resulting in edema and fibrosis. There may be some situations, however, where one should consider using a stent and nephrostomy tube. These would include a recent urinary tract infection or trauma resulting in a significant amount of residual mucosal edema, a very narrow caliber ureter, a floppy renal pelvis, or some degree of tension on the anastomosis. A stent providing both stenting and nephrostomy tube drainage in a single tube is very helpful under these circumstances for the pediatric population.

We have found it helpful to maintain an empty bladder during the first 24 to 48 hours postoperatively. This ensures drainage of the operated kidney without any impediment to flow due to a distended bladder. A distended bladder is not that uncommon postoperatively, particularly with the more common use of caudal anesthetics in the pediatric population. Bladder drainage over the first 24 to 48 hours, therefore, may reduce the amount of urinary extravasation and leakage from the newly created anastomosis.

Postoperative Evaluation

A failed pyeloplasty may or may not be an obvious determination to make. Indeed, if someone develops significant flank pain and/or pyelonephritis in the post-operative period, then one can be suspicious as to the etiology. However, persistent pelvocalyceal dilatation postpyeloplasty is not equivalent to failure. There may be months or even years before significant improvement in the appearance of the pelvocalyceal system as a result of the correction is evident. Indeed, in some cases, the dilatation may never seem to improve. However, one may detect increased uptake and more prompt excretion on excretory urogram or diuretic renogram. If, however, there does not seem to be a significant response on a diuretic renogram, then an antegrade pressure perfusion study would be indicated to determine whether obstruction has persisted despite correction (Fig. 5-2). In many instances, a poor response to the diuretic postoperatively may be the result of an inability of the renal parenchyma to response to the diuretic or simply a capacious pelvis that can result in a false-positive result. Therefore, the only reliable standard in determining postoperative obstruction is an antegrade percutaneous perfusion study.

Reoperative Pyeloplasty

Reoperative pyeloplasty can be a difficult and arduous task. One must deal with a significant amount of scarring and fibrosis in the peripelvic and ureteral regions. It is sometimes helpful to approach the kidney from a direction opposite to that used for the initial pyeloplasty, since one may encounter some virgin planes of

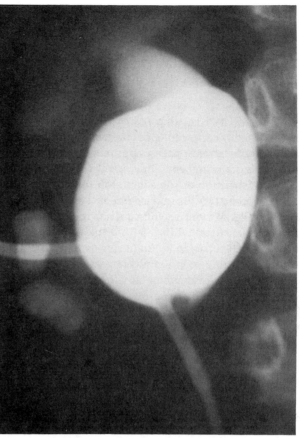

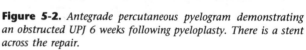

Figure 5-2. *Antegrade percutaneous pyelogram demonstrating an obstructed UPJ 6 weeks following pyeloplasty. There is a stent across the repair.*

dissection. A transperitoneal approach would not be out of the question in certain circumstances. Once again, the ureter must be handled very gingerly. It should be freed with as much periureteral tissue as possible, ensuring its blood supply. The pelvis must be dissected and mobilized extensively, since it is likely that a larger gap would need to be bridged for a tensionless repair. In freeing the pelvis, one should be particularly careful of the renal pedicle, since it too may be bound to the anterior renal pelvis.

A tensionless anastomosis into a widely spatulated ureter is essential. The details of the anastomosis are identical to those outlined in the section on intraoperative factors. Virtually all redo pyeloplasties should be stented and nephrostomy tubes used. In children, these can be brought out together percutaneously and therefore removed by that means without the use of an anesthetic. In a redo pyeloplasty, we generally ensure drainage around the stent before removal of the stent. This can be tested by means of the nephrostomy tube. Once drainage around the stent and down the ureter is ensured with no evidence of leakage, then the stent can be removed. The stent is generally left for approximately 5 to 7 days.

Ureteral Stenosis

When one is faced with a redo pyeloplasty in which there is a significant segment of ureteral stenosis affording little chance for a primary approximation of healthy spatulated ureter to pelvis, one might consider a spiral flap reconstruction or some variation thereof, as originally proposed by Culp and DeWeerd. This is only feasible, however, if there is significant pelvic dilatation and the pelvis is extrarenal (Fig. 5-3). If this is not possible due to a small pelvis, an intrarenal pelvis, a pelvis bound in scar inhibiting mobilization necessary to develop a spiral flap, or in cases where the ureter is stenotic for a more considerable distance, one might consider an ileal ureter. An additional option, however, particularly if there is a very large pelvis in a young child, would be to bring the pelvis of one kidney over to the pelvis of the contralateral kidney. This would work only in extremely unusual circumstances, but it is a technique that one should keep in one's armamentarium.

Ureterocalicostomy

Ureterocalicostomy is a procedure ideally suited to salvage a kidney that previously had undergone a failed pyeloplasty. While a repeat pyeloplasty would be the procedure of choice under most circumstances, this is not always technically feasible. When the renal pelvis is bound in very dense fibrosis due to the previous surgery, infection, or urinary extravasation, or when the renal pelvis is particularly intrarenal, then a primary ureteropelvic anastomosis may not be achievable. Similarly, if there is a small but significant segment of upper ureteral stenosis making it difficult for primary reapproximation without tension, then ureterocalicostomy should be considered.

The situation best suited for ureterocalicostomy

Figure 5-3. *Spiral flap urethroplasty. Anteriomedial projection of kidney shown. A. The projected flap is outlined on the renal pelvis and extending through the UPJ and proximal ureter. B. The cephalad extent of the flap is sutured to the apex of the ureteral incision. C, D. The anterior and then posterior walls of the anastomosis completed. (Reprinted with permission from DeWeerd, JH. Ureteropelvioplasty. In JF Glenn (ed),* Urologic Surgery, *3d ed. Philadelphia: Lippincott, 1983, chap 21, p 235.)*

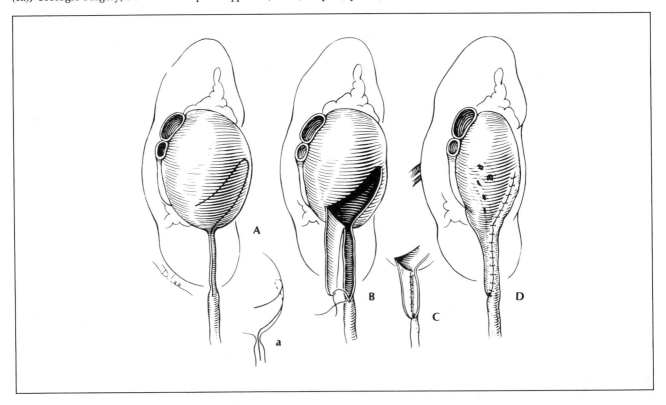

would be when there is significant thinning of the renal parenchyma in the lower pole. However, it also can be accomplished, although with less consistently satisfactory results, in the face of a normal amount of lower-pole parenchyma. Under the latter circumstance, a significant amount of renal parenchyma must be excised in order to expose the most dependent calyx without interfering renal parenchyma. This is best accomplished by raising capsular flaps that can later provide coverage over the ureterocaliceal anastomosis, and then a guillotine-type amputation of the cortex into the collecting system is made. The proximal ureter is widely spatulated, taking care to preserve the periureteral tissue and, therefore, its blood supply. Using blunt dissection, the edges of the calyx are dissected from the surrounding renal parenchyma, and a primary anastomosis is accomplished with interrupted dissolvable sutures. While a watertight closure is preferable, it is not absolutely necessary. This anastomosis is generally done over a stent of (8 French); a nephrostomy tube is also placed into the collecting system for postoperative drainage. The capsular flaps can then be used to provide a second layer of coverage over the anastomosis. Additionally, an omental pedicle graft can be brought through the peritoneum and wrapped around the anastomosis for additional coverage (Fig. 5-4).

Endourologic Approach to the Failed Pyeloplasty

Endourologic management of primary ureteropelvic junction obstruction has more recently come into vogue. Open reoperation for the failed pyeloplasty can sometimes be avoided employing these same endourologic techniques. These techniques are the extension of the intubated ureterotomy of Davis used in the treatment of long proximal ureteral strictures. With the advancements made in endoscopic instrumentation and stenting technology, these methods offer effective treatment without resorting to open reoperation.

A percutaneous nephrostomy also may be necessary to drain an obstructed infected kidney or to relieve pain. If an endourologic solution to the problem is to be entertained, then the percutaneous nephrostomy should be placed with this in mind. The straightest possible access to the ureteropelvic junction will dictate the appropriate calyx to enter, generally a middle or superior calyx in the posterior group. This allows for easier and smoother manipulation of not only rigid instruments such as the percutaneous nephroscope but also guidewires, balloons, and stents. If there is moderate to severe compromise of renal function at the time of percutaneous nephrostomy, then it is preferable to leave the tube to drainage for 4 to 6 weeks to allow for renal recovery.

Figure 5-4. *Ureterocalycostomy. A. Lower-pole vessel is ligated (if obvious). B. Lower-pole parenchyma is incised, leaving a margin of capsule anteriorly and posteriorly. Ureter is spatulated. C. Anastomosis of ureter to calyx and closure of the capsule. (Reprinted with permission from Lucas BA. Ureterocalycostomy. In JF Glenn (ed),* Urologic Surgery, *3d ed. Philadelphia: Lippincott, 1983, chap 40, p 436.)*

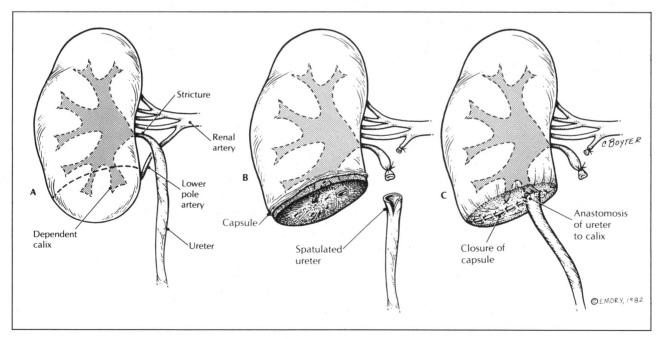

Choice of endourologic procedure to manage pyeloplasty failure will depend on the chronicity and severity of the stricture and the skills of the operators. Dilation of the strictured area is the simplest procedure and can be accomplished antegrade or retrograde. This method is most successful for short strictured areas (<2 cm) of short duration (<3 months).

Antegrade dilation of the ureteropelvic junction can be accomplished with rigid dilators (sequential or coaxial) or with balloon dilation. A guidewire must first be negotiated across the strictured area. Passage of the first few sizes of the rigid dilators may be necessary in order to allow the balloon to traverse the strictured area. The balloon dilator used will vary depending on the length of the stricture and the estimated caliber of the adjoining normal ureter. The balloons range in width from 4 to 10 mm and in length from 4 to 10 cm. Tolerance of the balloon is also important and should be in the range of 2 to 10 atm.

Once the balloon is placed across the stricture, it is inflated with dilute contrast material, and the form of the balloon is observed fluoroscopically for a waist. Sufficient inflation pressure must be exerted to lyse this waist. When the waist resolves, dilation is maintained for 5 to 10 minutes, and the balloon is then deflated. A stent that can be completely internalized or an external nephroureteral stent is then placed. The caliber of this stent should be large enough both to promote drainage and to act to hold the dilated area open. The stent is left for 4 to 6 weeks and, if external, can be switched to a nephrostomy to allow further study and/or drainage. Repeat dilation may be successful if the area restricts early on and the nephrostomy is still in place. An arbitrary limit of three such dilations is set before other methods are pursued.

Retrograde dilation by means of a transurethral approach also can be accomplished using balloon dilators. Application of this method is limited in infants and small children by urethral caliber and instrumentation size. Preliminary dilation of the ureteral orifice or other segment of the ureter may be needed prior to placement of the balloon. The balloon is placed across the narrowed area under fluoroscopic control and is inflated as previously described. An indwelling stent is placed and removed in 4 to 6 weeks.

Endopyelotomy involves the endoscopic incision of the strictured area similar to the method of visual internal urethrotomy. Endopyelotomy also may be accomplished by an antegrade or retrograde approach. In the antegrade method, a nephrostomy is established using the calyx that will provide the straightest course to the strictured area. The tract is dilated to accommodate an Amplatz sheath (Fig. 5-5). The endopyelotome is introduced, and the renal pelvis is inspected. Several different blades for the various manufacturers' endopyelotomes have been developed. A hooked blade that can capture the strictured area in the hook has been found to be very useful. Incision using electrocautery or lasers also has been described, but the cold knife incision remains the most commonly used. Once the pelvis has been inspected, the strictured area is visualized, and the area of incision is planned on the posterolateral aspect of the ureteropelvic junction. This area is inspected carefully to be certain that there are no pulsations from a lower-pole vessel. The strictured area is incised in one place with multiple short, shallow strokes of the endopyelotome. A full-thickness incision of the stricture down to fat is desired. Often, however, because of extensive scarring and reaction, fat may not be seen. In these cases, incision depth is gauged on the adequacy of the lumen created. Placement of a stent across the endopyelotomy is critical to success. The stent should be secure in its placement, extending from the pelvis to the bladder without a free end in the ureter, and the caliber across the incised area should be adequate enough to allow for healing around the stent without restricture (10–14 French). Several special stents meeting these criteria have been developed, both internal-external and completely indwelling types. The stent is left in place for 4 to 6 weeks and is removed or exchanged for a nephrostomy through which the repair can be evaluated radiologically and urodynamically.

Recent reports of retrograde ureteroscopic endopyelotomy have appeared. The method is similar to the antegrade approach but obviates the need for large-caliber dilation of a nephrostomy tract, and in some reports, no nephrostomy is used. Experience in ureteroscopy should be extensive before undertaking these challenging procedures. Even with extensive experience, one should allow 3 to 4 hours for completion of these cases. A no. 2 or 3 French electrode is used to incise the stricture. This requires use of the special operating ureteroscope that is insulated to avoid electrothermal damage to the ureter. A perineal urethrostomy may be necessary in male patients to allow rigid ureteroscopy to the level of the ureteropelvic junction. Again, placement of the stent is critical, and the same criteria for the stent apply. The stent may be placed antegrade or retrograde.

Complications of endopyelotomy include both intraoperative and late postoperative complications. Bleeding is the most common intraoperative complication and generally can be controlled with placement of a large-bore nephrostomy tube to tamponade the percuta-

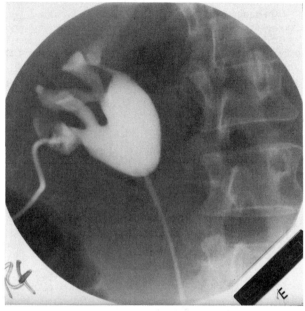

A

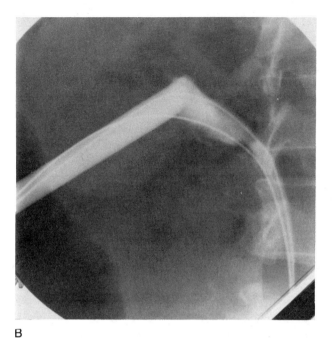

B

Figure 5-5. *A. Kidney with UPJ obstruction, nephroureteral stent in place. B. Operating nephroscope with two guidewires in place. UPJ has been incised. C. Final placement of stenting tube and nephrostomy drainage tube. Note expected extravasation of contrast material.*

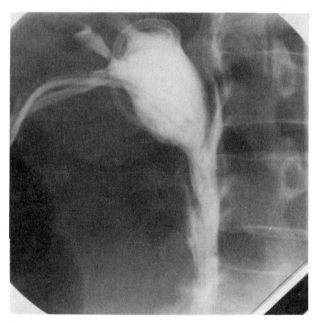

C

neous tract along with a pressure dressing and keeping the patient at rest in the supine position. If there is continued evidence of significant bleeding despite these measures, open exploration may be necessary. Damage to the ureter also can occur, to the point of avulsion, which would require open repair. This complication usually can be avoided if care is taken not to force instruments and tubes across ureter too small in caliber to handle them. Gentle gradual dilation of the ureter first

will generally allow for passage of larger materials. Absorption of fluid from venous entry or extravasation is possible, and saline should be used exclusively except when electrosurgical instrumentation is in use.

Late complications include failure of the procedure, which can be treated with repeat endopyelotomy, balloon dilation, or open surgical procedure. Injury to the ureter resulting in ureteral stricture can present late, requiring endourologic or open repair. This can be avoided for the most part by ensuring that the stent extends all the way into the bladder, since a free end of the stent presents a point of irritation in the ureter leading to potential stricture.

In summary, there are both open and endourologic options available to manage the failed pyeloplasty. Most would opt for an endourologic repair, resorting to a redo procedure if endopyelotomy fails.

Bibliography

Clayman, RV, Basler, JW, Kavoussi, L, and Picus, DD. Ureteronephroscopic endopyelotomy. J Urol 144:246, 1990.
Duckett, JW, and Pfister, RR. Ureterocalycostomy for renal salvage. J Urol 128:98, 1982.

Hendren, WH, Radhakrishnan, J, and Middleton, AW, Jr. Pediatric pyeloplasty. J Pediatr Surg 15:133, 1980.

Homsey, Y, Simard, J, Debs, C, et al. Pyeloplasty: To divert or not to divert? Urology 16:577, 1980.

Karlin, GS, and Smith, AD. Endopyelotomy. Urol Clin North Am 15:439, 1988.

O'Brien, WM, Maxted, WC, and Pahira, JJ. Ureteral stricture: Experience with 31 cases. J Urol 140:737, 1988.

Persky, L, and Tynberg, P. Unsplinted, unstented pyeloplasty. Urology 1:32, 1973.

Persky, L, McDougal, WS, and Kedia, O. Management of initial pyeloplasty failure. J Urol 125:695, 1981.

Stone Surgery

SAMUEL D. THOMPSON
MARTIN I. RESNICK

The management of urolithiasis has changed radically in the last 10 years. The perfection of percutaneous techniques, the miniaturization of instruments that has made ureteroscopy a safe procedure, and the introduction of extracorporeal shock wave lithotripsy (ESWL) has altered the method by which urologists treat stone disease. Open stone surgery has seemingly become obsolete for all but the most selected patients, but at times, the more severe complications of these newer technologies still require open surgical operations. This chapter will discuss the complications of ESWL, percutaneous manipulation, ureteroscopy, and open stone surgery that require an intervention or reoperation. The reoperative technique will be defined, as well as important patient preparation, potential problems, and contraindications to the technique or procedure.

Extracorporeal Shock Wave Lithotripsy

Extracorporeal shock wave lithotripsy (ESWL) is a nonsurgical method of treating upper urinary tract stones which has proven itself to be a safe and effective treatment for symptomatic patients. Wide experience with the complications involved in use of the Dornier HM-3 lithotripter in the United States has been reported, and this will serve as the basis for discussion (Fig. 6-1). Similar complications have been recognized to occur with the newer lithotripters as well. The complications of shock wave treatment that require intervention are rare and are usually related to bleeding or retained stones or stone fragments causing obstruction and/or infection.

Hematuria after ESWL is such a common occurrence that it is almost expected. The hematuria is minor

in character and responds to conservative therapy such as bed rest and oral hydration. The incidence of clinically apparent perirenal hematoma following ESWL has found to be approximately 0.66 percent. Experience has indicated that it is often associated with disorders in blood clotting not infrequently related to the ingestion of nonsteroidal anti-inflammatory agents and aspirin. It is manifested by flank pain and may require transfusion. Initial evaluation should include routine complete blood count, including coagulation studies, as well as a renal ultrasound or computed tomographic (CT) scan to establish the diagnosis and serve as a baseline for follow-up studies. The imaging study also will serve to rule out other causes of postprocedure flank pain, which will be discussed below.

Treatment consists of bed rest, correction of any coagulation defects, and blood product replacement until the clinical bleeding resolves. Frank hypotension is rarely seen with perirenal hematoma secondary to ESWL but would be an indication for angiography to serve as a diagnostic as well as a therapeutic measure. The majority of these hematomas resolve in 3 to 6 months, but a few may persist for over a year. For this reason, surgical drainage is rarely indicated and is most often performed when infection and sepsis are related to the extravascular collection of blood. No data on long-term follow-up of these hematomas are currently available.

Retained stone fragments following ESWL cause ureteral obstruction by a phenomenon called *steinstrasse*, or literally, "street of stone." The likelihood of developing this complication is directly related to the stone burden treated and the presence of a prophylactic stent. Approximately 5 to 10 percent of patients symptomatic for steinstrasse will require intervention. Stein-

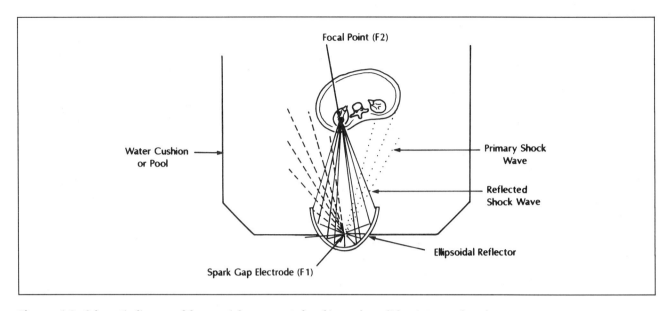

Figure 6-1. *Schematic diagram of the essential components found in spark-gap lithotripters, such as the Dornier HM-3. (From Resnick, MI, and Pak, CYC (eds).* Urolithiasis: A Medical and Surgical Reference. *Philadelphia: Saunders, 1990, p 324. Used with permission.)*

strasse of less than 5-cm length and not associated with infected urine can be managed ureteroscopically if a safety guidewire is passed beyond the obstruction to minimize the risk of ureteral perforation. A ureteral stent should be left in place for a week following endoscopic manipulation. These patients also can be managed with in situ ESWL to the area of steinstrasse. A 90 percent success rate with this technique has been reported. Large-volume steinstrasse (greater than a 5-cm length of ureter) or steinstrasse associated with urosepsis should be treated with primary drainage of the collecting system with percutaneous nephrostomy and antibiotic treatment. Experience has shown that in many instances, with adequate drainage, the steinstrasse will pass spontaneously by ureteral peristalsis. A knowledge of the complications of ESWL requiring intervention is essential for the urologist treating stone patients in order for the potential morbidity to be minimized.

Percutaneous Nephrostolithotomy (PCN)

Percutaneous treatment of renal stones is a rapidly evolving field that involves a number of puncture techniques to gain access to the intrarenal collecting system (Fig. 6-2). The instrumentation includes both rigid and flexible nephroscopes and the ability to perform ultrasonic, laser, and electrohydraulic lithotripsy. Indications for percutaneous procedures remain controversial

but typically include treatment of stones larger than 3 cm, most staghorn calculi, and urolithiasis associated with abnormal anatomy such as ureteral pelvic junction obstruction or horseshoe kidneys. Stones composed of harder material such as cystine and calcium oxalate monohydrate are more resistant to ESWL and are treated more successfully with percutaneous techniques. The major complications associated with this technique are bleeding, perforation, ureteral obstruction, and damage to contiguous structures.

Bleeding is the most common complication of PCN and has been noted to require transfusion in 2 to 12 percent of patients. Proper patient preparation, including reversal of any coagulation abnormalities and cessation of aspirin ingestion, cannot be overemphasized. Proper nephrostomy placement technique is beyond the scope of this chapter but likewise is essential to decrease the risk of bleeding as well as to complete a successful stone extraction.

If substantial bleeding occurs after dilation of the nephrostomy tract, balloon tamponade of the tract and termination of the procedure are indicated. The stone procedure can be postponed until the hemorrhage has ceased and blood replacement performed. The administration of aminocaproic acid is of value in controlling postoperative hemorrhage and can be used with bleeding associated with PCN. Aminocaproic acid acts by inhibiting the action of endogenous urokinase, which serves to break down fibrin clot in the urine. The drug is

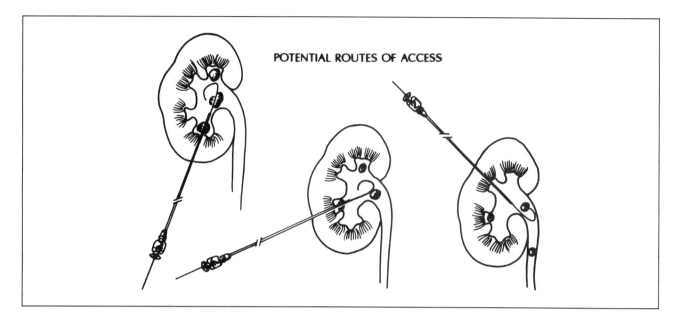

Figure 6-2. *Percutaneous extraction of renal calculi. Renal puncture site is selected based on the location of the stone. (From Resnick, MI, and Pak, CYC (eds).* Urolithiasis: A Medical and Surgical Reference. *Philadelphia: Saunders, 1990, p 295. Used with permission.)*

administered intravenously in doses that depend on the degree of bleeding and the response achieved and is followed by administration of the agent orally for several days after the bleeding has subsided. Disseminated intravascular coagulation (DIC) must be ruled out by the appropriate laboratory tests prior to administration of this agent. Aminocaproic acid will prolong and worsen the potentially devastating manifestations of DIC.

In the event that balloon tamponade of the nephrostomy tract along with conservative measures is unsuccessful or if hypotension presents, arteriography should be performed to further define the site of bleeding. If an actively bleeding vessel is identified, an experienced angiographer often can occlude the vessel by embolization of Gelfoam, coils, or autologous blood clot. The procedure can be repeated if the bleeding recurs, but some loss of renal parenchyma is experienced with each embolization. Delayed hemorrhage secondary to an arteriovenous fistula typically presents 1 to 2 weeks after the procedure and is particularly amenable to angiographic treatment. Rarely, life-threatening hemorrhage must be treated with open partial or simple nephrectomy. This obviously depends on the clinical situation and is a last-resort option.

Perforation or extravasation from the collecting system following PCN has been reported to occur in 5 to 25 percent of patients. If there is evidence of extravasation at the end of a percutaneous procedure or significant manipulation was performed in the area of the ure-

teropelvic junction, a universal stent should be inserted in addition to the nephrostomy tube. A nephrostogram can then be performed several days postoperatively to confirm healing of the perforation and absence of obstruction. The nephrostomy tubes can then be removed and the patient discharged, or the patient can be discharged with the nephrostomy tube in place as a precaution against secondary bleeding. Major perforation or disruption of the ureteropelvic junction must be managed with open surgical techniques, which will be described in a subsequent section of this chapter.

Unrecognized perforation with accompanying obstruction will develop into a urinoma. The patient will present with flank pain, flank mass, and, if infection intervenes, urosepsis. The size and location of the urinoma are best assessed by CT scan. Treatment consists of drainage of the urinary tract by ureteral stenting and percutaneous drainage of the infected urinoma.

Ureteral obstruction following PCN is a minor complication, since adequate drainage is provided by the nephrostomy tube, and access for further procedures to relieve the obstruction can be performed easily. Strictures and stenosis of the collecting system are possible following PCN and will be discussed in a subsequent section of this chapter.

Injuries to adjacent organs such as pleura, liver, spleen, duodenum, and colon can occur in the process of nephrostomy tube placement. Pneumothorax is possible whenever the puncture is made above the twelfth rib. It is commonly recognized on the postoperative chest radiograph or during the procedure under fluoroscopy. Management is straightforward, with the use of simple aspiration intraoperatively or tube thoracostomy postoperatively. Significant perforations to solid organs and a hollow viscous must be managed by exploratory laparotomy and open repair.

Colon injuries tend to occur during complicated PCN involving staghorn calculi, horseshoe kidneys, previous renal surgery, kyphoscoliosis, and hepatosplenomegaly, to name a few. The injury is usually recognized at the time of the intraoperative or postoperative nephrostogram. If the injury is recognized immediately, it can be managed by alternate decompression of the collecting system by a ureteral stent or additional nephrostomy tube and staged removal of the original nephrostomy tube. The original nephrostomy tube should be pulled back into the colon after an adequate cutaneous tract has formed. Once closure of the urocolonic fistula is demonstrated by nephrostogram, the original nephrostomy tube can be removed. During this healing phase, adequate urinary drainage must be maintained, and the patient should be kept NPO and sustained on intravenous hyperalimentation. Experience has shown that most perforations heal spontaneously; permanent fistulization is an unusual event.

Ureteroscopy

Ureteroscopy as a transurethral method of stone manipulation has become an accepted method of treatment as the instruments have improved and the morbidity has lessened over the last 10 years. Unlike urethral and bladder endoscopy, ureteroscopy involves using relatively fragile instruments within a delicate thin-walled structure, the ureter. The most common complication of ureteroscopy is perforation, although bleeding and strictures occur as well. Obstruction secondary to retained stones is a failure of this therapeutic modality and not, strictly speaking, a complication.

The degree of morbidity caused by perforation depends on the size of the instrument, catheter, or guidewire causing the perforation. Wires and catheters cause minor perforations that heal spontaneously within 8 to 24 hours; in these cases, stenting may not be necessary. Perforations caused by urethroscopes, baskets, or other ureteroscopic instruments are potentially more serious and always require ureteral stenting. When a significant perforation is recognized, the procedure should be terminated to minimize extravasation of the irrigant. A retrograde pyelogram must be performed before re-

moval of the stent postoperatively in order to ensure healing of the injured ureter.

The intramural portion of the ureterovesical junction is the narrowest part of the ureter and therefore is the most common site of stricture following ureteroscopy. Local trauma or vigorous dilation of this area predisposes to subsequent stricture formation. Operative management is discussed under complications of ureterolithotomy.

Hematuria following ureteroscopy is a common but rarely serious complication. Conservative measures consisting of hydration, bed rest, and rarely, ureteral stent placement are all that are necessary.

Open Stone Surgery

Open stone surgery is now a rare, but by no means obsolete method of treatment for stone disease. Indications include a large stone burden, stones in the presence of an abnormal, scarred, or previously operated renal unit that will need revision, as well as patients with contraindications to the other forms of treatment. The operations and techniques used in open stone surgery are important methods for the treatment of the complications of ESWL PCN, and ureteroscopy, as well as other types of renal and ureteral surgery. The complications of open stone surgery itself can be divided into two anatomic areas of interest. The operations used to treat upper tract stones, such as anatrophic nephrolithotomy (Fig. 6-3), pyelolithotomy, coagulum pyelolithotomy, and partial nephrectomy, are complicated by bleeding, renal infarction, and obstruction of the collecting system caused by stricture or retained stones. Ureteral stones are treated in an open fashion by ureterolithotomy, which is complicated primarily by stricture formation and extravasation of urine.

Open Surgery of the Upper Collecting System

The incidence of hemorrhage during upper tract stone surgery is often related to the surgeon's knowledge of the pertinent renal anatomy. Complete review of renal anatomy is beyond the scope of this chapter. However, renal hemorrhage will occur in less than 10 percent of anatrophic nephrolithotomy cases if well-placed nephrotomy incisions are made and precise closure of the collecting system and renal capsule is performed. Delayed bleeding is usually intrapelvic and occurs on the seventh to fourteenth postoperative day, and it will usually respond to hydration and blood transfusion. If bleeding persists, passage of a ureteral stent and intro-

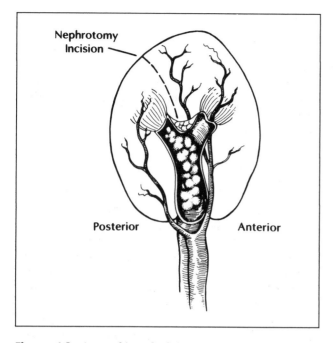

Figure 6-3. *Anatrophic nephrolithotomy. Renal incision is placed along a plane between the anterior and posterior vascular segments. (From Resnick, MI, and Pak, CYC (eds).* Urolithiasis: A Medical and Surgical Reference. *Philadelphia: Saunders, 1990, p 224. Used with permission.)*

duction of aminocaproic acid, as described previously, may be of benefit. Further bleeding or frank hypotension requires angiography and embolization of the bleeding site.

Temporary occlusion of the renal artery is a technique used to decrease the amount of intraoperative hemorrhage and reduce tissue turgor, which will facilitate access to the collecting system for extensive intrarenal reconstruction. When renal artery occlusion is anticipated, care must be taken to ensure adequate levels of hydration and maintenance of sufficient intraoperative blood pressure to produce constant renal plasma flow. The intraoperative administration of mannitol (25 gm intravenously) 5 to 15 minutes prior to arterial clamping will increase renal plasma flow and decrease vascular resistance. Renal cooling reduces the cellular metabolism of parenchymal cells, which enables them to better tolerate a period of ischemia. Warm ischemia time beyond 30 minutes is poorly tolerated by paired kidneys, but solitary kidneys may be able to withstand longer periods of warm ischemia. The method of renal cooling, whether it be packing in ice slush or application of eternal cooling devices, does not appear to make any clinical difference as long as the kidney is maintained at approximately 15 to 20°C.

Care must be used when clamping renal arteries in order to avoid direct injury. Atraumatic vascular clamps always should be used, and they should be applied carefully and gently. Thorough dissection of the artery should be performed prior to application of the clamp; care should be taken not to injure the adventitia and small blood vessels associated with the artery. Injury to a segmental artery during temporary occlusion of the main renal artery may go unnoticed because there will be no change in the appearance of the kidney. Obviously, arterial injury must be repaired and the severed vessel either ligated or reanastomosed with fine absorbable suture, because there is no collateral arterial circulation in the various renal segments. If a less extensive procedure is planned, occlusion of one or more segmental arteries will be sufficient to perform the nephrotomy. After occlusion of the segmental arteries, the ischemic portion of the kidney can be delineated by injection of methylene blue or cooling of the kidney and application of a thermocouple to map the area.

Venous injuries are uncommon, and typically, the main renal vein is not clamped during periods of renal ischemia and hypothermia. In this fashion, the kidney is drained of blood, and the resulting pliability makes reconstruction of the collecting system and identification of retained stones much easier. Venous thrombosis is very rare, even if occlusion of the renal vein is necessary secondary to elevated central venous pressure and back-bleeding.

If open stone surgery renders a stone-free kidney, postoperative obstruction secondary to retained stones is obviated. However, one cannot assume that a kidney has been successfully cleared of calculi intraoperatively until radiography of the entire parenchyma is performed. Radiopaque stones of greater than 2 mm in diameter can be detected consistently by intraoperative radiography.

Other modalities have been used as adjuncts to intraoperative radiography to identify retained stones. Rigid nephroscopy has been shown to visualize approximately 60 percent of calyces. Flexible nephroscopy raises this percentage considerably and is a useful tool in the stone surgeon's armamentarium. Intraoperative ultrasound is another technique that is widely available. It utilizes high-frequency transducers to assist in localizing retained stone fragments. A Keith needle is used as a probe to assist in localizing the stone, and a nephrotomy is made along its tract to remove the retained stone. Three-dimensional localization can be obtained with a hand-held transducer. Ultrasound is especially effective in localizing radiolucent calculi that might not otherwise be identified.

Detection of a retained stone postoperatively requires management decisions based on the type of calculi present and the clinical situation. Indications for ESWL, PCN, ureteroscopy, or open surgery for retained stones will be examined in a separate section.

Obstruction of the collecting system secondary to scarring may develop at the level of the calix, infundibulum, ureteropelvic junction, or ureter itself. The scarring will distort the anatomy of the collecting system and may cause obstruction at any level.

Obstruction at the level of the calix secondary to previous surgery can be revised by a calicorrhaphy, calicoplasty, calicocalicostomy, or diverticulectomy. The end result should yield a completely reepithelialized renal pelvis and calices.

Calicorrhaphy is a technique whereby the calix and its infundibulum are closed by simple suturing (Fig. 6-4). Care should be used to suture only the pelvic mucosa and not include renal parenchyma, which would predispose to arteriovenous fistula and postoperative hemorrhage. This is a rare procedure because most calices are obstructive in nature and can be surgically rebuilt.

Calicoplasty is the surgical modification of a calix and infundibulum to relieve obstruction. The mobile infundibula of the pelvis allow the application of plastic surgical techniques for enlarging lumens. Two or more infundibula may be combined into a single unit. The use of sliding flaps from an adjacent dilated calix or the renal pelvis can be combined with a V-Y plasty to enlarge a single infundibulum.

Calicocalicostomy is the joining of two calices and is used when an absent or rudimentary pelvis must be enlarged (Fig. 6-5). Side-to-side anastomosis of dilated calices and subsequent joining of these structures to the pelvis or ureter will serve to enlarge or create an adequate pelvis.

Before *diverticulectomy* is performed, a true diverticulum must be differentiated from a strictured calix with parenchymal atrophy. The thickness of the overlying cortex and identification of the papilla within the calyx will help with the differentiation. A strictured calix can be repaired with calicoplasty, whereas an obstructing diverticulum should be excised. The thick-walled diverticulum is bluntly "shelled out" of the renal parenchyma, and the stoma is sutured shut.

Every effort should be made to limit the extravasation of urine by closing the renal capsule and pelvis with continuous fine absorbable sutures in a watertight fashion. The use of microsurgical techniques is often necessary. Urinary drainage is accommodated by internal stents; nephrostomy or pyelostomy tubes are not necessary. Removal of functional renal parenchyma in order to achieve a closure must be kept to a minimum, even in

Figure 6-4. *Caliorrhaphy. Type of repair used for a single stenosed calyx. (From Resnick, MI, and Pak, CYC (eds).* Urolithiasis: A Medical and Surgical Reference. *Philadelphia: Saunders, 1990, p 225. Used with permission.)*

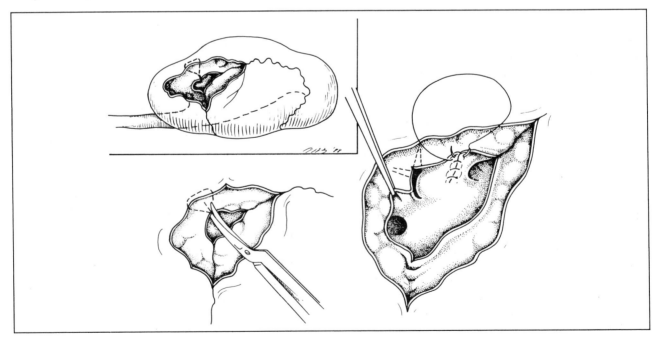

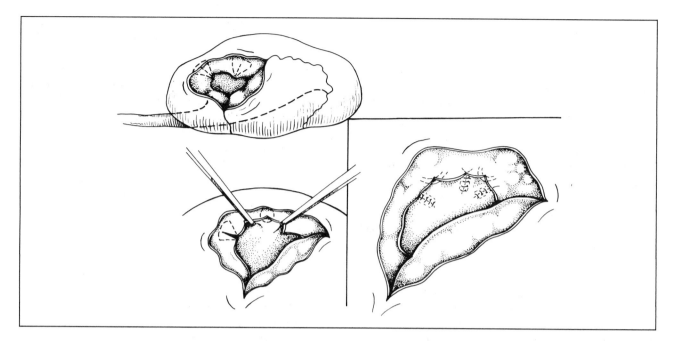

Figure 6-5. *Calicocalicostomy. Type of repair used for adjacent strictured calyces. (From Resnick, MI, and Pak, CYC (eds).* Urolithiasis: A Medical and Surgical Reference. *Philadelphia: Saunders, 1990, p 226. Used with permission.)*

the face of nephrocalcinosis. It should be remembered that resection of a papilla also requires resection of the entire involved arterial segment so that devitalized parenchyma is not left behind. It also should be remembered that nephrocalcinosis in the absence of obstruction or infection will not lead to further stone formation.

Scarring and stenosis of the ureteropelvic junction following open stone surgery can allow calculi to become impacted at this point. Inadvertent injury to the blood supply at this level will cause impaired healing and possible stenosis. It should be kept in mind that the blood supply to the renal pelvis and the superior segment of the ureter arises from the renal artery, runs anteriorly on the renal pelvis, and is closely applied to the proximal ureter. During mobilization of the ureter, it should not be denuded of its adventitial tissue, and occlusive tapes and clamps must be avoided. The ureter should be enveloped carefully in perirenal fat prior to closing, which can be anchored with small sutures. If perirenal fat has been removed, a sheet of omentum brought through the posterior peritoneum may be used for this purpose. A meticulous watertight closure cannot be overemphasized, because extravasation of urine, especially in the presence of infection, will increase the inflammatory response and the likelihood of stenosis. The technique of dismembered pyeloplasty to repair a strictured and obstructed ureteropelvic junction is well described in the sources listed in the Bibliography at the end of this chapter.

Ureterolithotomy

Various surgical approaches and techniques are used in ureterolithotomy, and all of them are designed to accomplish the same goal, that is, to remove the offending ureteral stone. Two surgical complications that all these techniques have in common are ureteral stricture and ureterocutaneous fistula.

Ureterocutaneous fistula is secondary to distal infection, foreign body, or a devascularized segment of ureter. Prolonged fistula drainage should prompt a thorough search for a causative agent. Correction of these underlying causative factors will lead to resolution. Any ureteral manipulation carries with it the risk of subsequent stricture formation. It should be emphasized that in order to avoid ureteral necrosis and subsequent stricture formation, a minimal amount of dissection should be employed in the presence of obstruction and infected urine in order to keep inflammation and scarring to a minimum.

Distal ureteral injuries are best managed by ureteroneocystostomy if sufficient length of ureter is available to perform an anastomosis without tension. An infraumbilical midline incision is used to gain exposure to the distal third of the ureter. The diseased ureter is resected to a point where the blood supply is deemed adequate, and a standard spatulated fishmouth end-to-side anastomosis with the bladder is performed. The apical ureteral suture anchors it to the detrusor muscle; the other sutures are interrupted and contain full-thickness ureter and bladder mucosa. A Silastic stent is used, and a Penrose drain is left in the extraperitoneal space.

A Boari flap is used when ureteroneocystostomy cannot be performed without tension and is usually required with a larger segment of strictured ureter. It is more difficult on a bladder that has been irradiated, traumatized, or has undergone previous surgery. A Gibson incision is used to expose the distal ureter and bladder. A bladder flap 2 to 4 cm longer than the ureteral defect must be raised. The base of the flap at the cephalad portion of the bladder must be 2 to 5 cm, and the distal portion of the flap gradually narrows and is angulated across the bladder to gain length (Fig. 6-6). The ureter is reimplanted in either a refluxing or nonrefluxing fashion as long as tension on the anastomosis is avoided (Fig. 6-7). A psoas hitch, performed by mobilizing the bladder and using absorbable suture to attach the bladder serosa to the psoas muscle, will yield an extra few centimeters of length.

A special mention should be made of transureteroureterostomy only to note that the presence of stone disease is a contraindication to this operation. The risk of obstruction at the anastomosis in the event of further stone formation is the rationale.

Creation of an ileal ureter is indicated when an extensive portion of the ureter must be replaced (Fig. 6-8). The intent of the operation is a proximal ileopyelostomy and a distal ileovesicostomy. Adequate exposure can be obtained through a midline or thoracoabdominal incision. A segment of well-vascularized ileum is selected and brought through the colonic mesentery or retroperitonealized. The continuity of the divided bowel is reestablished, and a single-layer ileopyelostomy is performed. The distal anastomosis is performed on the posterior bladder wall in combination with a psoas hitch to ensure a tension-free anastomosis. Redundant bowel should be avoided to prevent stasis. Because of the relatively high incidence of metabolic acidosis with this technique, renal insufficiency is a relative contraindication. Patients with short gut, small bowel disease, or previous abdominal radiation are poor candidates for this procedure.

Autotransplantation is used when total ureteral replacement is necessary and when other techniques are not feasible or are contraindicated. It carries the risks of renal artery stenosis and rare acute tubular necrosis and ischemic damage but avoids the use of bowel with its accompanying electrolyte and infectious complications. The procedure is contraindicated in patients with significant inflammation of the renal pelvis or hilum. Preoperative arteriography should be performed to determine the anatomy of the renal arteries. The surgeon performing the procedure should be well versed in the vascular and surgical techniques of homotransplantation.

Figure 6-6. *Creation of a Boari flap used for substitution of distal ureter. (From Resnick, MI, and Pak, CYC (eds).* Urolithiasis: A Medical and Surgical Reference. *Philadelphia: Saunders, 1990, p 246. Used with permission.)*

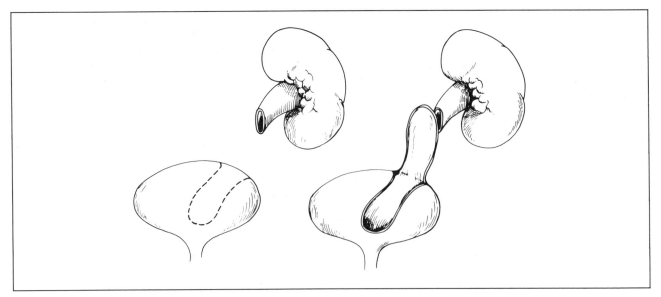

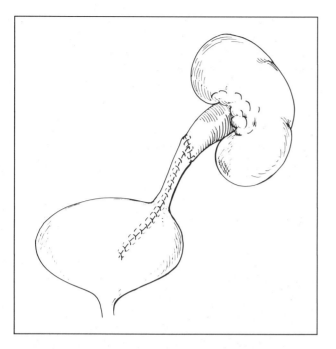

Figure 6-7. *Anastomosis of ureter to bladder flap in a refluxing m,anner. (From Resnick, MI, and Pak, CYC (eds).* Urolithiasis: A Medical and Surgical Reference. *Philadelphia: Saunders, 1990, p 247. Used with permission.)*

Retained Stones

Elimination of all stones and eradication of infection are the goals of the stone surgeon. Retained stones serve as a potential source of patient morbidity, the most serious of which is the need for reoperation. Stones composed of calcium oxalate, cystine, or uric acid may grow in size, but the growth is influenced by the concentration of the active products in the urine and the formation product of these substances and not by the presence of stone fragments alone. Residual fragments of struvite calculi represent a continued source of bacteriuria, a prerequisite essential for stone growth or new stone formation.

Retained stones following extracorporeal shock wave lithotripsy are more likely to occur with increasing stone burden. The stone fragments retained in the immediate postoperative period can cause obstruction in the form of steinstresse, as previously discussed. A patient with asymptomatic retained stone fragments which are neither struvite nor metabolically active need not be treated but must be followed on a regular basis. If infection or stone growth is detected, the patient can be evaluated at that time for repeat ESWL, chemolysis, or another type of stone treatment.

Chemolysis can be used as a primary treatment of

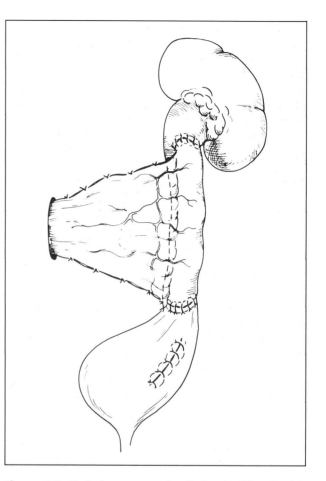

Figure 6-8. *Typical appearance of an ileal ureter. (From Resnick, MI, and Pak, CYC (eds).* Urolithiasis: A Medical and Surgical Reference. *Philadelphia: Saunders, 1990, p 249. Used with permission.)*

a stone or secondary treatment following a surgical or a fragmentation procedure. The choice of chemolysis as a treatment depends on the stone type and location, the clinical status of the patient, and the availability of the methods of treatment.

A number of solutions have been used to dissolve retained stones. Uric acid and cystine stones respond to systemic alkalinization, as well as irrigation with highly alkaline solutions such as sodium bicarbonate, one-sixth molar lactate, and tromethamine E (THAM-E). Struvite stones are treated with appropriate antibiotics and hemiacidrin irrigation. Hemiacidrin is a 10% solution with a pH of 4.0 that is composed of citric acid, D-glucuronic acid, glucuronolactone, magnesium citrate, magnesium gluconocitrate, magnesium carbonate, and calcium carbonate. Local irrigation with hemiacidrin results in complete chemolysis in 73 to 100 percent of patients.

Chemolysis is most effective when the irrigant is

infused directly onto the surface of the stone and complete drainage is available. Intrapelvic pressure during irrigation must be monitored and maintained below 20 to 25 cm H_2O to prevent systemic absorption and hypermagnesemia in the case of hemiacidrin. An overflow safety apparatus can be fashioned easily from a central venous pressure manometer to ensure that this pressure is not exceeded. Rate of infusion should generally not exceed 120 cc/hr. Sepsis is associated with infusion of hemiacidrin in an infected system; therefore, during irrigation, appropriate antibiotics must be used to render the urine sterile, and daily surveillance cultures from the nephrostomy tube must be followed. After open stone surgery, complete healing of the collecting system is imperative before irrigation is initiated. A negative nephrogram should be obtained to show free drainage of contrast material down the ureter without extravasation. The irrigation should be stopped immediately if the patient experiences discomfort, fever, or evidence of extravasation.

Residual stones following percutaneous nephrolithotomy or open stone surgery have been reported in 5 to 45 percent of cases and are related to stone burden, type of stone, location of stone, and stone composition. Struvite stones should be eliminated from the collecting system secondary to the risk of continued urinary tract infection and stone growth. Retained stones that are symptomatic or metabolically active likewise should be eliminated from the collecting system.

Retained stones frequently represent a smaller stone burden than that of the initial procedure and can be treated in a less invasive fashion. Patients are candidates for ESWL if a small stone burden is present in the face of nonobstructive, normal anatomy. Obviously, if a nephrostomy tube is still in place, repeat PCN or chemolysis is an option. Open stone surgery patients may not have anatomy amenable to ESWL and may require PCN, ureteroscopy, or in rare cases, when further revision of the collecting system is necessary, repeat open stone surgery.

Bibliography

Boyce, WH, and Harrison, LH. Complications of renal surgery. In RM Smith and DG Skinner (eds), Complications of Urologic Surgery: Prevention and Management. Philadelphia: Saunders, 1976.

Boyce, WH. Renal calculi. In JF Glenn (ed), Urologic Surgery, 3rd Ed. Philadelphia: Harper & Row, 1983.

Lineman JE, Smith LH, Woods JR, Newman DM. (eds). Urinary Calculi: ESWL, Endourology, and Medical Therapy. Philadelphia: Lea & Febiger, 1989.

Resnick, MI. Surgery of stone disease. Urol Clin North Am 10:4, 1983.

Resnick, MI, and Elkins, IB. Application of renal anatomy to intrarenal surgery. In MI Resnick and MP Parker (eds), Surgical Anatomy of the Kidney. Mount Kisko, NY, Futura, 1982, pp 165–176.

Resnick, MI, and Pak, CYC (eds). Urolithiasis: A Medical and Surgical Reference. Philadelphia: Saunders, 1990.

Ureteral Calculi

CULLEY C. CARSON III

Ureteral stones originate in the kidney and through urine flow are frequently transported into the ureter. Eighty percent of ureteral calculi less than 5 mm in diameter will pass spontaneously. Patients who have previously passed ureteral calculi without surgical intervention or ureteral scarring may be able to pass stones of ever-increasing diameters. Stones of 5 to 8 mm in diameter pass in only 15 percent of patients, and stones above 8 mm in diameter have a less than 5 percent chance of spontaneous passage without intervention. Because of smaller ureteral diameters, ureteral calculi in children should be considered for surgical intervention. The most common locations for ureteral calculi in the ureter that has not been operated previously are at the ureteropelvic junction, the level of ureteral crossing of the iliac vessels, and the ureterovesical junction. Patients who have had previous ureterolithotomies, previously impacted calculi, or traumatic ureteroscopy may have additional narrowed or scarred areas of the ureter that allow urine passage but impede the passage of a ureteral calculus. Thus, in a previously instrumented or operated ureter, calculi of smaller diameters may require open surgical or endourologic manipulation.

Diagnosis

Because patients who have had previously manipulated ureters may have a ureteral course that is outside normal radiographic limits, careful diagnostic investigation must be carried out prior to planning surgical, endoscopic, or lithotripsy treatment of ureteral calculi. Excretory urography remains the most important diagnostic procedure for the identification, localization, and surgi- cal planning of ureteral calculi. In patients with previous surgery, postvoid and oblique views may be necessary to ensure the presence of a calcification within the ureter. Delayed films and prone views also may enhance ureteral imaging and stone localization. Special attention should be paid to areas of previous surgery, ureterostomy, ureteral reimplantation, or ureteropelvic junction repair. If the excretory urogram is unclear and the presence or location of a ureteral calculus is in doubt, retrograde ureterography may further define a possible calculus or identify a nonopaque ureteral calculus. A computed tomographic (CT) scan of the abdomen and pelvis also may assist in the differentiation of nonopaque urinary calculi from lesions such as ureteral neoplasms or blood clots and is especially helpful in patients with nonopaque obstructive lesions of the ureter following bladder substitution procedures.

Expectant Treatment

Despite the technologic advances in stone management over the past decade, it is still appropriate to allow expectant management of many small ureteral calculi. This expectant treatment is especially important in patients with previous surgery, since further manipulation may result in ureteral scarring or injury. Expectant management with increased fluid intake, activity, and analgesics may result in passage of many stones less than 5 mm in diameter. Patients are instructed to strain all urine to determine stone passage. Antibiotics are administered if urinary tract infections are present. Continued expectant treatment with close follow-up is appropriate unless the stone is present in a solitary kidney, significant renal infection behind an obstructing stone is present, intractable renal colic occurs, or the stone fails to progress during a reasonable follow-up.

Choice of Surgical Procedure

Extracorporeal Shock Wave Lithotripsy

Since the advent of extracorporeal lithotripsy and the subsequent development of second-generation lithotriptors, initial treatment is usually attempted through extracorporeal lithotripsy. In patients who have been manipulated previously or whose ureters have been operated previously, ESWL may continue to be helpful. If distal ureteral obstruction from ureteral stricture or other distal ureteral pathology is present, ESWL alone is not an appropriate approach. Steinstrasse (as in Fig. 7-1) is more likely with distal ureteral stricture, impacted stone, or other obstruction. Most commonly, however, manipulation of a ureteral calculus into the kidney with subsequent ESWL achieves the highest success with the lowest number of treatments and the lowest morbidity. Shock wave lithotripsy for primary ureteral calculi is reported successful in more than 85 percent of patients. Success depends on stone size, position within the ureter, stone composition, impaction of the stone within the ureter, and ureteral tortuosity. Riehle reports an 88 percent overall success rate in fragmentation of ureteral calculi, with 84 percent success in ureteral stones treated in situ. Rassweiler and associates also report excellent results with in situ treatment, with 75 of 111 ureteral

Figure 7-1. *Steinstrasse complicating ESWL stone passage in a patient with previous ureteroneocystostomy.*

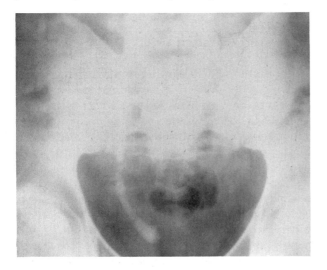

calculi satisfactorily fragmented by ESWL when treated in situ. Overall success was raised to 96 percent in this study by retreatment and subsequent postfragmentation manipulation. Hofbauer and associates report similar results, with an 85 percent stone-free rate at 3 months. Success rates from these authors were 98 percent in the upper, 71 percent in the middle, and 84 percent in the distal ureter. The majority of stones treated by these authors were, however, stones located within the proximal ureter and were not impacted. Newer extracorporeal lithotripsy devices without a water bath may be used for some distal ureteral calculi. The success rate of treatment of these lower ureteral stones in situ is, however, significantly less than those stones treated in the proximal ureter, especially if displaced into the kidney.

Impacted ureteral calculi, especially if in areas of ureteral narrowing from previous surgery, are especially difficult to fragment in situ. Antegrade extraction of these stones may be necessary when ESWL fails (Fig. 7-2). Since the success rate for ureteroscopy, fragmentation, and removal of calculi in the middle and distal thirds of the ureter approaches 100 percent, initial treatment with ureteroscopy may provide success with a single treatment and anesthesia.

Retrograde ureteral stone displacement for ESWL, especially in fixed ureters following surgery, requires some patience and a number of different techniques.

Fluoroscopy is essential in monitoring and assisting manipulation. A portable C-arm which rotates to various positions may be helpful in differentiating pelvic and other intraabdominal calcifications from ureteral calculi. As a result, I prefer the portable C-arm unit associated with a urologic operating table designed for radiographic procedures. This equipment is also quite helpful in percutaneous procedures, and in patients who have had previous surgery with tortuous ureters, intraoperative percutaneous access placement and antegrade manipulation may be necessary. With the patient in the lithotomy position, cystoscopic instrumentation is used to pass a 0.038-in. angiographic guidewire under fluoroscopic control to the level of the ureter. It is helpful to begin the procedure by administering lidocaine intravenously in an effort to promote ureteral relaxation. Using a Teflon-coated Benson guidewire or a hydrophilic-coated Torumo guidewire, attempts are made to pass the impacted ureteral calculus. If the distal ureter must be outlined with contrast material, it is most appropriate to use very dilute contrast material so that the ureteral calculus is not shrouded and can be visualized fluoroscopically during displacement. Careful passage

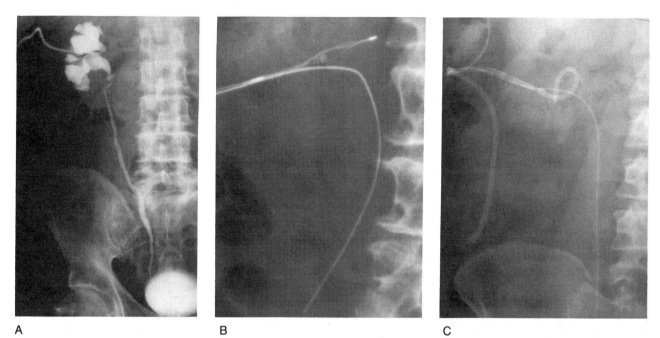

A   B   C

Figure 7-2. *Right proximal ureteral calculus impacted at area of previous ureterolithotomy. Two ESWL procedures failed to fragment the calculus. A. Percutaneous antegrade study. B. Stone in basket passed under vision beyond calculus. No fragment evident in proximal ureter. C. Postmanipulation percutaneous nephrostomy tube and antegrade stent.*

of a guidewire is then performed. It is essential that this guidewire have a soft, floppy tip to limit the risk of ureteral perforation or a submucosal tunneling of the guidewire.

If it is difficult to pass the guidewire, the ureter may be straightened by placing the patient in a steep Trendelenburg position with an assistant providing pressure beneath the ipsilateral costal margin in an effort to reflect the kidney cephalad (Mertz maneuver). Stones that are difficult to pass may require the use of a J-wire or angiographic catheters or the placement of lidocaine jelly around the calculus.

In some cases, however, a stone cannot be passed, and visualization with a small ureteroscope may be necessary to pass a guidewire beyond the calculus under direct vision. Once an angiographic guidewire has been passed beyond the stone, an additional small ureteral catheter can be placed below the stone with gentle flushing using normal saline or lidocaine jelly to displace the stone into the renal pelvis or collecting system. In order to avoid subsequent migration of the calculus, a ureteral stent is placed into the kidney.

Some authors recommend the use of a balloon occlusion catheter at the ureteropelvic junction to hold the stone within the kidney during transportation to the lithotripter. After ESWL treatment, the ureteral stent is maintained in position for 24 hours. If extravasation has been demonstrated during the manipulation procedure, a double-J ureteral stent is placed and maintained in position for 5 to 7 days. Proximal stones that cannot be displaced can be treated in situ with extracorporeal shock wave lithotripsy, but such stones may require other manipulative methods for removal. Documentation of fragmentation with fluoroscopy and subsequent tomography will ensure adequate lithotripsy.

Ureteroscopy

Fragmentation, extraction, and treatment of ureteral stones in the lower two-thirds of the ureter can be performed successfully with low morbidity using ureteroscopy. Stone removal from the lower third of the ureter approaches 100 percent, and that of the middle ureter is approximately 80 percent. These results are equivalent to or somewhat better than the results of lower ureteral ESWL treatment. Expected low morbidity and high success make ureteroscopy the treatment of choice for stones of the lower two-thirds of the ureter in most medical centers. In patients who have been manipulated previously or who have had previous surgical exploration of the ureter, ureteroscopy may be somewhat more difficult, since ureteral tortuosity and fixation may make access difficult. This access difficulty is especially marked in patients with previous traumatic ureteroscopy and resultant scarring (Fig. 7-3). In some such patients, the antegrade approach to the ureter may be more successful.

In patients with previous surgery and resultant tortuous ureters, a variety of techniques, instrumentation, and endourologic creativity may be necessary to help straighten the ureter. Initial passage of an angiographic guidewire through a tortuous but pliable ureter may result in straightening of the ureter and creation of a simple, straightforward ureteroscopic procedure. Initial placement of an angiographic guidewire using a floppy-tipped Benson guidewire, J-wire, or Torumo (glide) wire followed by placement of a stiffer Torque or Lunderquist wire using an open-ended ureteral catheter may further straighten the ureter. Similarly, use of the Mertz maneuver in combination with a steep Trendelenburg position also may help straighten a tortuous, previously operated ureter. Straightening a tortuous ureter also can be accomplished by placement of a dilation balloon or Finlayson ureteral access sheath into the ureter after angiographic guidewire placement. All procedures must be fluoroscopically controlled, and great care must be taken in passing these devices because ureteral perforation in a fixed tortuous ureter is a significant risk. The Finlayson sheath system incorporates a peel-away 60-cm sheath in sizes up to no. 18 French in association with a polyethylene introducer and a polytetrafluoroethylene (Teflon) sheath. This sheath also may be helpful in introduction of various instruments into the ureter during

a complicated calculus fragmentation procedure. Use of a flexible ureteroscope may aid in direct-vision passage of some tortuous areas in the ureter. If the ureter is fixed from previous retroperitoneal surgery, however, these techniques may be inadequate in reaching a stone proximal to a fixed, scarred ureteral curve or area of ureteral stenosis caused by postoperative fibrosis.

Ureteroscopy also may be difficult in patients with previous surgery at the ureterovesical junction. Such patients include those who have had previous ureteral reimplantation, especially if Cohen-type transtrigonal techniques have been used, psoas hitch and Boari flap procedures for shortened ureters, and often multiple ureteral stone passage. Initial guidewire passage in these situations is critical but may be especially difficult after these bladder and ureteral reconstructive procedures. It has been my experience that percutaneous nephrostomy with an antegrade passage of methylene blue or an angiographic guidewire may identify a ureteral orifice that is otherwise difficult to identify. Once an antegrade angiographic guidewire is positioned, it can be retrieved through the bladder and the ureteral orifice dilated in a standard retrograde fashion for subsequent ureteroscopy. Incision or resection of the ureteral orifice using endoscopic scissors, YAG laser, or Bugby electrode can further assist in ureteral orifice dilation prior to ureteroscopy. In patients who have undergone ureteroneocystostomy using the Cohen technique, access to the bladder using a percutaneous suprapubic approach may be necessary to achieve an angle at which the ureter can be accessed. This technique, described by Rich, is also useful in patients with ectopic ureteral orifices, Cohen reimplantations, and following renal transplantation.

Figure 7-3. Proximal right ureteral stenosis, tortuosity, and fixation after ureterolithotomy.

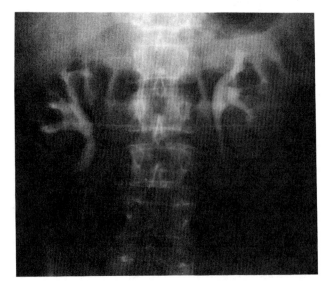

Percutaneous Antegrade Procedures

In those patients with proximal or middle ureteral calculi whose ureters cannot be accessed with a ureteroscope, with significant distal ureteral obstruction or tortuosity, or with urinary intestinal conduits, a percutaneous approach to ureteral calculi may be necessary. Using a percutaneous approach for removal of these ureteral calculi, the number of calculi, the site of obstruction, and the nature of the proximal ureter can be well defined prior to stone manipulation and extraction. With ureteral narrowing and scarring from previous ureteral surgery, adequate dilation may be impossible. In these patients, an antegrade approach may be possible (Fig. 7-4). Because most obstructing ureteral calculi produce proximal ureteral dilation, antegrade ureteral stone manipulation is frequently simpler than retrograde extraction through a nondilated ureter. Calculus fragmentation in these situations may not be necessary.

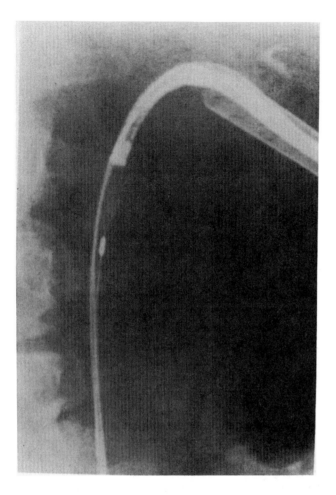

Figure 7-4. *Direct-vision proximal ureteral calculus extraction using flexible nephroscope. Note angiographic safety guidewire.*

The percutaneous approach for antegrade ureteral calculus extraction is designed primarily for use in the upper two-thirds of the ureter, since ureteral stones in the lower third of the ureter are usually best managed with ureterorenoscopy. The most significant difficulty in extracting ureteral calculi is overcoming the impacted ureteral stone and manipulating it into the renal pelvis. In some cases, a combined approach using ureterorenoscopy or retrograde flushing techniques to manipulate the stone into the renal pelvis may be helpful. The ureteral calculus that has been retracted into the pelvis is simpler to remove from the pelvis using standard endourologic techniques. In many cases, however, a percutaneous approach to renal calculi is associated with loss of fragments down the ureter or ureteral calculi in the presence of a large renal calculus. In these patients, a single procedure is useful for removal of not only the renal but also the ureteral calculi.

The most successful and least traumatic method for antegrade manipulation of ureteral calculi involves retrograde flushing of calculi from the ureter to the renal pelvis with subsequent retrieval of these calculi using previously described endourologic extraction techniques. This procedure may be performed using local anesthesia in the cystoscopic suite. First, a no. 7 French occlusion balloon catheter with a 3-mm balloon is manipulated into the ureter over a guidewire. The balloon is positioned just below the ureteral calculus, and the guidewire is removed from the central portion of the catheter. Contrast material, saline, lidocaine jelly, or carbon dioxide can be infused. This retrograde flushing technique will commonly displace the calculus into the renal pelvis without difficulty, even in tortuous or scarred ureters. Several attempts at flushing may be necessary to displace the stone, especially if it is impacted within the ureter. Severe stone impaction, however, may cause this retrograde flushing technique to fail. If the stone flushes easily into the renal pelvis, one-stage percutaneous extraction or extracorporeal shock wave lithotripsy fragmentation can treat the ureteral calculus.

If a stone cannot be displaced into the renal pelvis, it is frequently easier to pass a ureteral obstruction and obstructing ureteral stone in an antegrade fashion, since the reaction, inflammation, and induration of the ureter occur most significantly below the area of an obstructing ureteral calculus. It may be a simple matter, therefore, to pass a 0.038-in. angiographic guidewire such as a Benson J guidewire antegrade beyond this calculus. Once the guidewire has passed the stone, antegrade manipulation can be easily initiated.

In order to approach the upper ureter percutaneously for a ureteral manipulation or endopyelotomy, an ideal percutaneous access tract must be established to facilitate instrumentation of the ureter. Because the ideal placement of this access is so important in the final success of the procedure, careful discussion of its placement, goals of therapy, and renal anatomic sites must be undertaken with the radiologist placing the access tract prior to renal puncture. A lower-pole calyceal puncture, while easier to establish technically, frequently requires manipulation angles of greater than 90 degrees between the percutaneous tract and the ureteropelvic junction. This hampers rigid instruments from entering the ureter. Furthermore, any traction placed on a renal calculus that is to be manipulated is likely to produce trauma to the ureteropelvic junction and may result in ureteropelvic junction laceration and subsequent stenosis. Once an upper tract access has been established, a guidewire is advanced down the ureter past the stone or stricture. An additional guidewire is placed to act as a "safety guidewire'' and is maintained during the entire manipulation procedure.

The percutaneous tract is dilated in the standard fashion, and the nephroscope with or without working sheath is inserted. The ureteropelvic junction is then identified visually. Those calculi which are at the ureteropelvic junction can then be extracted primarily or fragmented using the ultrasonic lithotripter, laser lithotripter, or electrohydraulic lithotripter. Many of these calculi, however, can be extracted primarily despite their difficulty in manipulation without direct vision. Stones below the level of the ureteropelvic junction that cannot be visualized easily frequently can be accessed because the ureter above them is usually dilated. If the ureter is dilated, stones as low as L5 can be seen and directively manipulated through an antegrade-placed rigid nephroscope. Primary extraction of these stones using forceps or stone baskets under direct vision usually can be performed if impaction is not severe.

If the stone cannot be visualized or accessed using a rigid universal nephroscope or ureteroscope, a flexible nephroscope or ureteroscope can be used to follow a somewhat more tortuous and less dilated ureter to the area of the impacted calculus. Once the flexible endoscope is passed, however, rigid instruments can no longer be used, and one is limited to less effective graspers, baskets, or laser or electrohydraulic lithotripters. In most individuals with reasonable ureteral anatomy, the flexible nephroscope or flexible ureteroscope can be passed at least to the middle ureter and frequently to the distal ureter. This technique has been especially helpful in patients with calculi impacted at the ureterointestinal anastomosis after intestinal diversion procedures. Because of decreased irrigation fluid flow through the flexible nephroscope when instruments are inserted, vision may be obscured when one is at the area of the calculus to be manipulated. It may be helpful in this situation to pass an additional ureteral catheter in a retrograde or antegrade fashion to allow high flow of irrigation fluid to improve visibility. Similarly, use of high-pressure infusion aids such as the Ureteromat may further increase irrigation fluid through the flexible ureteroscope.

Once the ureteral stone is visualized, it can be extracted under direct vision using a flat wire basket such as the Segura stone basket or fragmented using the previously mentioned lithotripters. Extreme care and caution must be maintained to prevent ureteral injury or damage to the lens of the flexible ureteroscope during this lithotripsy procedure. A change in irrigation solution to one-sixth normal saline must be carried out prior to using the electrohydraulic lithotripter, since physiologic solutions will inhibit spark discharge. While in the ureter, only single-shot low-voltage settings should be used with the electrohydraulic lithotriptor to preserve ureteral integrity. In this situation, with a flexible ureteroscope, the pulse-dye laser is the most convenient, effective, and safe method for stone fragmentation. Once the stone has been fragmented or grasped in a basket, the nephroscope, basket, and calculus are removed under direct vision. If traction on the ureter appears to be excessive during extraction, further fragmentation must be carried out to eliminate the possibility of ureteral avulsion or injury.

If a flexible nephroscope or ureteroscope is not available or will not pass down a rigid, fixed postoperative ureter, additional techniques must be employed to pass an alternate scope or allow fluoroscopic stone basketing. Balloon dilation of the proximal ureter can be carried out if the flexible nephroscope will not pass. This can be performed using angiographic balloon dilators to dilate the ureter to approximately nos. 12 to 15 French under fluoroscopic control. Through an upper-pole renal access, a rigid ureteroscope can be passed in an antegrade fashion in some cases, allowing some additional options for ureteral manipulation.

If direct vision of the stone is not possible, fluoroscopic basketing in an antegrade fashion may be considered (Fig. 7-5). This option may be especially useful in those patients with fragments of a renal or ureteral calculus that are released beyond the ureter during nephrolithotripsy. If a guidewire has been placed beyond the calculus to be fluoroscopically manipulated, an over-wire stone basket can be employed with excellent expected results.

Once a stone has been removed in an antegrade fashion, the ureter must be stented for at least 48 hours. The stent must pass beyond the area of calculus dislodgment. The use of a no. 5 French Gensini catheter in an antegrade fashion is well suited to this task. For longer-duration stenting, a double-J pigtail stent may be placed through the percutaneous tract and retrieved cystoscopically in the outpatient setting.

Ureteral Stones and Urinary Diversion

Ureteral calculi frequently obstruct ureters that have been implanted into intestinal segments after intestinal diversion procedures. This is especially frequent in patients with chronic renal infection who have developed multiple infection-related calculi. In many of these patients, distal ureteral stenosis or narrowing makes ESWL with subsequent Steinstrasse at the ureteral ileal anastomosis a significant risk. Occasionally, one can insert a

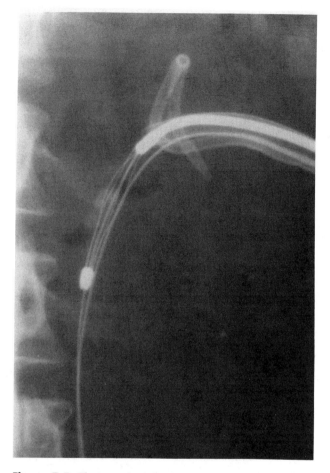

Figure 7-5. *Fluoroscopic-assisted antegrade calculus extraction using overwire basket.*

flexible ureteroscope into the ileal conduit and pass a stone basket in a retrograde fashion to retrieve this obstructing calculus. Most commonly, however, the ureterointestinal anastomosis cannot be visualized effectively in a retrograde fashion or satisfactorily dilated to allow retrograde stone removal. It is, however, possible to grasp and extract these calculi in an antegrade fashion using stone-basketing techniques previously described.

In these patients, an angiographic guidewire is placed using a percutaneous nephrostomy and manipulated down the ureter through the ureteroileal anastomosis. Once the wire is passed into the intestinal conduit, it can be retrieved using forceps, a stone basket, or a flexible endoscope. An angiographic catheter can be passed in an antegrade fashion over this guidewire and out the ileal stoma. This catheter can easily be attached to a no. 4- or 6-wire stone basket outside the ileal conduit. The stone basket is then passed into the stoma through the ureteroileal anastomosis and, using fluo-

roscopic control, is manipulated until the stone is grasped and retrieved. These calculi frequently can be extracted in a retrograde fashion once the ureteroileal anastomosis has been dilated. The stone can then be extracted easily from the conduit. If the ureteroileal anastomosis is stenotic or fixed, the stone must be retracted into the kidney and removed percutaneously, as previously described. Because constant access has been maintained through the ureteroileal anastomosis, a guidewire can be reinserted through the angiographic catheter to allow single-pigtail stent placement. Similarly, a Smith universal stent can be passed through the nephrostomy down the ureter and out the intestinal conduit to maintain through-and-through control for postoperative healing. Use of a self-retaining internal double-pigtail ureteral stent may be associated with mucous obstruction leading to sepsis and even death. Thus all stents in intestinal urinary diversions must be externalized to ensure adequate drainage.

Frequently, the ureterointestinal anastomosis will be stenotic, causing obstruction and allowing future calculi to lodge at this level. This is especially true after patients have had previously impacted stones at the ureteroileal anastomosis for prolonged periods of time. Dilation of these ureterointestinal anastomoses has met with limited success because of their severe internal cicatrization. Balloon dilation of these strictures seems to be effective for only a short period of time, with rapid return of ureteroileal anastomotic stricture. Smith and associates, however, have reported successful antegrade ureteroileal meatotomy in a number of patients. This technique is applicable primarily for short strictures of the distal ureter and is ineffective for malignant strictures, long, ischemic strictures, or other long, narrowed segments of the ureter. Meatotomy can be performed using a no. 5 French ureteral catheter modified with a steel stylet. Most of the stylet is insulated from the ureter within the ureteral catheter. The stylet, however, emerges from one side hole and reenters another side hole for total exposure length of approximately 1.5 cm. This area of guidewire can be placed fluoroscopically to the location of ureteral stricture, and with a brief application of cutting current from the electrocautery unit, controlled meatotomy may be performed. A newer device incorporating an electrocautery wire into a dilation balloon may further facilitate these procedures. After this meatotomy has been performed, the stenotic area will be open. Further opening may be carried out using post-meatotomy balloon dilation. At the conclusion of the incision and dilation procedure, a Smith universal stent or other stenting device must be placed and remain for at least 4 to 6 weeks to allow healing. This meatotomy also can be performed in an antegrade or retrograde fashion using the YAG laser under direct vision through a flexible or ureteral endoscope. This controlled direct-vision incision followed by balloon dilation and prolonged stenting for 6 weeks has been used successfully in three patients at Duke University Medical Center with low morbidity.

Using these percutaneous techniques, antegrade ureteral calculus extraction has been carried out successfully in over 90 percent of reported series. Thus stones in the proximal two-thirds of the ureter that cannot be managed in a retrograde fashion with ESWL or are associated with distal obstruction can be removed through percutaneous methods with a high expected success rate.

Ureterolithotomy

In some cases, however, ureteral stones associated with anatomic defects such as ureteral stricture, ureteropelvic junction obstruction, or an inability to access the upper tract percutaneously will require open classic ureterolithotomy. Open surgery for ureteral calculi is currently indicated for 1 to 5 percent of ureteral calculi too large to pass spontaneously. Similarly, ureterolithotomy may be most appropriate in small children, in whom ESWL and endourologic techniques are not possible as a result of ureteral size or patient size. In addition, some patients who have had multiple endoscopic or ureteroscopic procedures may choose open ureterolithotomy. In many of these patients, Foley or lumbotomy incisions may offer short hospitalization and reduced morbidity.

In patients with previous retroperitoneal surgery or ureterolithotomies, fixation of the ureter in the presence of an impacted ureteral stone may require treatment with open surgical intervention. When a stone lodges at the site of a previous ureterolithotomy or area of ureteral scarring from previous surgery, subsequent ureteral exposure may be difficult. If possible, a ureteral stent or guidewire should be placed preoperatively to facilitate ureteral palpation. Dense scarring and adhesions in these patients may preclude a totally retroperitoneal exposure. Thus it may be necessary to open the peritoneum and mobilize the cecum on the right or the sigmoid colon on the left to palpate the ureteral stone. The stone can then be removed intraperitoneally. A suction drain can be placed to exit the retroperitoneum and the peritoneum closed. In patients who have had previous ureteral surgery, prolonged urinary drainage can be expected, and ureteral stenting and suction wound drainage will facilitate healing of these scarred ureters without postoperative urinoma.

Newer laparoscopic techniques may be an alternative to open surgery for ureteral calculi that are not treatable with ESWL or ureteroscopy. Laparoscopic approach to the middle and upper ureter is frequently performed during laparoscopic procedures. Identification, stone removal, and closure of the ureter can be performed if ureteral tortuosity or stricture precludes ureteroscopy. Stone localization in these cases may be difficult, and fluoroscopic localization will facilitate accurate ureteral incision. Prior to beginning laparoscopy, a ureteral catheter can be placed to the stone, and fluoroscopic guidance can assist with the laparoscopic incision of the ureter. The previously placed catheter can then be advanced past the ureterotomy for stenting, and a suction drain can be placed through the abdominal access port for external drainage. While laparoscopic ureterolithotomy is not standard therapy for patients with ureteral calculi, it may eliminate a large incision and resulting postoperative morbidity in selected patients.

Summary

Surgical treatment of calculi in ureters that have had previous surgical manipulation, especially ureterolithotomy, presents challenging situations for ureteroscopy, percutaneous antegrade calculus stone manipulation, and even ESWL. The endourologist must be experienced in standard techniques and well supplied with skills and a variety of equipment to address these problems. Approaching these calculi from both antegrade and retrograde may be necessary to solve an especially difficult clinical dilemma. After stone removal, stenting is essential in these situations and should be maintained for a minimum of 4 to 6 weeks. An integral part of endourologic experience is knowing when to abandon these techniques and remove the ureteral stone with a standard open surgical approach.

Bibliography

Anderson, EE. The management of ureteral calculi. Urol Clin North Am 1:357, 1974.

Aronson, WJ, Barbanic, ZL, Fain, JS, and Fuchs, GJ. Fluoroscopically guided incision of ureteral strictures in pigs with the cautery-wine balloon catheter: A phase I study. J Endourol 2:241, 1990.

Bagley, DH, Huffman, JL, and Lyon, ES. Flexible ureteropyeloscopy: Diagnosis and treatment in the upper urinary tract. J Urol 138:280, 1987.

Carson, CC. Percutaneous antegrade approach to ureteral calculi. Urol Clin North Am 15:399, 1988.

Carson, CC, Braun, S, Weinerth, JL, and Dunnick, NR. Modified Johnsons stone basket for antegrade stone extraction. Urology 24:359, 1984.

Cass, AS. Extracorporeal shock wave lithotripsy for ureteral calculi. J Urol 147:1502, 1992.

Dretler, SP, Keating, MA, and Riley, J. An algorithm for the management of ureteral calculi. J Urol 136:1190, 1986.

Dunnick, NR, Carson, CC, Moore, AV, et al. Percutaneous approach to nephrolithiasis. AJR 144:451, 1985

Grasso, M, Shalaby, M, el Akkad, M, and Bagley, DH. Techniques in endoscopic lithotripsy using pulsed dye laser. Urology 37:138, 1991.

Hofhauer, J, Turck, C, Hobartl, K, et al. ESWL in situ or ureteroscopy for ureteric stones? World J Urol 11:54, 1993.

Hulbert, JC, Reddy, PK, Gonzalez RT et al. Percutaneous management of ureteral calculi facilitated by retrograde flushing with carbon dioxide or diluted radioopaque dye. J Urol 134:29, 1985.

Kahn, RI. Endourological treatment of ureteral calculi. J Urol 135:239, 1986.

Kapoor, DA, Leech, JE, Yap, WT, et al. Cost and efficacy of ESWL versus ureteroscopy in the treatment of lower ureteral calculi. J Urol 148:1095, 1992.

Kavoussi, LR, Clayman, RV, Brunt, LM, and Soper, NJ. Paparoscopic ureterolysis. J. Urol 147:426, 1992.

Kressel, K, Hoffmann, H, and Butz, M. Long term experience with transurethral rigid ureteroscopy as a complementary method to ESWL. Urol Int 48:76, 1992.

Lingeman, JE. ESWL for ureteral stones above the pelvic brim. Probl Urol 1:630, 1987.

Meteryk, S, Albala, DM, Clayman, RV, et al. Endoureterotomy for treatment of ureteral strictures. J Urol 147:1502, 1992.

Miller, GA, Dunnick, NR, and Carson, CC. Radiographic percutaneous manipulation. In CC Carson and NR Dunnick (eds), Endourology. New York: Churchill-Livingstone, 1985, p 71.

Morse, RM, and Resnick, MI. Ureteral calculi: Natural history and treatment in an era of advanced technology. J Urol 145:263, 1991.

Perez, LM, Friedman, RM, and Carson, CC. Endoureteropyelotomy in adults: Review of procedure and results. Urology 39:71, 1992.

Psihramis, KE. Laser lithotripsy of difficult ureteral calculus: Results in 122 patients. J Urol 147:1010, 1992.

Raboy, A, Fenzli, GS, Ioffreda BT, and Albert, PS. Laparoscopic ureterolithotomy. Urology 39:223, 1992.

Rossweller, J, and Eisenberger, F. ESWL of distal ureteral calculi. In RA Riehle (ed), Principles of ESWL. New York: Churchill-Livingstone, 1987, p 185.

Rich, MA. Ureteroscopy of the abnormal ureter. Urol Clin North Am 15:407, 1988.

Riehle, RA. Extracorporeal shock wave lithotripsy: Patient selection and results. Probl Urol 1:609, 1987.

Smith, AD, Lange, PH, Miller, RP, et al. Controlled ureteral meatotomy. J Urol 121:587, 1979.

Walther, PJ, Robertson, CN, and Paulson, DF. Lethal complications of standard self-retaining ureteral stents in patients with ileal conduit urinary diversion. J Urol 133:851, 1985.

Weinberg, JJ, Snyder, JA, and Smith, AD. Mechanical extraction of stones with ureteroscopes. Urol Clin North Am 15:339, 1988.

Ureteral Strictures

DAVID ESRIG
JEFFRY L. HUFFMAN

The failed repair of a ureteral stricture is an important and often difficult problem in urologic practice. Although commonly believed that gynecologic and general surgical procedures account for the greatest numbers of ureteral injuries and consequently the highest rate of strictures, a recent review demonstrated that only 13 percent of strictures are secondary to nonurologic procedures.

The most common urologic causes for ureteral strictures are stenosis of a ureteral ileal anastomosis, ureteral lithotomy, and ureteroscopy. As indications for flexible and rigid ureteroscopy are expanding, we may be faced with an even higher incidence of these complications.

The management of *recurrent* ureteral strictures following an attempt at unsuccessful repair may be a surgical dilemma. In the past decade, the refinements in endourology have fast become a therapeutic alternative to surgery in the management of these strictures.

The preoperative evaluation of a patient with a recurrent ureteral stricture must delineate the entire extent of ureteral involvement for optimal results. Antegrade and retrograde pyelography in conjunction with a triple-phase renal isotope study, including furosemide washout, is necessary for morphologic evaluation. A Whittaker test also might be considered, especially if a nephrostomy tube is in place. The patient's physical condition, of course, will influence therapeutic options. For example, the debilitated or end-stage cancer patient may best be managed conservatively with either an indwelling stent or percutaneous nephrostomy.

Etiology

Nonurologic Surgery

Trauma to the ureter during intraabdominal and pelvic surgery may result in ureteral stricture. Gynecologic surgery followed by colorectal surgery ranks as the most frequent nonurologic procedure resulting in this problem. Devascularization, ligation, crush injury, fulguration, and perforation with fistula formation are all possible causes of stricture disease created by intraoperative injury.

Within the boundaries of the true pelvis, the ureter is in close proximity to the ovarian pedicle, is crossed anteriorly by the uterine vessels, and runs lateral to the cervix. It may be injured at any of these locations. Radical hysterectomy has the highest incidence of ureteral injury. The injury usually occurs during ligation of the uterine pedicle or might result after devascularization of the ureter during dissection within the broad ligament. Bleeding can obscure the operative field, resulting in inadvertent clamping or ligation of the ureter. Inadvertent injury to the ureter also may occur during vaginal hysterectomy when surgical exposure is suboptimal or during oophorectomy when the ureter lies in close proximity to the ovarian pedicle.

General surgical procedures involving the rectum and sigmoid colon are occasionally associated with ureteral injury leading to subsequent stricture formation. The left ureter is injured more frequently because it is closer to the sigmoid colon, which may be involved in disease processes such as tumor and diverticulitis. The inflammatory phlegmon caused by diverticulitis may result in significant periureteral fibrosis and ureteral stricture. If the surgeon believes the inflammatory process is extensive or significant tumor burden exists, then a preoperative ureteral stent should be placed for easier identification of the ureter.

Abdominal aortic aneurysm can cause a significant inflammatory reaction with fibrosis and narrowing of the ureter. Repair of the aneurysm may be associated with ureteral fistula or stenosis. The location of the ureteral stricture following this type of vascular surgery limits the surgical options for repair. The position is too proximal for a psoas hitch or Boari flap, and the surrounding inflammation would make a ureteroureterostomy or transureteroureterostomy difficult. Therefore, ileal ureter substitution, autotransplantation, and nephrectomy would be options in management.

Urologic Surgery

Ureterolithotomy and pyelolithotomy are associated with stricture disease for a variety of reasons. Stone impaction causes an inflammatory reaction with subsequent fibrosis. Impairment of blood supply secondary to vigorous tissue manipulation during surgery or excessive traction on the anastomosis may result in stricture formation. The type of ureterotomy used, transverse versus longitudinal, can be implicated as the causative factor.

Smith reported 94 patients with ureteral strictures secondary to urologic procedures. Fifteen were the result of pyelolithotomy. Of these, 13 were managed successfully by endopyelotomy and 2 by open repair. We believe that endopyelotomy should be the initial option for repair of all secondary ureteral pelvic junction (UPJ) strictures. Conservative measures for treating upper ureteral strictures with dilation have been unsuccessful. Smith reported 4 patients with midureteral strictures following ureteral lithotomy managed by balloon dilation. All these procedures failed. Three patients were managed successfully by Boari flap and one by transureteroureterostomy.

Banner and Pollack reported a series of 27 benign ureteral strictures treated by balloon dilation, including 3 following ureterolithotomy. All 3 responded to balloon dilation. The authors hypothesized that these patients became symptomatic early with hydronephrotic pain, and intervention was performed before the stricture became densely fibrotic.

The ureteral orifice may be injured during transurethral resection of bladder tumors or the prostate gland. The ureteral stenosis may be managed initially conservatively with balloon dilation or meatotomy;

however, if the stricture returns, reimplantation should be considered. Dilation of the ureteral orifice and intramural tunnel for ureteroscopy do not seem to cause stricture disease. In a series of 300 patients, Bagley reported no ureteral-vesical junction strictures. He attributes the lack of stenosis to adherence to strict guidelines for adequate dilation and passage of the smallest practical instrument.

Diagnosis

The patient with a recurrent ureteral stricture usually presents with symptomatic ureteral obstruction. Generally, these patients have abdominal or flank pain and often urinary infection. In addition, stone formation secondary to stasis also may complicate the clinical picture. Occasionally, a patient may present with "silent" obstruction noted on follow-up studies.

The intravenous urogram (IVU) will be the initial imaging study in most instances. Delayed excretion with or without an obstructed nephrogram effect reflects both the severity and the acuteness of the obstruction. Calicectasis is usually present, but this finding is not a reliable indicator of recurrent obstruction, since postobstructive atrophy may have occurred, characterized by permanent dilation of the intrarenal collecting system. The site of ureteral narrowing should be viewed on multiple images before concluding that it represents the location of obstruction.

Cystoscopy with retrograde ureteropyelography should be performed in order to evaluate the distal extent of the stricture. The initial contrast film should be taken after instillation of 3 cc of contrast material, followed by more films with larger volumes of contrast material if necessary to opacify the upper ureter and renal pelvis. Care should be taken to avoid high-pressure injection and overdistension of the ureter and collecting system. Partial obstruction from a recurrent ureteral stricture will be seen as narrowing with little contrast material in the proximal ureter or renal pelvis depending on the location of the stricture. Delayed images demonstrating impaired drainage from the upper urinary system confirm the presence of obstruction. Complete obstruction is indicated by the failure of any contrast material to flow proximal to the area of stricture.

The presence of incomplete obstruction may be equivocal by standard radiographic studies. The diagnosis may be obscured by the fact that the patient has already undergone one operation for repair of the stricture. The urinary system, previously blocked and dilated, may not have returned to normal anatomically.

Therefore, use of the renal isotope scan with either diethylenetriamine pentaacetic acid (DTPA) or glucoheptonate (GHA) becomes invaluable for the diagnosis of obstruction and the evaluation of individual kidney function. A normal renal scan should demonstrate bilaterally symmetrical isotope uptake with visualization of the collecting systems on the 3- to 6-minute images. Initial activity in each kidney (T_{max}) should be reduced by at least 50 percent ($T_{1/2, max}$) at 9 to 12 minutes. Diuresis-induced renal isotope scanning attempts to distinguish between anatomic dilation and functional obstruction. This test becomes a crucial part of the preoperative evaluation of the recurrent ureteral stricture. A loop diuretic, usually furosemide, is administered intravenously at the plateau of isotope activity. Obstruction is considered to be present if it takes longer than 15 minutes to wash out 50 percent of the tracer activity from the renal pelvis. The major limitation to the renal isotope scan is its interpretation in the face of renal insufficiency, often present with chronic stricture disease.

If the initial stricture was treated percutaneously, or if a nephrostomy tube was required for relief of obstruction, then antegrade pyelography may be performed to better evaluate the upper ureter and renal pelvis. In this situation, the antegrade instillation of contrast material through a nephrostomy tube provides information on ureteral anatomy proximal to the stricture. It is important to know that the upper ureter transports contrast material promptly to the point of narrowing or if there is additional stricture disease.

The percutaneous tube also allows for the use of the Whittaker test. The Whittaker test, like the diuresis renal scan, attempts to distinguish urinary dilation from obstruction. Through a nephrostomy tube, fluid is instilled at a rate of 10 cc/min, and the pressure is measured in the renal pelvis and bladder. If the system is completely obstructed, the pelvic pressure will continue to rise at any flow rate. Significant obstruction is diagnosed with a pressure difference greater than 20 cm H_2O.

As the indications for ureteroscopy expand, the numbers of ureteral strictures encountered may increase. Thus far, however, postprocedure strictures are exceedingly rare. Biester and Gillenwater report 4 cases of ureteral stricture following ureteroscopy, 2 of which were located in the upper ureter. Lyon and associates reported 3 strictures in 240 patients following ureteroscopy and ultrasonic lithotripsy. Possible mechanisms for these ureteral injuries include stone extraction that involved prolonged stone fragmentation with either electrohydraulic or ultrasonic lithotripsy. Also, perforation with urinary extravasation may cause periureteral fibrosis and subsequent stricture.

One of the more frequent causes of ureteral strictures in urologic surgery involves stenosis of the ureteral-intestinal anastomosis in ileal conduits. This complication has an incidence of approximately 4 percent. Continent diversion is gradually replacing the ileal conduit as the preferred method of diversion and maintains a similar anastomotic stricture rate. The cause of these strictures is stripping of the adventitial blood supply to the ureter during its mobilization. An important point to remember is that recurrent tumor must be ruled out as the cause for an anastomotic narrowing in a patient whose cystectomy is performed for carcinoma.

The standard treatment for this stricture is exploratory laparotomy with revision of the ureteral-intestinal anastomosis. However, Kramolowsky and associates reported on seven patients with strictures in whom endoscopic incision and balloon dilation were performed. They compared this group to nine patients undergoing open revision and found an 89 percent success rate compared with 71 percent for the endoscopically managed group. In comparing these two techniques, the authors found that the group managed endoscopically had fewer intraoperative and postoperative complications. Three of the procedures also were performed under local anesthesia.

Considerations Prior to Reoperation of a Ureteral Stricture

The urologist faced with a recurrent stricture must consider a variety of therapeutic alternatives before proceeding with repair (Figs. 8-1 and 8-2). The surgeon also must realize that the choice of procedure should be definitive and long lasting. The patient may be anxious or even angry; has undergone a multitude of tests, radiographic studies, and hospitalizations; and desires intervention that will solve the problem. Only after a detailed preoperative workup as outlined above can this be accomplished.

One of the basic decisions is whether repair will be performed by endourologic techniques or open surgery. The success of endourologic repair of ureteral strictures ranges from 48 to 63 percent and depends on a variety of factors. Beckman and Roth report a 66 percent success rate for percutaneous incision and balloon dilation for secondary ureteropelvic-junction strictures. Most investigators agree that strictures of short duration and short length are more amenable to endoscopic manipulation. Chang and associates reported that ureteral strictures of 2 cm or less responded well to balloon dilation and stenting. They described the radiographic distinc-

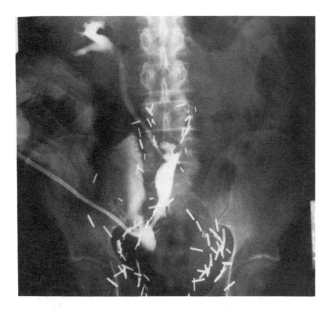

Figure 8-1. *An 80-year-old patient presented 6 years after radical cystectomy and continent urinary diversion because of left flank pain and urinary tract sepsis. IVU demonstrated left hydronephrosis, and CT scan showed the left hydronephrosis but no evidence of retroperitoneal disease. A left percutaneous nephrostomy tube was placed initially, and the patient's infection resolved. Unfortunately, the nephrostomy tube became dislodged. Therefore, an endoscopic procedure was performed in a retrograde route through the Kock pouch stoma. This radiograph shows a flexible nephroscope passed through the efferent and afferent valve of the Kock pouch reservoir and into the afferent limb. Free reflux is noted into the right collecting system but none in the left.*

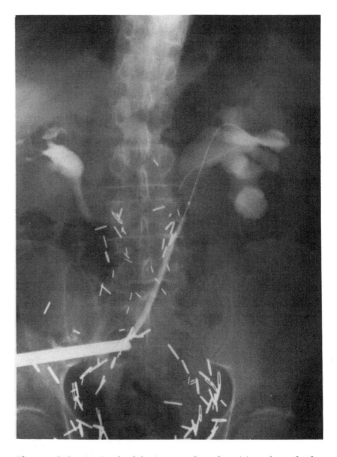

Figure 8-2. *A wire had been passed under vision through the flexible instrument into the upper urinary tract, and a catheter passed over the wire was used to instill contract material, opacifying the dilated left urinary system. The catheter was removed after a wire was replaced, and over the wire a 10 cm × 6 mm balloon dilating catheter was passed and inflated to dilate the ureteral-ileal stricture. This radiograph demonstrates the balloon dilating catheter across the region of the ureteral-ileal stricture with the floppy-tip guidewire coiled in the dilated left renal pelvis. A diversionary stent was left in place, and follow-up Lasix washout renal scan showed improved function of the left kidney without obstruction.*

tion between short and long strictures. Short strictures on antegrade pyelography demonstrate a dilated ureter proximal to the stenosis with abrupt narrowing at the stricture site. Long strictures show a gradual tapering of the ureter to the narrowed segment because of the limited distensibility of the ureter proximal to the stricture.

A short interval between ureteral surgery or injury and the dilation procedure is associated with a higher success rate. Investigators postulate the reason for this to be associated with less organized fibrous tissue and a more "elastic" scar.

Important consideration should be given to the type of previous surgery that resulted in ureteral stricture. Strictures secondary to radical hysterectomy are usually not amenable to endoscopic dilation because of ureteral hypoxemia and frequent use of preoperative radiation. Strictures that result from ureteral perforation with fistula formation also do not respond as well to endoscopic techniques secondary to extensive periureteral fibrosis. Stenoses at the ureteral-intestinal anastomosis are unlikely to remain patent after dilation

alone, but good results have been obtained with endoscopic incision and stenting. Strictures occurring after ureteral lithotomy are often managed successfully with dilation only.

Endoscopic techniques are less invasive and associated with fewer complications compared with open surgery. They are also associated with a shorter hospital stay. These facts make them more attractive as first-line treatment for strictures. However, little data exist on their effectiveness and their degree of safety in managing recurrent ureteral stricture. Most investigators admit to a higher success rate for open surgery. However, with these better results come more frequent complications such as bleeding, intestinal injury, small bowel obstruction, and abscess formation. In addition, open repair frequently requires extensive ureteral mobilization. Complications of endoscopic incision and dilation are infrequent but may include ureteral perforation and urinoma formation and creation of new and multiple strictures. Management of the recurrent stricture also should be dictated by the skill and expertise of the urologist at endoscopic techniques.

The medical condition of the patient also should play an important role in the decision process. The debilitated or elderly patient may be managed most appropriately with simple ureteral stenting. If a more definitive procedure is necessary, percutaneous techniques are advantageous because they frequently are performed under local anesthesia with intravenous sedation only. If at all possible, the cancer patient with metastatic disease should be managed by nonsurgical means.

Finally, the degree of function of the involved renal unit is an important consideration. If little function remains and it is associated with pain or infection, then nephrectomy should be performed. A patient with marginal renal function or stricture disease in a solitary renal unit should be managed with the procedure with the highest possibility for success.

Procedures for Treatment of Recurrent Stricture

Endoscopic Balloon Dilation

Development of the Gruntzig balloon catheter dilation for coronary arteries, in addition to refined ureteroscopic and percutaneous techniques, has changed the approach to ureteral strictures. Most investigators agree that balloon dilation may be used with a moderate chance of success for strictures of short length (less than 2 cm) and short duration (less than 3 months). This would apply to primary and secondary strictures. If these criteria exist, then a stricture that has already undergone open repair may be approached with dilation or endoscopic incision.

Endoscopic balloon dilation may be approached antegrade through a percutaneous nephrostomy or retrograde by means of the cystoscope. A 0.035-in. Bentson guidewire is passed beyond the stricture site. A 4- to 6-mm balloon catheter is then inserted over the guidewire and its position confirmed fluoroscopically. The balloon is then inflated until no waist is visualized, confirming complete balloon expansion. An indwelling ureteral stent, usually a no. 6 to 10 French, is left in place

for 4 to 6 weeks to allow time for healing around the stent.

Endopyelotomy

Management of a recurrent stricture at the ureteropelvic junction after failed pyeloplasty or other types of open surgery may be accomplished by endoscopic incision (Figs. 8-3 to 8-6). This procedure is based on the work of Davis with an intubated ureterotomy and has recently been popularized by Smith through a percutaneous nephrostomy access. Endopyelotomy also may be performed through a transurethral ureteroscopic route, but this procedure is technically more difficult. The technique for endopyelotomy has been described in detail by Smith. In summary, after dilation of the percutaneous nephrostomy tract, a guidewire is passed under vision through the ureteropelvic junction stenosis. If unsuccessful, an attempt should be made to pass the guidewire in a retrograde manner to be grasped with a nephroscope. An endopyelotomy blade is passed by

Figure 8-3. *A 29-year-old woman had suffered a ureteral injury at the time of vaginal hysterectomy treated by right ureteral implant and stent placement. Following this procedure, obstruction of the right ureteropelvic junction was noted on follow-up IVU. This condition did not exist on studies done prior to the ureteral reimplantation surgery. This x-ray demonstrates a right retrograde ureterogram with complete obliteration of the ureter at the level of the right ureteropelvic junction.*

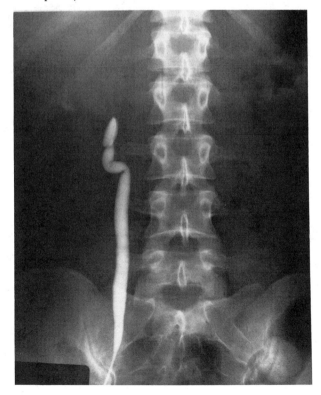

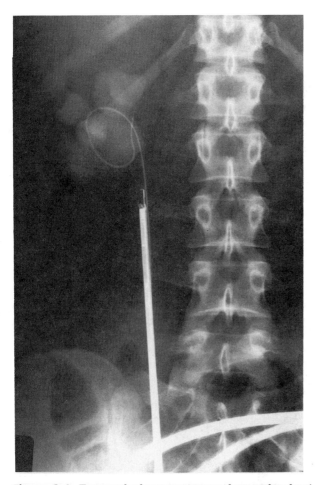

Figure 8-4. *Transurethral ureteroscopy was done, and under vision, the opening into the renal pelvis was identified. The flexible-tip guidewire was passed and contrast material instilled. This radiograph demonstrates the rigid ureteroscope in the proximal ureter with the endoscopic stricture blade extended from the tip of the instrument. The guidewire is noted to be coiled in the renal pelvis with marked hydronephrosis present.*

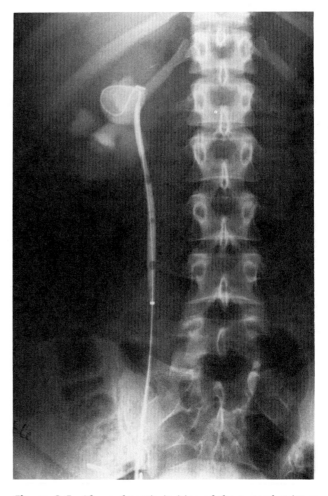

Figure 8-5. *After endoscopic incision of the ureteral stricture, which was done laterally, a 5 mm × 10 cm balloon dilating catheter was passed and the balloon inflated. This radiograph demonstrates partial expansion of the balloon dilating catheter across the area where the stricture had been incised.*

means of the working sheath of the rigid nephroscope, and an incision is made posterior and lateral in the ureter/pelvis until periureteral fat is visualized. This incision avoids anterior and medial blood vessels. A no. 6 French ureteral stent bypasses the incision site, is brought out through the nephrostomy tract, and is left indwelling for approximately 4 to 6 weeks. A nephrostomy tube is placed and left to gravity drainage for 3 days. At that time, an antegrade nephrostogram is obtained, and if no extravasation is demonstrated, the nephrostomy tube is removed. Repeat IVU or renal scan is obtained at 3 months.

Potential complications from endopyelotomy include intraoperative bleeding, ureteral avulsion, urinoma, and problems associated with nephrostomy access. Badlani and associates report an intraoperative

complication rate of 3.1 percent. Two complications occurred in 64 cases, both requiring open surgery for bleeding and ureteral avulsion. McEvoy and Huffman reported an 83 percent success rate for endopyelotomy for failed pyeloplasty and 93 percent in all cases where stricture length was 1 cm or less. Contraindications to endopyelotomy for ureteropelvic junction stricture include a large redundant pelvis and some instances of high insertion of the ureter.

Endoscopic Incision of Ureteral-Intestinal Strictures

Ureteral-intestinal strictures have been reported to be managed successfully with balloon dilation in approx-

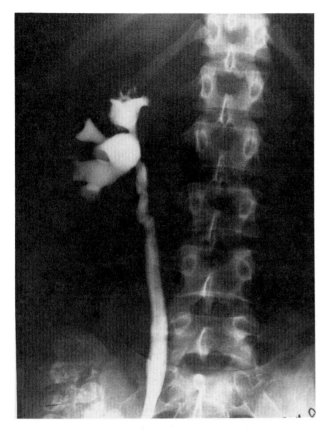

Figure 8-6. *Follow-up contrast studies demonstrated improved right renal function with less dilatation and patency of the ureteropelvic junction. This x-ray is a selected film from a cystogram done with an internal stent still in position demonstrating free reflux into the right kidney and patency of the right ureteropelvic junction.*

imately 60 percent of patients. A ureteral-intestinal stricture greater than 2 cm should be managed by open revision of the anastomosis. Strictures less than 2 cm may be approached with endoscopic incision. Most investigators agree that a stricture that initially failed endoscopic balloon dilation or incision may be repaired successfully by open revision. Serious consideration may be given to chronic internal drainage or nephrectomy in the management of strictures that recur following multiple open revisions.

The endoscopic incision can be performed in a retrograde or antegrade manner. A guidewire is passed beyond the strictured site. The narrowed segment is then visualized with a flexible cystoscope or nephroscope, and a "cold knife" ureterotome or electrode is passed through the working element. The stricture is incised posteriorly until retroperitoneal tissue is visualized. Following the incision, a 6- or 10-mm high-pressure balloon is passed, and the segment is dilated until no waist

is seen fluoroscopically. A ureteral stent is then passed over the guidewire and left indwelling for approximately 4 to 6 weeks.

Example

A 65-year-old man underwent radical cystectomy and Indiana pouch continent urinary diversion for pathologic stage P1N0 transitional cell carcinoma of the bladder. He did well for approximately 6 months until he developed recurrent urinary tract infections with left pyelonephritis. IVU revealed delayed function of the left kidney with left hydroureteronephrosis. He then underwent endoscopy of the pouch. The right ureteral orifice was visualized, but the left ureteral orifice could not be identified. A left percutaneous nephrostomy was performed under the same anesthetic, and the guidewire was negotiated passed the stricture into the pouch. An open-ended catheter was then placed over the guidewire and into the pouch. The patient was then placed in the supine position, and endoscopy was performed, using the "cold knife" ureterotome to incise the strictured area. A 6-mm balloon catheter was then used to dilate the stricture until no waist was seen fluoroscopically. A no. 7 French single-J catheter was placed and brought out through the stoma. The stent was left indwelling for 4 weeks. IVU performed 3 months postoperatively revealed improved drainage of the left kidney. The patient is now 14 months from the procedure and asymptomatic.

Ureteroureterostomy

Ureteroureterostomy is performed for persistent strictures of the middle third of the ureter and for short strictures of the proximal third of the ureter. The proximal ureteral stricture usually requires extensive mobilization of the kidney and peripelvic tissues to gain adequate length. The important considerations for successful ureteroureterostomy are adequate debridement of damaged tissues and creation of an anastomosis without tension. Care must be taken to preserve as much of the blood supply to the midureter as possible. After adequate dissection, a spatulated anastomosis is created with interrupted 5-0 absorbable sutures. The sutures should be placed closely for a watertight anastomosis, and the ureter should not be handled directly with forceps. This helps prevent necrosis of the end of the ureter, which has the most tenuous blood supply. After completion of the ureteroureterostomy, a vascularized segment of omentum may be used to wrap the anastomosis. A Penrose drain is also left in place. If an indwelling stent is used, a double-J catheter works well and should be left for a minimum of 2 weeks. A retrograde study can then be performed to document absence of extravasation prior to removing the stent. Follow-up radiographic studies should include an IVU at 3 months to look for evidence of stricture recurrence.

Transureteroureterostomy

Transureteroureterostomy (TUU) has come under scrutiny as the initial procedure for middle and distal third ureteral injuries after the report by Ehrlich and Skinner describing significant complications. The primary drawback of this procedure is the risk to the normal recipient renal unit from the anastomosis. Hendren and Hensle remain strong proponents of this procedure, especially for cases of undiversion and reimplantation of megaureters if strict attention to detail is maintained.

Through a midline incision and after reflection of the peritoneum lateral to the colon on the donor side, the ureter is mobilized above the stricture. Great care is taken to preserve its blood supply. With extensive mobilization, the spermatic or ovarian vessels may be divided distally and preserved in the periureteral tissue for collateral supply to the ureter. The posterior peritoneum over the recipient ureter is divided, and a tunnel beneath the sigmoid mesentery and inferior to the mesenteric artery is created for the donor ureter. Angulation beneath the inferior mesenteric artery should be avoided. A 1.5-cm incision is made on the medial aspect of the recipient ureter, and the donor ureter is spatulated to an equal length. The anastomosis is performed with interrupted 4-0 or 5-0 absorbable sutures with the knots tied on the outside. A large Penrose drain is placed to drain the area of anastomosis. The use of intraureteral stents remains controversial. When used, they should be of small caliber in order to prevent undue pressure on the anastomosis.

In the report by Ehrlich, five complications developed following TUU, resulting in two ileal ureters, one ureteral stricture, and one persistent hydronephrosis of the recipient renal unit. Also, three nephrectomies and one ileal ureter were required in the donor renal unit. The common denominators in these complications were poor blood supply and anastomotic tension. Contraindications to TUU include prior high-dose pelvic radiation, calculus disease, retroperitoneal fibrosis, and reflux of the recipient ureter.

Psoas Hitch Ureteral Reimplantation

Injuries to the pelvic portion of the ureter are frequently secondary to gynecologic surgery and result in fistulas and strictures. Adjuvant radiation, frequently indicated

for pelvic malignancy such as cervical and bladder carcinoma, also can cause stricture and certainly complicates reoperation. In these instances, it is advisable to resect the affected ureter and create a healthy anastomosis between viable ureter and bladder brought up to the psoas muscle. This mobilization of the bladder is accomplished by dividing the contralateral superior vesical vascular pedicle. It is also important to remain extraperitoneal if at all possible.

The technique of ureteral reimplantation with psoas hitch begins with a lower midline incision. After sharply dissecting the peritoneum off the superior and anterior bladder wall, a vertical or horizontal cystotomy is made. The ipsilateral posterior bladder wall is mobilized to the psoas muscle and attached to it with three sutures of 2-0 Vicryl. A tunneled ureteral reimplantation (Leadbetter-Politano) is then created to this fixed portion of the bladder. This prevents angulation of the ureter, which might occur if an anastomosis were performed on a more mobile portion of the bladder. A diversionary stent is left indwelling for 10 to 14 days. The bladder is closed in three layers with 3-0 absorbable suture in the mucosa followed by a 2-0 suture in the serosa and muscularis and then an inverting suture of interrupted 2-0. An extravesical drain should be left in place along with a Foley catheter for a minimum of 5 days. Depending on the clinical circumstances, a suprapubic cystostomy tube is utilized.

Boari Flap

In 1894, Boari described this reconstructive surgical technique in four canines, and in 1947, Ockerblad popularized the method for bridging a 10- to 15-cm length of ureteral defect. Usually, the Boari flap is used when the ureteral stricture involves the middle or distal third of the ureter and a psoas hitch is not feasible. Complications are greater with the Boari flap than with the psoas hitch. When bridging extensive ureteral gaps, it is important to maintain a good blood supply from the superior vesical artery to the flap. Necrosis at the tip of the flap can occur with resulting urine leak and fistula. This can lead to stenosis and hydronephrosis. It is important to create a ureteral and vesical anastomosis that is free of tension with intact vascular arcades. Controversy exists regarding the method of anastomosis. Ideally, the ureteral-vesical anastomosis should be tunneled and antirefluxing. However, this requires an additional 3 to 4 cm of ureteral length, which may result in an anastomosis under tension. Therefore, an end-to-end anastomosis must be created. Thompson and Ross reported 23 patients who underwent ureteral-vesical anastomosis in an end-to-end fashion. One patient did not have a normal or improved urogram. This patient's kidney had already suffered significant damage preoperatively. This procedure should be performed extraperitoneally. After careful measurement of the ureteral defect, a trapezoidal pedicled flap is created. Most authors recommend a base width of approximately 4 cm. The longer the flap, the wider the base should be in order to preserve blood supply. The flap should be on the posterior bladder wall and spiraled to the anterior wall. In creating the bladder flap, its ultimate location should be kept in mind so that it is spiraled in an appropriate direction to prevent angulation. The entire flap should be fixed to the psoas muscle lateral to the iliac vessels.

Closure of the vesical defect and tubularizing of the flap are accomplished with two layers of continuous absorbable suture. The first row incorporates the mucosa, and the second layer incorporates the serosa and muscularis of the bladder. Prior to creating the bladder tube, the ureteral-vesical anastomosis is created in an antirelux manner. A 3- to 4-cm submucosal tunnel is made at the end of the flap, the ureter is brought through the tunnel with a right-angle clamp, and a spatulated anastomosis is created with fine absorbable suture. Ureteral stents should be employed for a minimum of 10 days, and an extravesical drain should be placed. Suprapubic cystostomy drainage should be employed along with a Foley catheter.

Ileal Ureter

When ureteroneocystostomy, Boari bladder flap, and TUU are not feasible for repair of a ureteral stricture injury, an ileal ureter should be considered. Boxer and associates reported 89 patients who underwent ureteral replacement with ileum, and 80.9 percent were successful. Serum electrolytes and creatinine were not adversely affected if the preoperative serum creatinine was less than 2 mg/dl. Of 11 patients with a preoperative creatinine greater than 2 mg/dl, 45 percent had progressive renal failure postoperatively. The ileal ureter should be considered especially in the management of recurrent upper ureteral strictures because of its high success rate.

After preoperative bowel preparation with Neoloid, neomycin, and erythromycin, a thoracoabdominal approach is used through the bed of the eleventh or twelfth rib. This provides excellent exposure to the renal pelvis and kidney. This exposure is especially necessary when previous percutaneous, ureteroscopic, or open procedures have caused extensive perinephric and peripelvic inflammation. When ureteral stricture disease is associated with renal calculi, the ileal segment should be

anastomosed to the pelvis, lower-pole infundibulum, and lower-pole calyx to provide dependent drainage of the kidney.

After entering the peritoneal cavity, the lateral peritoneal reflection to the ascending colon is incised, and the mesentery of the small intestine is mobilized to the duodenum. A suitable segment of ileum is measured, usually based on the ileal colic artery or the terminal ileal artery. The incision in the proximal mesentery should be sufficiently long to allow the proximal portion to reach the kidney. An opening is made in the colonic mesentery, and the segment is passed through the opening and rotated 180 degrees to lay in an isoperistaltic position.

The proximal anastomosis is created between renal pelvis and ileum with a running 3-0 absorbable suture. If the proximal ureter is anastomosed to the ileum, then the proximal bowel is closed with a running 3-0 chromic catgut Parker-Kerr suture in two layers.

A psoas hitch is then created, and the distal ileum is anastomosed to the posterior bladder wall. This is the most immobile portion of the bladder and prevents angulation during bladder emptying. The anastomosis is performed with a running 3-0 absorbable suture, which may be placed from inside or outside the bladder. The psoas hitch allows the minimum amount of bowel to be used, thereby limiting reabsorption problems. The ileal-vesical anastomosis is refluxing, which has not been shown to be detrimental to the kidney and seems beneficial in recurrent stone disease (Fig. 8-7). Nephrostomy and cystostomy tubes are placed, and both anastomotic sites are drained with Penrose drains. Stents are generally not used but can be attached to the end of the cystostomy tube or Foley catheter for eventual removal.

Mucus formation by the ileal ureter has not been found to be a major problem. Preoperative knowledge of the patient's voiding history is important, especially if there is a question of bladder outlet obstruction. Occasionally, male patients require simultaneous transvesical open prostatectomy.

Autotransplantation

Extensive ureteral strictures require either autotransplantation or ileal ureter for preservation of renal function. Autotransplantation was first described by Hardy in 1963 and performed for ureteral loss. The primary indication today for autotransplantation is renal vascular disease.

Bodie and associates described their experience in

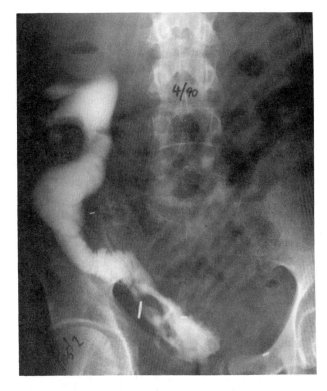

Figure 8-7. *The ileal ureter substitution is an excellent form of reconstructive surgery for patients with recurrent ureteral strictures and stone disease. This radiograph is a film from a cystogram study done immediately following creation of a right ileal ureter. Free reflux of contrast material is noted from the bladder to the right kidney, where there is a very patent pelvoileal anastomosis. Distortion of the bladder is due to the psoas hitch procedure that stabilizes the distal anastomosis, thus preventing angulation. The psoas hitch also decreases the amount of bowel needed to complete the reconstruction.*

23 patients in whom autotransplantation was performed to replace a major portion of the ureter. They reported no postoperative mortality, and all but one of the kidneys functioned immediately postoperatively. Twelve percent of the autotransplanted kidneys ultimately were lost, but 88 percent were successful. Relative contraindications to autotransplantation include a kidney with severe parenchymal disease, severe atherosclerotic disease of the iliac vessels, or severe retroperitoneal fibrosis. The advantages of autotransplantation over ileal substitution are the avoidance of mucus production and the occasional electrolyte problems created by urine contact with the small bowel mucosa.

Summary

Recurrent ureteral strictures may result following a variety of urologic and nonurologic procedures. Similar to the initial assessment of a stricture, one must document stricture site, extent, and renal function prior to proceeding with reoperation. There are several open surgical approaches to the repair of a recurrent stricture, as discussed above, depending on the stricture site and extent. Endourologic methods may be therapeutic options, and initial reports of success rates are encouraging.

Bibliography

Badlani, G, Karlin, G, and Smith, AD. Complications of endopyelotomy (abstract). J Urol 137:175A, 1987.

Bagley, DH. Dilation of the ureterovesical junction and ureter. In JL Huffman, DH Bagley, and ES Lyon (eds), Ureteroscopy. Philadelphia: Saunders, 1988, p 51.

Banner, MP, et al. Catheter dilation of benign ureteral strictures. Radiology 147:427, 1983.

Beckman, CF, and Roth, RA. Secondary ureteropelvic junction stricture: Percutaneous dilation. Radiology 164:365, 1987.

Biester, R, and Gillenwater, JY. Complications following ureteroscopy. J Urol 136:380, 1986.

Bodie, B, et al. Long-term results of autotransplantation for ureteral replacement. J Urol 136:1187, 1986.

Boxer, RJ, et al. Replacement of the ureter by small intestine: Clinical application and results of the ileal ureter in 89 patients. J Urol 121:728, 1979.

Buchsbaum HJ. The urinary tract and radical hysterectomy. In HJ Buchsbaum and J Schmidt (eds), Gynecologic and Obstetric Urology. Philadelphia: Saunders, 1982.

Chang, R, Marshall, FF, and Mitchel, S. Percutaneous management of benign ureteral strictures and fistulas. J Urol 137:1126, 1987.

Davis, DM. Intubated ureterotomy. Surg Gynecol Obstet 76:513, 1943.

Ehrlich, RM, and Skinner, DG. Complications of transureteroureterostomy. J Urol 113:467, 1975.

Fine, EJ, and Blaufox, DM. Urological applications of radionuclides. In HM Pollack (ed), Clinical Urography. Philadelphia: Saunders, 1990, vol 1, pp 518–523.

Gruntzig, AR, Senning, A, and Siegenthaler, WE. Nonoperative dilation of coronary artery stenosis: Percutaneous transluminal coronary angioplasty. N Engl J Med 301:61, 1979.

Hardy, JD. High ureteral injuries: Management by autotransplantation of the kidney. JAMA 184:97, 1963.

Hendren, HW, and Hensle, TW. Transureteroureterostomy: Experience with 75 cases. J Urol 123:826, 1980.

Kramolowsky, EV, Clayman, RV, and Weyman, PJ. Management of ureterointestinal anastomotic strictures: Comparison of open surgical and endourologic repair. J Urol 139:1195, 1988.

Kramolowsky, EV, Tucker, RD, and Nelson, CM. Management of benign ureteral strictures: Open surgical repair or endoscopic dilation? J Urol 141:285, 1989.

Lyon, ES. Complications of ureteroscopy. Presented at the Third World Congress in Endourology, Sept. 21, 1985.

McEvoy, KM, and Huffman, JL. Experience with endopyelotomy. Presented at the annual meeting of the Western Section, American Urological Association, Monterey, California, Oct. 4, 1990.

Schmidt, JD, et al. Complications, results and problems of ileal conduit diversions. J Urol 109:210, 1973.

Skinner, DG, Boyd, S, and Lieskovsky, G. Creation of continent Kock ileal reservoir as alternative to cutaneous urinary diversion. In DG Skinner and G Lieskovsky (eds), Genitourinary Cancer. Philadelphia: Saunders, 1988, p 653.

Smith, AD. Management of iatrogenic ureteral strictures after urological procedures. J Urol 140:1372, 1988.

Spence, HM, and Boone, T. Surgical injuries to the ureter. JAMA 176:1070, 1961.

Thompson, IM, and Ross, G. Long-term results of bladder flap repair of ureteral injuries. J Urol 111:483, 1974.

Weinberg, SR, and Rosenberg, JW. Injuries of the ureter. In H Bergman (ed), The Ureter, 2d ed. New York: Springer-Verlag, 1986, pp 427–436.

Whittaker, RH. Methods of assessing obstruction in dilated ureters. Br J Urol 45:15, 1973.

Extrinsic Ureteral Obstruction (Including Retroperitoneal Fibrosis)

LOUIS L. PISTERS
MARC S. COHEN

The decision to reoperate on a patient for extrinsic ureteral obstruction can be difficult for both the surgeon and the patient. It may take months or even years before recurrent or persistent ureteral obstruction is appreciated. It can be difficult for both surgeon and patient to accept that a well-planned, carefully executed, and perhaps initially successful operation has failed. The prospect of a potentially more difficult second operation raises the stakes for both the surgeon and the patient. In select cases, depending on the patient's relative age and overall medical condition, long-term conservative management with ureteral stents or nephrostomy tubes may be a viable option. Recent data suggest a significant failure rate for indwelling ureteral stents in patients with extrinsic as opposed to intrinsic ureteral obstruction. This implies that a subset of patients with extrinsic ureteral obstruction may not respond to indwelling ureteral drainage and may require nephrostomy tube drainage for adequate renal decompression. This also emphasizes that patients treated conservatively for extrinsic ureteral obstruction with indwelling ureteral stents will require close scrutiny for evidence of stent failure. When surgeon and patient have decided to proceed with a second attempt to manage the extrinsic ureteral obstruction, thorough preparation with an awareness of all possible operative solutions will create the greatest chance for success. This chapter reviews the tests for ureteral obstruction, preparing the patient for reoperative ureteral surgery and the various operative possibilities.

Diagnostic Tests

A combination of anatomic and functional studies is needed in the evaluation of a patient with recurrent or persistent extrinsic ureteral obstruction. Several reports emphasize the pitfalls of using a single diagnostic modality such as ultrasonography to diagnose obstruction as a possible cause of renal failure. Ultrasound, computed tomographic (CT) scans, and antegrade and retrograde pyelograms provide mainly anatomic information. Functional information can be provided by diuretic renography, dynamic fluoroscopic examination of peristalsis, and the Whitaker test. Excretory urography can provide both anatomic and functional information.

Ultrasound

Renal ultrasound is an excellent way of evaluating patients with extrinsic obstruction (such as retroperitoneal fibrosis) over long periods of time. Serial ultrasound examinations following an initial procedure for extrinsic ureteral obstruction may demonstrate worsening hydronephrosis and hydroureter, suggesting recurrent or persistent obstruction. In addition to detecting hydronephrotic changes of the upper tracts, ultrasound has been used to monitor the inflammatory mass of retroperitoneal fibrosis following surgery and during medical therapy with steroids. The ultrasonic appearance of retroperitoneal fibrosis is a smooth-bordered and relatively echo-free mass anterior to the sacral promontory. Patients with severe baseline dilation of their collecting systems may be difficult to evaluate with serial ultrasound because a pattern of progressive dilation of the collecting system with recurring obstruction may not be appreciated. Patients also may retain significant anatomic dilation of their collecting systems despite adequate repair of a severe ureteral obstruction. In these patients, periodic diuretic renograms may be of more value than ultrasound in long-term follow-up after surgery.

Excretory Urogram (EXU)

The EXU traditionally has been the standard imaging study of the upper collecting system (particularly the ureter) in cases of extrinsic obstruction. The adverse consequences of intravenous contrast material will not be discussed here, but it should be recognized that with ureteral obstruction, poor visualization in patients with poor renal function may be encountered and that increased risk of contrast-induced renal failure may occur. The newer non-ionic contrast agents do not lower the incidence of contrast-induced renal failure. In patients who have previously reacted adversely to contrast material, one may opt to use other diagnostic methods or to proceed with the intravenous pyelogram following a steroid/antihistamine prep (see Table 9-1). Obstruction is suggested by a column of contrast material present on the delayed films. Delayed films taken 2 or more hours after the infusion of contrast material are useful in establishing the anatomic level of obstruction. The entrapped ureter may become involved in the inflammatory process of retroperitoneal fibrosis, leading to a combination of extrinsic as well as intrinsic ureteral obstruction. Subtle mucosal irregularities on the EXU may suggest intrinsic obstruction due to tumor, stone, blood clot, fungal infection, or an inflammatory process such as ureteritis cystica or extrinsic processes such as retroperitoneal fibrosis.

Antegrade Pyelogram

Many patients with persistent or recurrent symptomatic ureteral obstruction following an operative procedure will have unilateral or bilateral nephrostomy tubes in place. Antegrade pyelography provides anatomic information similar to the excretory urogram, with the exception that the collecting system can be filled and opacified better with a much lower risk of adverse reaction to contrast material. Antegrade pyelography is extremely useful in determining the anatomic level and degree of ureteral obstruction.

Retrograde Pyelography

Retrograde pyelography can be the best way to demonstrate the distal extent of the extrinsic ureteral compression when antegrade access has not been established.

Combined Antegrade and Retrograde Pyelography

Together, these two techniques performed simultaneously combine to give the best anatomic picture of ureteral compression and demonstrate the exact level and length of ureteral obstruction (Fig. 9-1).

CT Scan

Retroperitoneal fibrosis can be seen as an elliptical retroperitoneal mass encasing one or both ureters on CT scans. CT scan is useful to define the extent and anatomic location of the inflammatory mass in retroperitoneal fibrosis.

Table 9-1 *Pretreatment Recommendations for Patients Who Previously Had Reactions to Intravascular Contrast Material (ICM)*

Prednisone
50 mg PO q6hr for 3 doses beginning 13 hr before ICM
Diphenhydramine
50 mg PO or IM 1 hr before ICM
Non-ionic lower-osmolality contrast medium
(Optional)
Cimetidine 30 mg PO 1 hr prior to ICM

Figure 9-1. *Combination retrograde/antegrade pyelography. The study demonstrates a 7-cm ureteral defect in the middle third of the left ureter.*

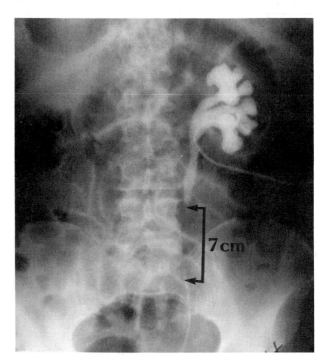

7 cm

Renography

Many radionuclides have been used to image the kidneys. The commonly used compounds include technetium diethylenetriamine pentaacetic acid (Tc-DTPA) for glomerular function and excretory imaging, radioiodine orthoiodohippuric acid (^{131}I hippuran) for tubular function, and technetium dimercaptosuccinic acid (Tc-DMSA) for cortical imaging and total functional renal mass. We have found diuretic renography with a Lasix DTPA scan to be the most useful in evaluating patients for obstruction. Using this radionuclide, split renal function and renal plasma flow can be estimated (ERPF) to provide a quantitative estimate of renal function. This quantitative estimate of renal function along with a creatinine clearance determination may be useful in deciding whether a kidney should be salvaged or an ipsilateral nephrectomy may be the best option.

Care must be taken in the nuclear medicine suite to perform all renogram studies in a uniform manner to minimize the effects of a number of variables that affect the washout rate of the radionuclide. These variables include the patient's renal function, state of hydration, timing of radionuclide administration, ability to respond to the diuretic, distensibility and volume of the collecting system, and intravesical pressure. Patients should be adequately hydrated so that intravascular volume contraction after administration of the diuretic does not diminish the response to the diuretic and result in a false-positive pattern for obstruction. Some authors recommend intravenous hydration throughout the entire renogram study, although intravenous hydration is not performed routinely at our institution. The diuretic needs to be administered only after sufficient time has elapsed for the collecting system to be filled with radionuclide or a false pattern for obstruction may result. In addition, a patient with poor renal function may not respond to the diuretic, potentially resulting in a false-positive renogram. Diuretic renography is unreliable in kidneys with a creatinine clearance below 25 ml/min $\times$ 1.73 m^2, even if the dose of diuretic is greatly increased. A noncompliant bladder can result in increased intravesical pressures and a false-positive test. Some authors feel that an indwelling urethral catheter should be placed prior to the renogram study in all patients, although at our institution a Foley catheter is placed prior to the renogram study only in those patients who are felt to have a noncompliant bladder. Lastly, patients with indwelling ureteral stents should have a urethral catheter placed prior to the performance of a diuretic renogram.

The results of diuretic renography have been categorized according to four basic patterns shown in Figure 9-2. These basic patterns were described initially and

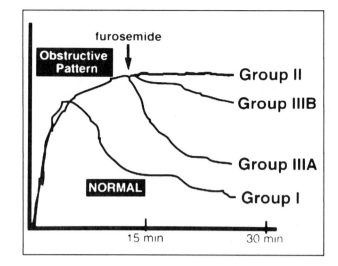

Figure 9-2. *Diuretic renogram demonstrating normal (group I) and obstructive patterns (group II). Response to furosemide (groups IIIa and IIIb) is demonstrated. (See text for explanation.)*

assigned numbers by Lupton and associates and have been confirmed by others. Pattern I is a normal tracing, with rapid spontaneous excretion of the radionuclide occurring before infection of the diuretic. In pattern II, there is no excretion of radionuclide either spontaneously or after injection of diuretic, and this is interpreted as showing obstruction. In pattern IIIa, although the radionuclide lingers in the renal area, it disappears rapidly after injection of the diuretic. This pattern is interpreted as showing dilation without obstruction. Finally, in pattern IIIb, the clearance of the radionuclide after administration of furosemide occurs at a slow rate, and this pattern is considered as representing partial obstruction. The diuretic renogram accurately and reliably rules out obstruction in cases were a type I pattern is observed. Similarly, in cases where renal function of the involved kidney is preserved and a type II pattern is observed, obstruction is invariably present.

In addition, the time required to excrete half the radioactive counts from the region of interest of injection of the diuretic ($T_{1/2}$) has been helpful in judging obstruction on a renogram. In an individual with normal or near-normal renal function, a $T_{1/2}$ of greater than 20 minutes indicates that some degree of obstruction exists. A $T_{1/2}$ of less than 15 minutes generally indicates no obstruction, and a $T_{1/2}$ of between 15 and 20 minutes is equivocal for obstruction. Several studies have compared diuretic renography with urodynamic (pressure/flow) studies, with the latter being used as the gold standard for obstruction. Gonzalez has shown that only 40 percent of patients with a partially obstructive (IIIb) pattern are obstructive on urodynamic studies. In addition, up to 25 percent of patients with a IIIa pattern, which is usually interpreted as indicating stasis, actually have obstruction by urodynamic parameters. This latter situation may be due to a noncompliant pelvis that requires high pressures to be generated for adequate flow to result in the excretion of the radioisotope.

Dynamic Fluoroscopic Assessment of Urinary Peristalsis

The excretory phase of a conventional excretory urogram can be performed under fluoroscopy to visualize ureteral peristalsis in great detail. This method has been described but involves significant radiation (mean fluoroscopy time 5 minutes), which limits its usefulness. Ureteral peristalsis also can be studied using a radionuclide method, although not in as great detail as with the fluoroscopic method.

Urodynamic Studies (Whitaker Test)

In urodynamic terms, obstruction describes a system in which high pressures are necessary to generate urine flow. Urodynamic testing of the upper urinary tract is the best way to demonstrate an alteration between renal pelvic pressures and urine flow rates and as such is probably the best test for obstruction. As initially described, the Whitaker test involves the infusion of saline or contrast material into the renal pelvis at a constant rate of 10 ml/min while the pressure difference between the renal pelvis and the bladder is monitored. If the pressure differential between the renal pelvis and the bladder is less than 15 cm H_2O, then no obstruction is said to be present. If the pressure differential between the renal pelvis and the bladder is greater than 22 cm H_2O, then obstruction is said to be present. A pressure differential of between 15 and 22 cm H_2O is equivocal, and some suggest that perfusion at high flow rates may be justified. Whitaker's findings and conclusions have been supported by others. In addition, the compliance of the renal pelvis can be assessed by the slope of increase in intrapelvic pressure during the infusion of saline or contrast material into the renal pelvis. In general, low compliance is present when there is a steep rise in intrapelvic pressure and is often associated with high differential pressures between the renal pelvis and the bladder and decreased renal function.

Bullock and associates described a two-needle modification of the Whitaker test such that infusion of saline or contrast material can occur through one 22-gauge needle while intrapelvic pressure is measured through another 22-gauge needle. This technique avoids some of the artificial fluctuations in pressure that occur when the same needle is used for infusion and pressure measurement. Woodbury and associates have described a constant-pressure perfusion method to determine obstruction in the upper urinary tract in which urine flow is measured while the renal pelvis is filled at a constant pressure. This latter method deserves more study, since it attempts to evaluate obstruction at physiologic renal pelvic pressures.

The major advantage of pressure/flow studies of the upper urinary tract is that they are independent of renal function. As already mentioned, the diuretic renogram is not valid in patients with decreased renal function, making the Whitaker test the only valid test for obstruction in these patients. The greatest disadvantage of the Whitaker test is its invasiveness; although it may be performed as an outpatient, anesthesia or significant sedation is often required for pediatric patients. In patients who already have a nephrostomy tube in place, a Whitaker test may offer definitive information about possible obstruction without any significant additional morbidity.

Several potential pitfalls exist that may lead to inaccurate interpretation of the Whitaker test. Several of these potential problems can be avoided if the study is done with contrast material under fluoroscopic control. Extravasation of the infusion material outside the collecting system can occur and, if undetected, may result in a false-negative test. In addition, patients with massively dilated collecting systems may require significant amounts of infused fluid before the renal pelvis is full. If the infusion of fluid is terminated before the renal pelvis is full, a rise in pressure will not be noted even if obstruction is present, also potentially resulting in a false-negative test.

The Whitaker test is a provocative test for obstruction, and as such, the parameters of this test may not be appropriate in certain patients. For instance, an infusion rate of 10 ml/min in a neonate or infant may be unduly stressful. If an infusion rate of 10 ml/min were maintained over 1 hour, 600 ml would be infused. Certainly, most of us never approach a urine output of 600 ml/hr, or 14.4 liters/day, under normal conditions. In this regard, constant-pressure perfusion methods may represent a more physiologic test for obstruction. Despite the preceding physiologic concerns, the Whitaker test as originally described accurately separates obstructed from nonobstructed systems in over 90 percent of patients.

Preparing the Patient and Surgeon for Reoperative Ureteral Surgery

After a decision has been reached by the surgeon and the patient to reoperate for extrinsic ureteral obstruction, the next steps necessary for a successful outcome relate to preparation of the patient for surgery. In a timely fashion, the patient should participate in a predeposit autologous blood donation program at the community blood bank or hospital and be placed on oral iron. A nutritional assessment should be made of the patient, and if necessary, the patient should be started on enteral nutritional support preoperatively. The patient should undergo an aggressive bowel preparation with intravenous hydration. We place patients on a clear liquid diet 24 to 48 hours prior to surgery and then give them 1 gallon of a polyethylene glycol electrolyte solution (e.g., Colyte) followed by two bottles of magnesium citrate on the day prior to surgery. Many patients will have indwelling nephrostomy tubes or ureteral stents and will have bacteriuria. We obtain a urine culture approximately 2 weeks prior to surgery and start patients on appropriate intravenous antibiotics 1 day prior to surgery when they are admitted to the hospital for their bowel preparation. We maintain patients on subcutaneous heparin sulfate (5000 units SC bid) perioperatively and use sequential lower extremity compression stockings intra- and postoperatively until patients are ambulating well. Even if the chance of autotransplantation is fairly low, a consultation with a transplant or vascular surgeon should be obtained preoperatively. It is important to review the old operative reports if available, with attention to several specific details: the indication for the original procedure (especially if the original procedure was done elsewhere), the operative approach (intra- versus extraperitoneal, flank versus transabdominal, etc.), the operative findings, and the consent for surgery. It is also important to discuss with the patient in simple terms the fact that the operation performed will depend on the operative findings and that several different reconstructive possibilities exist.

Surgical Options for Recurrent Ureteral Obstruction

Multiple surgical options are available for recurrent extrinsic ureteral obstruction, including ureteroureterostomy, psoas hitch, Boari flap, ureterolysis, ureteral substitution, renal displacement, autotransplantation, and nephrectomy. In difficult cases, transperitoneal exposure with subsequent extraperitoneal drainage may be

much faster and technically easier than difficult dissection through retroperitoneal scar tissue. In these cases, the ureter is often densely adherent to the peritoneum, and it may be easier to take a thin strip of peritoneum with the ureter instead of trying to dissect the peritoneum off the ureter. In a recent large series by Jain and associates, in patients undergoing unilateral or bilateral upper urinary tract operations through an anterior transperitoneal approach, exposure was found to be excellent, and there was no increased incidence of peritonitis or paralytic ileus due to urinary leak. At the time of surgery, it is important that the patient be in a position on the operating table that will accommodate as many reconstructive options as possible. This may involve positioning the patient in a supine as opposed to a lateral decubitus position. In large patients, a thoracoabdominal approach with the patient just slightly rotated (about 30 degrees from the horizontal) may give the surgeon many of the benefits of both flank and abdominal approaches. If the anticipated operating time is long, the patient should be positioned on a heating blanket. The patient should, of course, be prepped and draped in a wide fashion. An autotransfusion machine should be available in the operating room if anticipated blood loss is significant.

In our opinion, ureteral stents are very helpful in finding and identifying the ureter intraoperatively because they allow the ureter to be palpated even in the presence of significant amounts of scar tissue. Despite their aid in identifying the ureter, it has been shown that the use of interoperative ureteral stents actually does not lower the incidence of ureteral injury secondary to dissection. We generally leave the ureter stented after ureteral reconstruction for at least 1 week. We usually place a large-bore suprapubic tube if the bladder has been opened. We uniformly drain the area of reconstruction with two or more no. 10 Jackson-Pratt drains.

Ureteroureterotomy

Ureteroureterotomy is a simple and effective operation for short-segment ureteral obstructions of the middle and upper third of the ureter. Obstructions of the lower third of the ureter may be better treated with a ureteroneocystostomy with a psoas hitch. The importance of a tension-free anastomosis cannot be understated. In order to achieve a tension-free anastomosis, the kidney should be completely mobilized with Gerota's fascia in order to obtain 3 to 5 cm of additional length of the upper ureteral segment. The anastomosis should be completed over a no. 6 to 8 French ureteral stent, and the region of the anastomosis should be drained. Our preference is to use closed-suction Jackson-Pratt drains in the region of the anastomosis.

Bladder Elongation Psoas Hitch Procedure

The psoas hitch procedure is indicated for obstruction of the lower ureter (Fig. 9-3). As Turner-Warwick points out, "it is not so much the lateral mobilization and the hitch as it is the elongating incision [Fig. 9-3*B*] that makes it work." The bladder can be significantly elongated in this simple procedure by closing an obliquely oriented cystotomy longitudinally (Fig. 9-3*C*). By elongating the bladder in this fashion, the psoas hitch enables the bladder to reach a comparable level to the Boari flap. We have found this to be a highly satisfactory alternative for recurrent obstruction in the distal ureter. It is very important to mobilize the peritoneum from the dome of the bladder and free the vas in a male patient or divide the round ligament in a female patient. In addition, the superior vesical pedicles may be divided bilaterally while an excellent blood supply is maintained to the bladder by means of the inferior vesical trunk and branches. The kidney also may be mobilized from within Gerota's fascia to achieve greater ureteral length,

Figure 9-3. *Psoas hitch. A. Semioblique incision in the bladder* (dotted line). *B. With traction on the ipsilateral side of the bladder. Transverse incisions* (heavy lines) *allow for additional length to be obtained by creating a partial flap. C. Completed hitch* (dotted line) *shows original bladder configuration.*

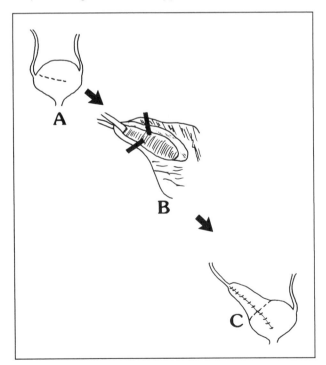

as mentioned in the preceding section on ureteroureterostomy. The anchoring sutures should be placed through the psoas muscle and tendon above and lateral to the iliac vessels with care not to include the genitofemoral nerve. This procedure should allow for a nonrefluxing ureteral reimplantation. We uniformly leave the reimplanted ureter stented and place a large suprapubic tube at the time of surgery.

The psoas hitch has many advantages over the Boari flap procedure. The psoas hitch is technically much simpler to perform, much easier to close, and therefore probably faster in most surgeons' hands. The Boari flap closure involves a full-length suture line, and the base of the flap can be very difficult to close properly. The effective width of the elevated bladder is much greater with the psoas hitch. If the bladder capacity is reasonable, the psoas hitch may still be performed with a thickened, hypertrophied bladder, which may preclude the tubularization of a Boari flap. The longitudinal closure of a slightly oblique cystotomy does not impair the bladder's vascularity compared with the delicate blood supply to the Boari flap. Finally, the reimplanted ureter following a psoas hitch procedure is much more accessible to endoscopic manipulation than following a Boari flap.

Boari Flap

The Boari flap and psoas hitch, as described above, achieve a similar end result—the bladder is molded into an elongated tubular structure that is brought upward and laterally to reach the ureter. This procedure is also indicated for obstruction of the distal ureter. This procedure is relatively contraindicated in patients who have received pelvic radiation therapy or those who have intrinsic disease of the bladder wall preventing the bladder flap from being tubularized. It is important to make the base of the flap at least 4 cm wide and even wider in cases where a longer flap is needed. It is important to use stay sutures to fix the bladder and flap as the flap is being cut. The ureter should be tunneled submucosally into the upper end of the flap, and then the flap should be anchored down to the psoas muscle in a fashion similar to the psoas hitch. The reimplanted ureter should be stented, and a large-bore suprapubic tube should be placed. The flap should be tubularized and the bladder closed in two layers. Urine leakage following this procedure most often is related to the bladder closure and not the ureteral reimplantation. For the reasons mentioned previously, our experience has shown that the psoas hitch usually suffices in the face of the Boari flap.

Renal Displacement

Renal displacement is a technique that allows one to mobilize and displace the kidney further inferiorly by transecting the renal vein and reanastomosing it to a point lower on the inferior vena cava. This procedure differs from renal autotransplantation in that the renal artery is not divided. This procedure allows the kidney to be displaced a significant distance further inferiorly than by simple mobilization within Gerota's fascia. The right kidney can be moved a greater distance lower with this technique than the left because of the longer right renal artery. In preparation for renal displacement, the renal artery should be occluded and the kidney cooled with an ice slush. Two Satinsky clamps are then placed on the inferior vena cava at the origin of the renal vein. The renal vein is then transected flush with the inferior vena cava to preserve as much renal vein length as possible. One Satinsky clamp is then removed, and the cavotomy is closed with a running 5-0/arterial monofilament suture (/) Prolene suture. The Satinsky clamp is then reapplied to the inferior vena cava at a lower level, and a cavotomy is made equal in length to the diameter of the renal vein. The posterior aspect of the renal vein to inferior vena cava anastomosis should be carried out

first by sewing on the inside. The anterior aspect of the anastomosis is then completed.

Ureterolysis

Ureterolysis is most commonly performed for obstruction of the upper and middle ureter related to retroperitoneal fibrosis and is usually accompanied by an omental sleeve (Fig. 9-4). This procedure is usually performed through a midline transperitoneal approach. After the ureter and the inflammatory mass have been identified, deep biopsies of the mass should be taken to rule out malignancy. Retroperitoneal fibrosis is related to malignancy in 8 percent of cases, with the most common malignancies being lymphoma and breast and colon cancer. It is helpful to start the dissection low, where the caliber of the ureter is normal and the risk of inadvertent ureteral injury is lower. A combination of blunt and sharp dissection is used to free the ureter in a cephalad direction. Care should be taken to avoid injury to the inferior vena cava and aorta, which are much closer to the ureter than under normal conditions. Significant bleeding also can result from inadvertent transection of the gonadal vessels. After the ureter has been mobilized

Figure 9-4. *Omental sleeve of ureters for retroperitoneal fibrosis. A. Separation/preparation of two omental segments* (O) *supplied by the gastroepiploic arch (S = demonstrates posterior aspect of stomach). B. The omental pedicle* (O) *is brought lateral to the colon, and the ureters* (U) *are wrapped. The omentum is tacked with chronic catgut sutures.*

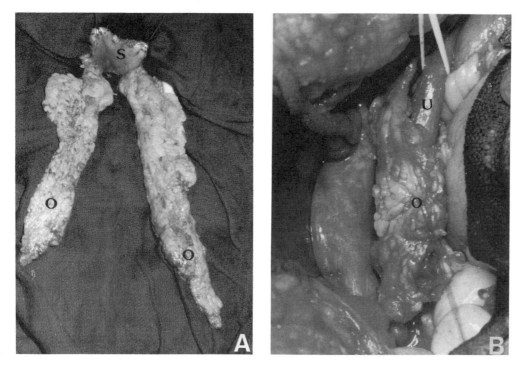

to a level several centimeters above the obstruction, the peritoneum should be closed behind the ureter with fine absorbable sutures with care not to compromise the ureter at an entry or exit site through the peritoneum. Next, an omental pedicle should be mobilized based on one of the gastroepiploic vessels and swung lateral to the colon (Fig. 9-4A). The omental pedicle is then brought posterior to the ureter and wrapped medially anterior to the ureter to envelop it. The omentum should be tacked in place with fine absorbable sutures.

Endourologic Management for Recurrent Ureteral Obstruction

Despite the fact that extrinsic obstruction has been managed traditionally by open operative techniques, extraordinary technological changes have made available an array of endourologic techniques as well. Because these frequently represent "minimally invasive" techniques, it has been our custom to employ these prior to some of the more aggressive open surgical techniques, such as bowel interposition or renal displacement. With regard to the endourologic approaches, we have tended to reserve those procedures which utilize permanent indwelling stents for individuals in whom open surgery is contraindicated or has been tried without success. Such techniques negate the use of chronic external drainage (e.g., nephrostomy tube).

Ureteral Dilation

Particularly in cases utilizing retrograde access, this is an integral part of achieving access to and treatment of the ureteral obstruction. Depending on the stricture location and its density, ureteral dilation sufficient to allow passage of a ureteroscope is frequently possible. Although pressure-controlled hydraulic dilation is possible using an automatic device (Uromat, Karl Storz, Culver City, Calif.), hand-held syringe dilators (Single Action Pumping System, Microvasive, Watertown, Mass.) are also available. These devices ease endoscopic instrument insertion and help define areas of stricture formation. Ureteral balloon dilation may be used to obtain ureteral access, and it also represents a method of treating obstruction. The balloon is passed over the guidewire under fluoroscopic guidance until it traverses the area of obstruction. Using a high-power inflation syringe (Leveen Inflator, Microvasive, Watertown, Mass.), the balloon is inflated and observed fluoroscopically. A "wasp waist" is observed initially that usually disappears with balloon inflation. Although this may be used

as the solitary means of managing ureteral strictures, success rates vary (48 to 79 percent). When possible, we usually try to include endoureterotomy in our treatment regime because success rates are somewhat better (57 to 82 percent).

Cold Knife Ureterotomy

We currently prefer this technique for ureterotomy (Fig. 9-5). It is our custom to maintain a safety wire in the ureteral lumen alongside the ureteroscope. When the obstruction is encountered, the endoscope is placed distally, and the knife is advanced proximally under direct vision, either over or along a guidewire. Hydraulic distension improves visualization and can help determine the success of incision by spreading when the stricture is released. Where the ureter is incised is determined by the ureteral segment, its blood supply, and the relationship to other vital structures. In the distal ureteral ($\leq$5 cm above the ureteral orifice), incisions are usually placed at the 12 o'clock position in the supine-positioned patient. In the proximal ureter ($\geq$3 cm below the ureteropelvic junction), incisions should be located posterolaterally. In the midureter, the incision sites are directed posterolaterally in the more proximal segment to avoid the medial gonadal vessels anteriorly at the level of the common iliac vessels and medially at the level of the internal iliac artery.

When treating proximal obstructions, the technique often involves marsupialization of the ureter into the renal pelvis. We most frequently approach these strictures in an antegrade fashion, and we commonly stent with an endopyelotomy (no. 14 to 17 French) nephroureteral stent. When incising distal strictures, our goal is to marsupialize the ureter into the bladder. We have had some success in this area with a blind ureterotome (Olympus Corp., Lake Success, N.Y.) in which the blade is "sheathed" within a no. 16 French shield. The device is positioned fluoroscopically over a wire in a retrograde manner (see Fig. 9-5). A no. 7 to 14 French stent may be placed in an inverted fashion so that the larger portion traverses the stricture. Midureteral strictures are treated most frequently with balloon dilation and, when possible, endoureterotomy. A "hot knife" positioned with the aid of a flexible or rigid ureteroscope also may be used to perform the needed incision.

Self-Expanding Ureteral Stents in the Treatment of Ureteral Obstruction

Implantation of self-expanding metal stents (Fig. 9-6) has been effective in the treatment of malignant bile

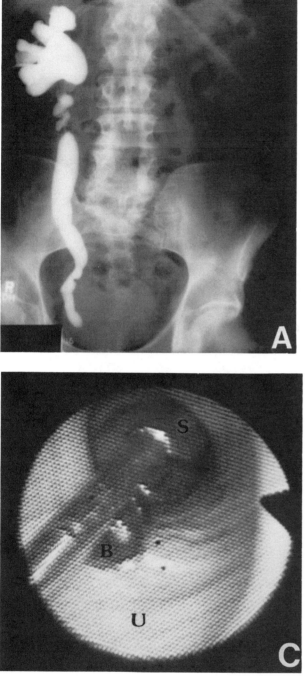

Figure 9-5. *Total obstruction of the distal right ureter after transureteral resection of the prostate. A. Antegrade nephrostogram with distal obstruction, proximal ureteritis, and tortuosity. B. Fluoroscopic view of flexible nephroureteroscope (N) above and ureterotome (U) below (W = ureteral guidewires). C. Endoscopic view of ureterotome (S = ureterotome sheath; B = ureterotome blade; U = dilated proximal ureter).*

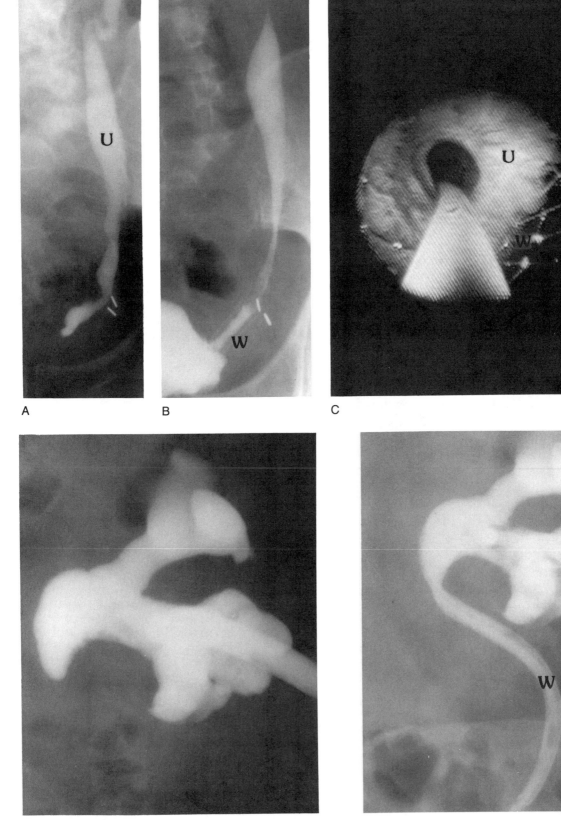

A

B

C

D

E

duct obstruction, urethral strictures, and benign prostatic hyperplasia. The use of similar devices in the treatment of ureteral obstruction would, with certain reservations, seem logical. The Wallstent (Medinvert, Lausanne, Switzerland) consists of a biomedical stainless steel alloy monofilament wire that is braided in a tubular mesh configuration. It is flexible and has an expanded diameter of 7 to 10 mm. The stent is mounted on a no. 7 French coaxial deployment catheter that follows a 0.035-in. guidewire. The stent is flexible and able to conform to ureteral contours. As with permanently implanted stents in the biliary tree and the urinary tract, the epithelium (urothelium) grows through the interstices of the stent, resulting in its incorporation into the ureteral wall, reducing the likelihood of encrustation.

Technique

The stenotic ureter is crossed by a guidewire under fluoroscopic and, when appropriate, endoscopic control. Both retrograde and antegrade access has been used with success. After successful negotiation of the stenotic segment, the ureter is balloon dilated (5 to 7 mm). The introducer sheath is placed across the strictured area, and the stent is deployed by retraction of an overlying protective catheter, allowing free stent expansion. Ureteral edema is managed by placement of a double-J or pigtail catheter through the stent lumen for approximately 4 weeks to prevent obstruction by early urothelial hyperplasia. Stents come in two lengths (4.2 and 6.8 cm) and may be "stacked" in order to accommodate longer strictures (Fig. 9-6E).

Results

In limited study, implantation of ureteral wall stents has been successful in 97 percent of attempted placements. Reported complications include hematuria (4 percent), stent encrustation (8 percent) (treated with endoscopic manipulation), occlusion by hyperplastic urothelial reaction (8 percent), and tumor overgrowth (2 percent). Overall, patency was 81 percent after 6 months and 61 percent after 8 months.

Balloon Dilatation/Incision Catheters

Recent reports of endoureterotomy with a specially designed no. 7 French catheter combining a no. 24 French ureteral dilating balloon with a 3 × 150 cm cautery wire have been encouraging. The Accucise (Applied Urology, Laguna Hills, Calif.) endopyelotomy endoureterotomy catheter is usually positioned after a no. 7 French indwelling ureteral stent has been in place for 1 week. The catheter is placed over a stiff, nonconducting guidewire (e.g., Terumo). The balloon and wire are positioned fluoroscopically. The cautery wire, when properly positioned, is activated with 75 watts of electric current, and the balloon is inflated with 1.5 cc of contrast material. Following incision, contrast is used to ensure adequate incision. The catheter is replaced with a no. 7 to 14 French endoureterotomy stent. Early studies suggest patency rates equal to those of other endoscopic techniques. Current contraindications consist of obstructions greater than 2 cm, use in the midureter, and use in ureteroenteric obstructions near crossing vessels.

Bibliography

Bannerm, MP, and Pollack, HM. Dilatation of ureteral stenosis techniques and experience—44 patients. AJR 143:789, 1984.

Bush, WH, and Swanson, DP. Acute reactions to intravascular contrast media: Types, risk factors, recognition, and specific treatment. AJR 157:1153, 1991.

Curatola, G, Mazzitelli, R, and Monzani, G. The value of ultrasound as a screening procedure for urological disorders in renal failure. J Urol 130:8, 1983.

Docimo, SG, and Dewolf, WC. High failure rate of indwelling ureteral stents in patients with extrinsic obstruction: Experience at 2 institutions. J Urol 142:277, 1989.

Eshgli, M. Endoscopic incisions of the urinary tract, part II. In AUA Update Series, vol. VIII, lesson 21. Houston: American Urological Association Office of Education, 1989.

Hinman, F. Atlas of Urologic Surgery. Philadelphia: Saunders, 1989, sec 15, pp 637–693.

Kass, EJ, and Majd, M. Evaluation and management of upper urinary tract obstruction in infancy and childhood. Urol Clin North Am 12:133, 1985.

Figure 9-6. *Wire mesh ureteral stents. A–C. A 70-year-old man with left ureteral obstruction following ureteral reimplant. A. Total ureteral (U) obstruction on an antegrade nephrostogram. B. Ureteral patency 3 months after placement of a wire-mesh stent (W). C. The endoscopic appearance of the stent 3 months after placement. D–E. A 75-year-old man with proximal right ureteral obstruction after a complicated ureterolithotomy. D. An antegrade nephrostogram showing total occlusion of the right ureter. E. Stenting of a 6-cm ureteral obstruction by "stacking" two wire-mesh (W) stents. The arrow indicates the points of stent overlap.*

Kelly, JF, Patterson, R, and Lieberman, P. Radiographic contrast media studies in high-risk patients. J Allergy Clin Immunol 62:181, 1978.

Kogan, BA, and Hattner, RS. Radionuclide imaging. In EA Tanagho and JW McAninch (eds), General Urology, 12th ed. Norwalk, Conn: Appleton & Lange, 1989.

Kogan, BA. Disorders of the ureter and ureteropelvic junction. In EA Tanagho and JW McAninch (eds), General Urology, 12th ed. Norwalk, Conn: Appleton & Lange, 1989.

Lang, EK, Glorioso, LW. Antegrade transluminal dilatation of benign ureteral strictures: Long-term results. AJR 150:131, 1988.

Lupton, EW, et al. Pressure changes in the dilated upper urinary tract on perfusion at varying flow rates. Br J Urol 57:622, 1985.

Meretyk, S, et al. Endoureterotomy for treatment of ureteral strictures. J Urol 147:1502, 1992.

Meretyk, S, et al. Endosurgery: Noncalculus applications in the upper urinary tract. In TA Stamey (ed), Monographs in Urology. Montverde, Fla: Medical Directors Publishing, 1991, p 4.

Milroy, EJC, et al. A new treatment for ureteral strictures. Lancet 1:1424, 1988.

Netto, NR, Jr, et al. Urological management of ureteral strictures. J Urol 144:631, 1990.

O'Brien, W, Maxted, WC, and Pahira, JJ. Ureteral stricture: Experience in 31 cases. J Urol 140:737, 1988.

Skeel, DA, et al. Retroperitoneal fibrosis with intrinsic ureteral involvement. J Urol 113:166, 1975.

Sosa, RE, Vaughan, ED, and Gibbons, RP. Retroperitoneal fibrosis. In *AUA Update Series*, vol VI, lesson 21. Houston: American Urological Association Office of Education, 1987.

Turner-Warwick, R. The use of the omental pedicle graft in urinary tract reconstruction. J Urol 116:341, 1976.

Wentzell, PG, et al. Two-needle modification of the Whitaker test. Br J Urol 62:388, 1988.

Whitaker, R. Methods of assessing obstruction in dilated ureters. Br J Urol 45:15, 1973.

Woodbury, PW, et al. Constant pressure perfusion: A method to determine obstruction in the upper urinary tract. J Urol 142:632, 1989.

Recurrent Vesicoureteral Reflux

EVAN J. KASS

Vesicoureteral reflux occurs in less than 1 percent of neurologically normal children who have never had a urinary tract infection; however, it can be detected in up to 50 percent of children with a single episode of urinary tract infection and in approximately 30 percent of children with neurogenic bladder disease. The management of children with vesicoureteral reflux remains controversial, and a consensus is lacking, thereby allowing for considerable variation in the surgical indications. However, it is important to note that the majority of children with reflux do not require surgery and can be managed medically with continuous antimicrobial prophylaxis to prevent urinary tract infection. This protocol for the medical management of vesicoureteral reflux is based on the observation that renal damage in children with reflux only occurs in association with urinary tract infection and that reflux can disappear spontaneously as the child grows. Therefore, if one can prevent urinary tract infection with a daily dose of a urinary antibiotic, it is possible to defer surgery for several years with the expectation that the reflux may resolve without surgery.

The possible complications of the nonsurgical management of reflux include the potential side effects of continuous antimicrobial therapy, the risk of urinary tract infection and renal damage, the trauma of periodic cystograms and other imaging studies, and the possibility that despite years of treatment the reflux will not disappear spontaneously. The major complications of antireflux surgery are obstruction at the ureterovesical junction and failure to correct the reflux. While the goal of this chapter is to delineate the potential complications of antireflux surgery and suggest a protocol for their management, not to discuss the indications for

surgery, it is obvious that poor judgment in the initial management of the child with reflux may increase the potential for surgical complications. In general, it is reasonable to manage the majority of patients with reflux medically for at least 1 year. The only absolute indication for early antireflux surgery is the occurrence of a symptomatic breakthrough urinary tract infection while on a program of medical management. Each year, imaging studies are repeated, and management options are, again, reviewed with the family. The presence of high-grade reflux, previous renal damage, poor compliance with medical management, and a duplex collecting system; age of the child; and persistent reflux despite years of successful medical management are relative, not absolute, indications for surgery. This period of medical management also facilitates the effective control of urinary tract infection and allows infection-induced bladder inflammation to resolve, thereby reducing potential surgical complications related to these problems.

The various surgical techniques for the correction of reflux are standardized and, in general, when performed by surgeons with considerable pediatric urologic experience, produce excellent results, with reported success rates varying from 95 to 98 percent in children with normal bladder function. The most common complications of antireflux surgery resulting in reoperation are persistent reflux and ureterovesical junction obstruction. The complication rate increases substantially (10 to 30 percent of cases) when this surgery is performed on a child with an abnormal bladder secondary to a posterior urethral valve or neurogenic bladder function and in children with grade 5 vesicoureteral reflux, particularly when ureteral tapering is required. The complication rate also may be higher when the surgery is performed by an individual who does not regularly perform antireflux procedures in children.

Etiology of Complications Resulting in Reoperation

The complications of antireflux surgery that result in reoperation may be categorized as either conceptual or technical. A *conceptual complication* is one that arises because of a failure to properly evaluate an individual prior to surgery or to perform the surgical procedure according to accepted principles. These complications should, for the most part, be preventable. *Technical complications* are those which occur even when the surgeon adheres to the accepted principles and may not be avoidable.

The preoperative evaluation of a child with reflux should attempt to identify those individuals with a significant voiding dysfunction, because if this abnormality is not identified and controlled effectively, even an expertly performed surgical procedure may fail. In addition, when the reflux is secondary to a voiding dysfunction (Fig. 10-1), there is a greater than usual expectation that it may resolve spontaneously when the bladder dysfunction is managed effectively. Usually, individuals with a posterior urethral valve or a neurogenic bladder are easily identified; however, identification of a child

with a nonneurogenic voiding dyssynergia may be more problematic. Urodynamic testing should be considered prior to surgery in children with day and night wetting, frequent and urgent urination, Vincent's curtsy sign, or encopresis. It is essential to maintain a high index of suspicion for this problem when evaluating any child with voiding symptoms and reflux, because children with bilateral high-grade vesicoureteral reflux may manifest only subtle voiding symptoms due to the dampening effect of the upper collecting system, which may mask the involuntary bladder contractions.

The essential surgical principles that must be followed to reduce postoperative ureteral obstruction include (1) delicate handling of the ureter, employing traction sutures rather than grasping of the ureter with forceps in order to minimize any potential traumatic or ischemic injury as well as postoperative edema, (2) avoiding angulation of the ureter around an extravesical structure when bringing it through a new muscular hiatus, (3) ensuring that the muscular hiatus or submucosal tunnel does not constrict the ureter or kink it, and (4) securing the ureter to the immobile posterior portion of the bladder so that it does not angulate when the bladder fills. The technical problems that may produce kinking of the ureter at the new hiatus or angulation of the ureter with bladder filling are associated primarily with the Leadbetter-Politano technique. In order to reduce the potential for persistent postoperative reflux, it is of critical importance to construct the new submucosal tunnel so that it is four to five times as long as the diameter of the ureter and to ensure that the ureterovesi-

Figure 10-1. *This 9-year-old boy presented with day and nighttime enuresis and recurrent UTIs. The VCUG demonstrates a thick-walled, elongated bladder and high-grade vesicoureteral reflux on the right. The reflux resolved on a program of anticholinergic medication and intermittent catheterization.*

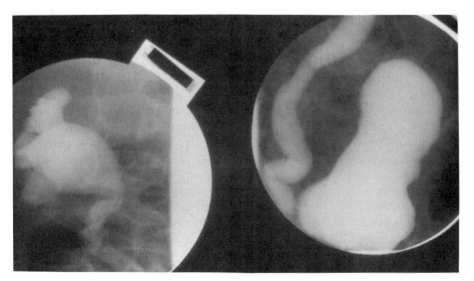

cal anastomosis is tension-free. Postoperative vesicoureteral reflux may result either from a failure to achieve an adequate tunnel length at the time of surgery or because the ureter does not remain fixed to the bladder muscle and becomes detached, thereby resulting in a shortening of a previously adequate tunnel.

Compromise of the ureteral blood supply or ureteral perforation during intravesical ureteral mobilization may result in a ureteral stricture or distal ureteral stenosis. This complication can occur with any ureter if the proper tissue plane is not established during the initial ureteral mobilization but is more common in patients with periureteral inflammation or fibrosis secondary to a recent urinary tract infection or large paraureteral diverticulum. Whenever there is difficulty in establishing the proper plane of dissection intravesically, it is often helpful to approach the ureter extravesically, and usually by alternating intra- and extravesical dissection, the ureter can be mobilized without injury. Ischemic stenosis also can occur following ureteral tapering for megaureter with either an excisional or a folding technique.

Postoperative Complications

Obstruction

Postoperative ureteral obstruction is the most serious complication of antireflux surgery because it can result in the loss of significant renal function, even in the absence of clinical signs and symptoms. The diagnosis is often suggested by the presence of hydronephrosis on the routine postoperative imaging studies; however, these may be difficult to interpret, since some degree of hydronephrosis may occur normally immediately following surgery (Fig. 10-2). A renal ultrasound or excretory urogram is generally obtained 4 to 6 weeks after surgery unless the child has symptoms suggestive of a possible obstruction, such as abdominal or flank pain, palpable mass, febrile urinary tract infection, decreasing urinary output, or rising serum creatinine level. In this setting, an urgent renal ultrasound is performed. During the first few months following antireflux surgery, the degree of upper tract dilatation should be no greater than that observed on the preoperative voiding cys-

Figure 10-2. A. Preoperative IVP. B. Postoperative IVP demonstrating bilateral hydroureteronephrosis similar in degree to the dilatation seen on the VCUG. A repeat IVP 2 months later demonstrated an image identical to the preoperative study.

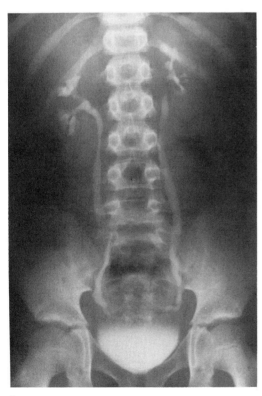
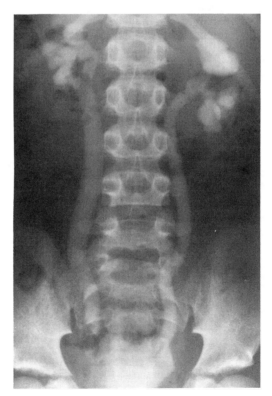

A

B

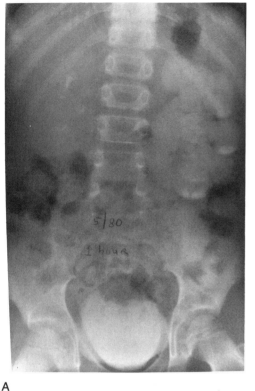

A

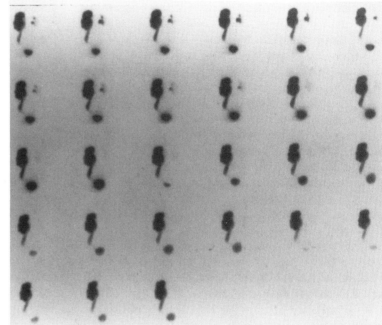

B

Figure 10-3. *A. Postoperative IVP demonstrating hydronephrosis that exceeds the dilatation observed on the preoperative VCUG. B. The diuresis renal scan demonstrates no washout of the radiopharmaceutical, and the half-time exceeds 20 minutes. C. An antegrade pressure perfusion study confirms an obstruction at the ureterovesical junction. At surgery, the distal ureter was stenotic. Following the second operation, the hydronephrosis improved considerably, and the diuretic renal scan demonstrated prompt washout of the tracer.*

C

tourethrogram (see Fig. 10-2*A* and *B*). However, when the hydronephrosis exceeds this degree of upper tract enlargement, or if it is still present 6 months after surgery, the possibility of an obstruction must be considered, and additional imaging studies should be performed (Fig. 10-3*A*).

When an obstruction is suspected, a diuresis renal scan should be obtained, and if this demonstrates diminished renal function and/or prolonged drainage of the radiopharmaceutical from the collecting system after diuretic administration, an obstruction is diagnosed (see Fig. 10-3*B*). An obstruction within 3 months of the original surgical procedure in a symptomatic patient or one with reduced renal function usually requires the placement of a percutaneous nephrostomy to decompress the kidney. However, when the renal function remains unchanged from preoperative studies and the patient's condition is stable, it is possible to temporize in order to determine if the obstruction will resolve spontaneously. When it is necessary to insert a percutaneous nephrostomy tube, urinary tract infection should be controlled before antegrade pyelography is performed to identify the site of obstruction. When the obstruction is related to postoperative edema, it will generally resolve within a few weeks, and the nephrostomy tube can be removed after appropriate imaging studies demonstrate a return of renal function to preoperative levels and patency of the ureterovesical junction. When the studies indicate a persistent obstruction after an appropriate period of healing (usually 3 to 6 months), reoperation should be considered (see Fig. 10-3*C*).

Delayed ureteral obstruction can occur even several years after apparently successful antireflux surgery, and therefore, annual imaging studies are usually performed for 4 to 5 years following apparently successful surgical correction of the reflux. Obstruction usually is the result of a narrow constricting ureteral hiatus, ureteral angulation at the inferior hiatal edge, or stenosis of the ureter (intra- or extravesically) (Fig. 10-4). The most difficult circumstance to evaluate is the asymptomatic patient with persistent postoperative hydronephrosis (Fig. 10-5*A* and *B*). In this setting, a diuresis renal scan can be very helpful. When renal function, as determined by nuclear renal scintigraphy, remains unchanged from preoperative levels and the drainage half-time is less than 20 minutes, no surgery is recommended, but the patient is followed with periodic ultrasound examinations and renal scans. However, when renal function is diminished postoperatively or the drainage half-time is prolonged, surgical intervention is considered. Antegrade or retrograde pyelography in this circumstance is often very helpful in precisely defining the anatomic circumstances.

Postoperative ureterovesical obstruction also can be intermittent, as a result of angulation of the ureter as the bladder fills. In this circumstance, the diuresis renal scan may be unobstructed with an empty bladder, and the diagnosis may only be established by performing an antegrade pyelogram combined with gradual bladder filling. The ureter will be seen to kink at the new ureteral hiatus, producing progressive ureteral dilatation. This type of obstruction does not typically occur following the Cohen technique because the ureteral hiatus is not moved to a new position.

Persistent Vesicoureteral Reflux

Failure to correct the reflux is the most common complication of antireflux surgery and is more likely with high-grade reflux, particularly when a wide lower ureter was present initially. In most instances, the reflux persists because an adequate ratio of tunnel length to ureteral diameter was not achieved at the initial surgery or be-

cause the ureter retracted from the intended trigonal attachment due to inadequate fixation resulting in a shortened tunnel length. However, occasionally, the reflux persists despite a technically perfect surgical procedure because ureteral peristalsis is poor as a result of either a primary congenital muscular deficiency or a secondary inflammatory or ischemic ureteral muscle injury.

Postoperative vesicoureteral reflux also can be transient, and occasionally, resolution of the reflux may not occur until 2 to 3 years following surgery. Reflux of this type tends to be of lesser degree than the original, but this is not always the case, so, in general, it is not possible to distinguish between postoperative reflux that will resolve and reflux that will require reoperation. In addition, following a unilateral antireflux operation, reflux into the nonoperated contralateral ureter may occur and also, tends to be transient, particularly when it is of low grade. However, since it may not resolve spontaneously in all children, some have recommended operating on the contralateral ureter whenever there is a history of bilateral reflux or the ureteral orifice on that side is at all abnormal. I have not routinely reimplanted the contralateral nonrefluxing ureter unless there has been a history of a least grade 3 vesicoureteral reflux in that ureter previously or the orifice is "golf hole" in appearance. This conservative approach to the contralateral ureter has resulted in some children having postoperative reflux on the nonoperated side (Fig. 10-6*A* and *B*); however, thus far, a second surgery to correct persistent contralateral reflux has not been necessary, although some children have required several years of antimicrobial prophylaxis.

My usual protocol following antireflux surgery is to place the child on antimicrobial prophylaxis and obtain a nuclear cystogram 6 months following surgery. When the reflux has resolved, the prophylaxis is discontinued; however, if the reflux persists, the child should remain on low-dose antimicrobial therapy and a cystogram repeated annually for as long as the reflux persists. In general, all children with postoperative vesicoureteral reflux are followed nonoperatively for at least 2 or 3 years before a decision to reoperate is made. When the grade of reflux has improved significantly postoperatively, reoperation has not usually been necessary; however, when high-grade reflux persists, reoperation usually will be required.

Patient Preparation

After a decision has been made to reoperate, it is important to obtain as much information as possible about the

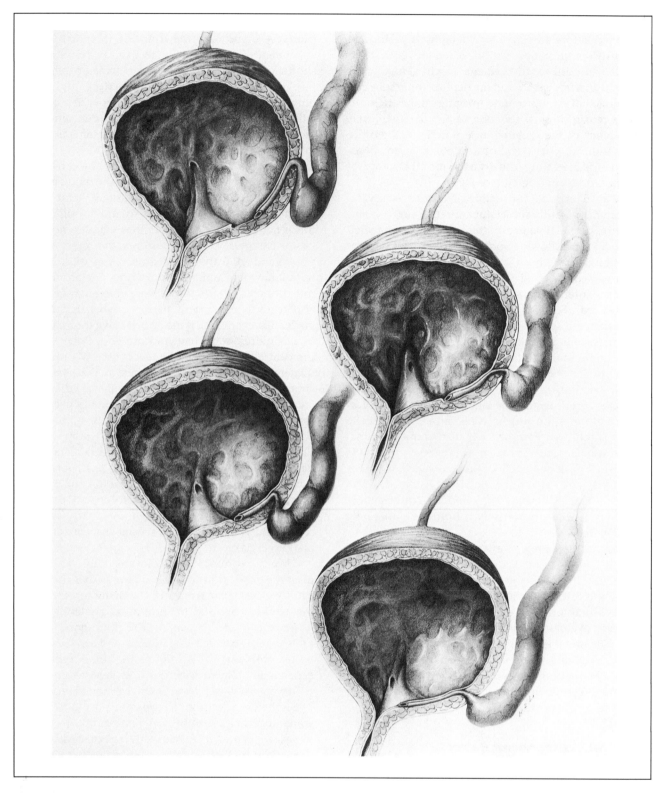

Figure 10-4. *Sites of ureteral obstruction after ureteroneocystostomy. Suprahiatal obstruction* (above, left), *hiatal obstruction due to narrow constricting hiatus* (center, right) *and to ureteral angulation at inferior hiatal edge* (center, left), *and infrahiatal obstruction* (below, right). *(Reproduced with permission from Dunne, EF, Jr, and Gibbons, MD, Ureteroneocystostomy. In JE Fowler, Jr (ed),* Mastery of Surgery: Urologic Surgery. *Boston: Little, Brown, 1992, p 204.)*

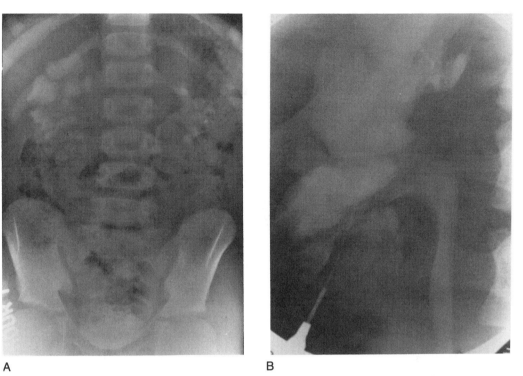

A   B

Figure 10-5. *A. Persistent right hydroureteronephrosis 3 years following antireflux surgery. The diuresis renal scan demonstrated good washout with a half-time of less than 20 minutes. B. A pressure-perfusion study confirmed the absence of obstruction.*

anatomy of the ureterovesical junction and bladder function and, hopefully, determine the reason for failure of the original operation. Intravenous urography and contrast voiding cystourethrography are performed routinely prior to secondary ureterovesical surgery, and retrograde or antegrade pyelography often helps to further define the distal ureter in those individuals with a secondary ureterovesical junction obstruction. Urodynamic testing to exclude an occult voiding dysfunction should be performed whenever there is a history of bowel or bladder control problems, if bladder wall thickening has been observed on previous imaging studies or at the time of the original surgery, and whenever there is a concern about diminished functional bladder capacity. Cystoscopy performed just prior to reoperation facilitates evaluation of the bladder and urethra for a subtle anatomic abnormality that may have been missed as well as evaluation of the ureteral orifices and tunnel length achieved by the initial surgery.

If the ureteral tunnel length is too short, reoperation will almost invariably be successful as long as a 4 or 5:1 ratio of ureteral width to tunnel is achieved at surgery. However, if the tunnel length achieved at the initial surgery is of sufficient length, the failure to correct

the reflux may be secondary to ureteral muscular dysfunction, and the secondary surgery also may fail unless an extremely long tunnel length is achieved.

Surgical Technique

The standard techniques for reoperation on the ureterovesical junction have been well described by Hendren. A vertical midline incision is preferred because it facilitates access to either or both ureters at the level of the iliac vessels. A no. 5 or 8 French pediatric feeding tube is introduced into the ureter and secured at 3 and 9 o'clock to the ureteral orifice with 4-0 or 5-0 chromic sutures. The orifice is circumscribed, leaving a 2- to 3-mm cuff at the bladder mucosa.

The ureter is mobilized intravesically as well as extravesically utilizing a "minimal touch" technique by using the feeding tube for traction, taking great care to preserve the periureteral blood supply and adventitia. Typically, a much more extensive extravesical mobilization is required for secondary procedures because it is important to expose the ureter to a level beyond the original operation in order to ensure that there will not

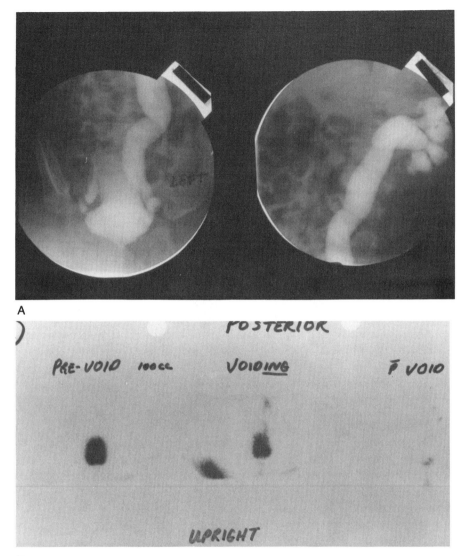

A

B

Figure 10-6. *A. Preoperative VCUG demonstrating high-grade left reflux and grade 1 right reflux; subsequent nuclear cystograms failed to demonstrate the right reflux. B. A left reimplantation was performed because of recurrent febrile UTIs, and postoperatively, the right reflux was again noted. The patient remains on antimicrobial prophylaxis 2 years later.*

be any kinking or angulation from fibrous adhesions. After the ureter is mobilized completely, it should be examined carefully for evidence of ischemic injury or previous scarring, and any abnormal segments should be trimmed, leaving only well-vascularized ureter. Wide ureters are tapered over a no. 10 French catheter utilizing a folding rather than an excisional technique, if possible, to minimize ischemia. Tailoring is typically required only when the ureteral width is the limiting factor in achieving the creation of a tunnel length at least four or five times greater than the width of the ureter.

The Politano-Leadbetter technique is generally preferred for most repeat ureteroneocystostomies because, when combined with a psoas hitch procedure, it allows one to create a long, tension-free submucosal tunnel that should not kink. The new hiatus is created by placing a right-angle clamp through the old hiatus and dissecting in a superolateral direction under direct vision along the posterior surface of the bladder wall. Right-angle retractors placed within the hiatus often facilitate the dissection. The new hiatus is created by incising the mucosa and muscle over the top of the clamp, again under direct vision to avoid inadvertent entry into the peritoneum or intestinal injury. The new hiatus should be of sufficient caliber to avoid constricting the ureter. Extravesical dissection should be sufficient to release any bands of tissue that could cause kinking of the ureter and ensure that the ureter follows a smooth, tension-free course.

The use of a psoas hitch facilitates the creation of a long, tension-free tunnel and helps to prevent the kinking that may occur when the ureter is reimplanted into a mobile portion of the bladder. An additional benefit of this technique is that sometimes it may be possible to create a tunnel of sufficient length that tapering may not be required for all-wide ureters. Use of the psoas hitch also makes it possible to bridge moderate defects in ureteral length without creating undue tension on the anastomosis that may result in retraction of the ureter and recurrent reflux. Longer defects in ureteral length may require a Boari flap or a transureteroureterostomy if it is not possible to achieve an adequate tunnel length without placing tension on the anastomosis.

In most cases, a standard approach either with or without a psoas hitch can be employed when perform-

ing a bilateral reimplantation; however, there are occasions when it is not possible to reimplant both ureters into the bladder and achieve an adequate tunnel length. In this circumstance, the better of the two ureters should be reimplanted into the bladder with a long tunnel utilizing a psoas hitch. The opposite ureter can then be trimmed to an appropriate length, spatulated, and a transureteroureterostomy performed utilizing a running 5-0 or 6-0 polyglycolic acid suture. A ureteral stent is usually placed across the anastomosis.

The management of persistent reflux in an abnormal bladder deserves special attention because these cases may not be easily amenable to reoperation. When a child has a small-capacity noncompliant bladder (regardless of the etiology), postoperative reflux or a ureterovesical junction obstruction may be secondary to unphysiologically elevated bladder pressures, and in this setting, a second ureteral reimplantation also may fail despite a technically adequate operation. In children with a noncompliant bladder and a suspected ureterovesical junction obstruction, the diuretic renogram may help to determine whether or not the obstruction is

Figure 10-7. *A. Preoperative IVP in a child with a neuropathic bladder and bilateral vesicoureteral reflux managed by anticholinergic medication and intermittent catheterization. Because of recurrent UTIs, antireflux surgery was performed. B. Postoperative IVP demonstrating bilateral hydroureteronephrosis. A diuretic renal scan with the bladder empty did not demonstrate an obstruction. Urodynamic studies demonstrated a small-capacity noncompliant bladder that did not improve with conservative therapy. C. Following bladder augmentation, the upper tracts returned to their preoperative status.*

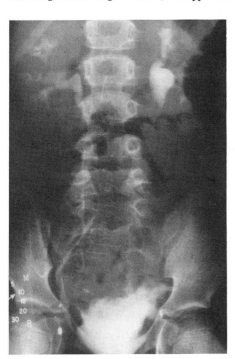
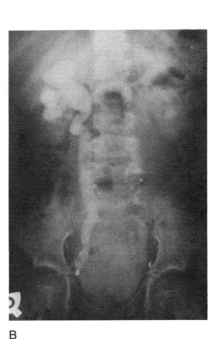
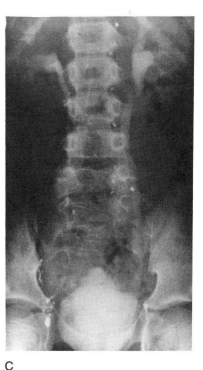

A   B   C

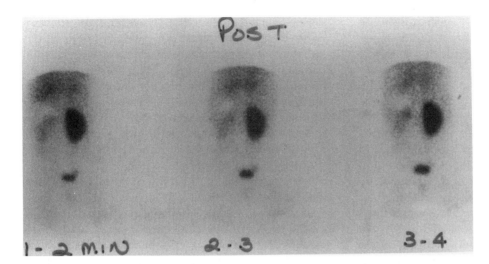

Figure 10-8. *A technetium-99m DMSA renal scan in a child with high-grade left reflux. Despite tapering and reimplantation, the reflux persisted. Since the left kidney provided less than 10 percent of the total renal function and the right kidney was normal, a left nephrectomy, rather than a repeat antireflux procedure, was performed.*

primary or secondary. The scan is performed with a catheter in the bladder, and if this study demonstrates normal washout with the bladder decompressed, the obstruction is secondary to elevated bladder pressures, and consideration is given to bladder augmentation without ureteral revision (Fig. 10-7). Similarly, in the child with persistent reflux, if the cystoscopic evaluation indicates that the ureteral tunnels are of adequate length, bladder augmentation alone may solve the problem in a child with a small-capacity, high-pressure bladder.

When there is reasonable bladder compliance in a child with a neurogenic or valve bladder, reoperation to correct reflux is the usual option; however, the potential for a successful correction of persistent reflux in children with abnormal bladders is considerably less than in a child with a normal bladder. In my opinion, this setting is the only one in which at the present time endoscopic correction of the reflux may be of value.

Although all urologists consider the preservation of renal tissue to be their primary goal in children, there are some occasions when a simple nephrectomy may be preferred. When the kidney in question has 15 percent or less of total renal function (as determined by technetium-99m DMSA renal scan) in a child with a normal contralateral kidney, consideration should be given to nephrectomy rather than a second attempt at antireflux surgery (Fig. 10-8). This option is even more attractive when the ureter in question will require tapering.

Summary

The majority of children undergoing antireflux surgery will have a successful result; however, in 2 to 5 percent of

cases, complications may occur. The potential for surgical complications may be diminished with appropriate preoperative selection and evaluation of patients, by adhering to well-defined surgical principles of antireflux surgery, and with a surgeon who has considerable pediatric urologic experience. Increased postoperative complications can be expected in children with abnormal bladder function and ureters requiring tapering. Transient obstruction and reflux may be noted postoperatively; however, as long as renal function and upper tract drainage remain stable, a conservative nonoperative approach is warranted. Secondary surgery is indicated for reflux that does not resolve after 2 to 3 years and when there is evidence of persistent obstruction, as manifested by diuretic renography 6 months or more after the initial surgery.

The surgical approach to reoperation should include an intravesical and extravesical mobilization of the ureter and reimplantation of the ureter with a long submucosal tunnel and a psoas hitch. All patients with apparently successful antireflux surgery should be followed for at least 5 years to detect potential late complications.

Bibliography

Ehrlich, RM. The ureteral folding technique for megaureter surgery. J Urol **134**:668, 1985.

Hendren, WH. Reoperative ureteral reimplantation: Management of the difficult case. J Pediatr Surg **15**:770, 1980.

Hendren, WH. Reoperation for the failed ureteral reimplantation. J Urol **101**:403, 1969.

International Reflux Study Committee. Medical versus surgical treatment of primary vesicoureteral reflux. Pediatrics **67**: 392, 1981.

Kass, EJ, Koff, SA, and Diokno, AC. Fate of vesicoureteral reflux in children with neuropathic bladders managed by intermittent catheterization. J Urol **125**:63, 1981.

Mesrobian, H-GJ, Kramer, SA, and Kelalis, PP. Reoperative ureteroneocystostomy: Review of 69 patients. J Urol **133**:388, 1985.

O'Donnell, B, and Puri, P. Technical refinements in endoscopic correction of vesicoureteral reflux. J Urol **140**:1101, 1988.

Poltitano, VA, and Leadbetter, WF. An operative technique for the correction of vesicoureteral reflux. J Urol **79**:932, 1958.

Riedmiller, H, et al. Psoas-hitch ureteroneocystostomy: Experience with 181 cases. Eur Urol **10**:145, 1984.

Siegelbaum, MH, and Rabinovitch, HH. Delayed spontaneous resolution of high grade vesicoureteral reflux after reimplantation. J Urol **138**:1205, 1987.

Bladder Cancer

MICHAEL J. DROLLER

The term *reoperation* implies the need for an additional surgical procedure when the initial surgery did not completely eradicate the original condition or when the original condition has recurred. Possibly implicit in this as well is the concept of surgery when some other form of therapy for a particular condition has failed. There are several situations in bladder cancer that merit consideration in this context.

The most common form of bladder cancer is superficial disease. This comprises those tumors which are mucosally confined and those which have invaded the lamina propria. The former are usually treated successfully by transurethral resection, but they can be expected to recur in 75 percent of instances. If they recur in superficial form, usually they can be managed successfully by repeat transurethral resection. The latter may have a more aggressive biologic potential; although they may recur in superficial form, in which case transurethral resection can be repeated, they may become invasive of the muscularis in 25 to 30 percent of instances. In these cases, more extensive surgery will be necessary (see below).

In those types of bladder cancer which present initially in a more advanced, albeit regionally confined, form, or in those which recur in progressive form after having appeared initially as superficial disease, the reoperative procedure that usually needs to be considered is radical cystectomy.

There are also instances in which more advanced regional bladder cancer is treated with "definitive" radiation therapy alone, chemotherapy alone, or the two in conjunction with one another after initial transurethral resection. Reoperation in these instances either to cure or palliate cancer persistence or recurrence may involve either extensive transurethral resection or radical cystectomy.

In this chapter we will discuss those factors which help determine decisions regarding reoperative surgery for various forms of bladder cancer, the situational context in which they are diagnosed, and how each type of surgery can be approached. We will also describe techniques that we have found useful in each setting to provide a safe and effective approach in the surgical management of that particular condition.

Recurrent Superficial Transitional Cell Carcinoma

The most common approach in the management of recurrent mucosally confined or lamina propria–invasive transitional cell carcinoma is repeat transurethral resection of the recurrent lesion(s). In addition, voided urinary cytology and cup biopsies either at random or in areas of erythema as well as at the margin of the recurrent tumors are important in assessing the extent and potential aggressiveness of the tumor diathesis.

If the recurrent cancer appears papillary, the superficial portion of the tumor should be resected flush with the mucosa (Fig. 11-1). Special care should then be taken in resecting more deeply to avoid perforating the bladder wall, which is likely to be very thin in these instances. If the recurrent tumor appears to be more nodular, a more extensive tumor resection can be undertaken with less concern for perforation, since the bladder wall in these instances is usually much thicker. Both specimens, superficial and deep, should then be sent for separate pathologic analysis.

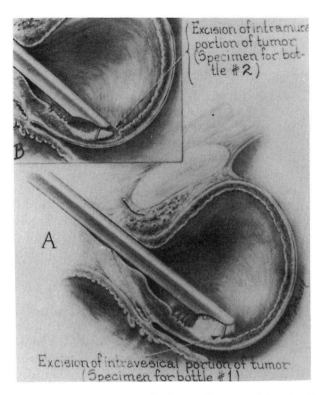

Excision of intramural portion of tumor (Specimen for bottle #2)

Excision of intravesical portion of tumor (Specimen for bottle #1)

Figure 11-1. *All tumors, whether papillary or nodular, should have their superficial components resected flush with the remainder of the bladder mucosa. Deeper resection should then be done to determine the depth of infiltration if invasion has occurred. With papillary superficial cancers, a very deep resection is usually not necessary, since for the most part these tumors are not accompanied by a thickened bladder wall, and bladder perforation can more readily occur. (From Jewett, HJ, Carcinoma of the bladder: Development and evaluation of current concepts of therapy. J Urol 82:92, 1959, with permission.)*

Electrocautery at the margin of tumor resection and of any focal bleeding points is sufficient to obtain hemostasis. A urethral catheter is generally left indwelling to prevent bladder distension and hemorrhage.

Repeated or rapid recurrence of mucosally confined tumors often can be controlled by intravesical therapy with a variety of agents (Table 11-1). Since most recurrences in low-grade mucosally confined disease are not progressive and do not become life-threatening, it is often possible to treat such a recurrence by simple cau-

terization. Laser therapy also can be performed. It is imperative, however, to monitor recurrent disease with urinary cytology. Any indication of an increase in grade will require repeat biopsy and resection to determine if more aggressive surgery is necessary.

Recurrent Muscle-Infiltrative Transitional Cell Carcinoma

When a diagnosis of deeply infiltrative cancer is made and cystectomy is not considered an option, extensive transurethral resection and cautery can be used to provide palliation for recurrent disease. Extensive resection generally can be accomplished in these instances with little risk of bladder perforation, since the bladder wall is usually thick. The superficial portion of the cancer should be resected flush with the bladder mucosa. Deeper resection will then possibly permit removal of a major part of the infiltrative portion of the cancer.

Radical Cystectomy for Infiltrative Bladder Cancer

Radical cystectomy is generally the treatment of choice for deeply invasive cancer or when a recurrent cancer has characteristics that suggest a high risk for progression (e.g., high-grade tumors that extensively invade the lamina propria, diffuse carcinoma in situ, and continued failure to respond to intensive intravesical therapy). In males, radical cystectomy encompasses removal of the bladder, pelvic lymph nodes, prostate, and in certain instances, the urethra. In females, radical cystectomy includes removal of the bladder, uterus and adnexa, anterior vaginal wall, and urethra.

Following a mechanical bowel preparation and appropriate antibiotic treatment, the patient is draped with the entire abdomen and perineum in the operative field. The legs are elevated and abducted in a modified lithotomy position to permit access to the perineum and room for an assistant to stand during the surgery (Fig. 11-2). A urethral catheter with a 30-cc balloon is inserted

Table 11-1 *Intravesical Treatment for Recurrent Bladder Cancer*

Agent	Dosage	Regimen	Complications
Thiotepa	30 mg in 30 cc H_2O	Weekly 6–8 weeks	Marrow suppression
Mitomycin C	40 mg in 40 cc H_2O	Weekly 6–8 weeks	Skin rash
Adriamycin	50 mg in 50 cc H_2O	Weekly 6–8 weeks	Urgency
BCG*	1 ampule in 40 cc saline	Weekly 6 weeks	Hematuria, frequency

*Connaught (120 mg), Pasteur (75–150 mg), Tice (50 mg), Armand-Frappier (120 mg).

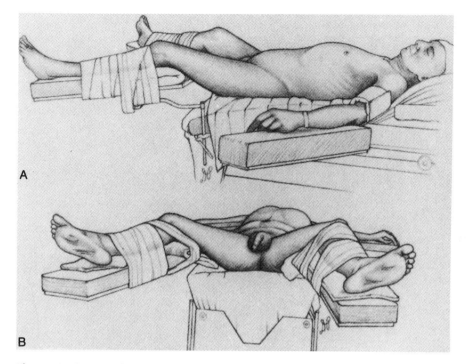

Figure 11-2. *For radical cystectomy, the patient should be placed in a supine position with the legs extended and abducted on cradle stirrups so that the perineum is accessible. (From Fair, WR, and Atlas, I, Radical cystectomy. In MJ Droller (ed),* Surgical Management of Urologic Disease: An Anatomic Approach. *St Louis: Mosby–Year Book, 1992, with permission.)*

under sterile conditions and kept in the operative field on continuous drainage.

A midline incision is made from just above the umbilicus to the symphysis pubis. Depending on the type of diversion that is selected, a paramedian incision also can be made to accommodate the stoma of a planned conduit or the orifice of a continent pouch.

The peritoneal cavity is entered, and the intraperitoneal organs are palpated and inspected for metastases. A Balfour clamp is placed to retract the abdominal sidewalls. A moist laparotomy pad is placed to protect the intestines, and a rolled towel can then be used to retract the small intestines cephalad. This can be facilitated by cephalad retraction of the right colon after incising the posterior peritoneum at the line of Toldt around the cecum and lateral to the ascending colon (Fig. 11-3).

An incision is made in the peritoneum along the obliterated umbilical vessels to the internal ring on each side. This is extended cephalad along the external iliac arteries to the bifurcation of the aorta. This permits identification and mobilization of the ureters and initial exposure of the pelvic lymph nodes. The urachus is divided, and a Kocher clamp is placed for retraction and manipulation of the bladder during the dissection (Fig. 11-4).

Fibroadipose and lymphatic tissues are dissected from the external iliac arteries and swept medially from the external iliac artery and vein and from the obturator nerve toward the bladder. In males, the vas deferens is divided between ligaclips.

The ureters are divided as they approach the posterior wall of the bladder approximately 3 cm after crossing the common iliac arteries (Fig. 11-5). Ligaclips or ligatures are placed on the ureter to prevent potential seepage of tumor cells from the distal cut end and to permit proximal dilation that will facilitate later anastomosis of ureter to bowel. A section of the proximal margin on each side is sent for frozen-section analysis to exclude carcinoma in situ.

After dissection of the posterolateral bladder pedicles is begun, the superior and middle vesical arteries are divided between 0 silk ligatures as they are encountered (Fig. 11-6). It may be useful to divide the hypogastric arteries distal to their gluteal branches and incorporate them with the surgical specimen. This may facilitate the dissection if prior radiation therapy has obscured the vesical arteries through the development of large amounts

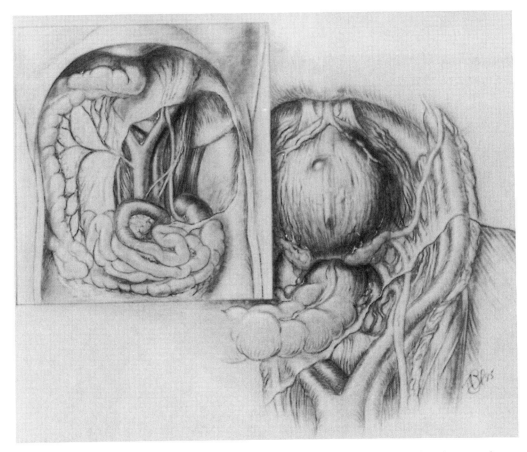

Figure 11-3. *After a midline abdominal incision has been made and the peritoneal cavity entered, exposure of the pelvic retroperitoneum can be accomplished by incising the posterior peritoneum in the line of Toldt just lateral to the ascending colon and around the cecum and retracting the cecum, ascending colon, and small intestine cephalad. (From Skinner, DG, Lieskovsky, G., Technique of radical cystectomy. In DG Skinner and G Lieskovsky (eds),* Diagnosis and Management of Genitourinary Cancer. *Philadelphia: Saunders, 1988, with permission.)*

Figure 11-4. *An incision should be made along the obliterated umbilical arteries anteriorly and then along the external iliac arteries toward the bifurcation of the aorta. The urachal remnant can be grasped in the midline with a Kocher clamp and used for retraction through its attachment to the dome of the bladder. (From Fair, WR, and Atlas, I, Radical cystectomy. In MJ Droller (ed),* Surgical Management of Urologic Disease: An Anatomic Approach. *St Louis: Mosby–Year Book, 1992, with permission.)*

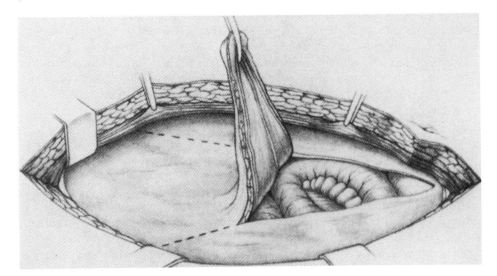

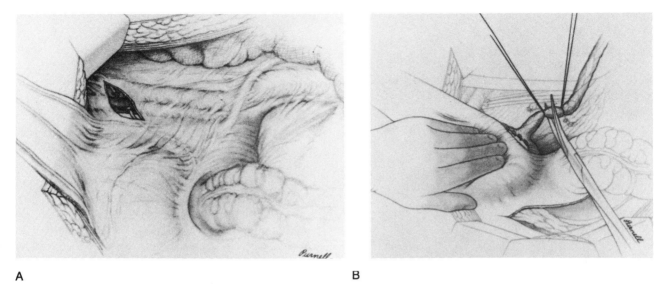

A   B

Figure 11-5. *The ureters are dissected as they cross the common iliac arteries (A) and are divided 3 to 4 cm distal to that point (B). A specimen of the proximal end should be sent for frozen-section analysis to ensure that no cancer is present. (From Fair, WR, and Atlas, I, Radical cystectomy. In MJ Droller (ed),* Surgical Management of Urologic Disease: An Anatomic Approach. *St Louis: Mosby–Year Book, 1992, with permission.)*

Figure 11-6. *Dissection of the bladder proceeds along the lateral bladder pedicles on either side. Superior vesical and middle vesical arteries should be divided between 0 silk ligatures. Corresponding veins should be similarly controlled and divided. (From Skinner, DG, and Lieskovsky, G, Technique of radical cystectomy.* Urol Clin North Am *8:353, 1981, with permission.)*

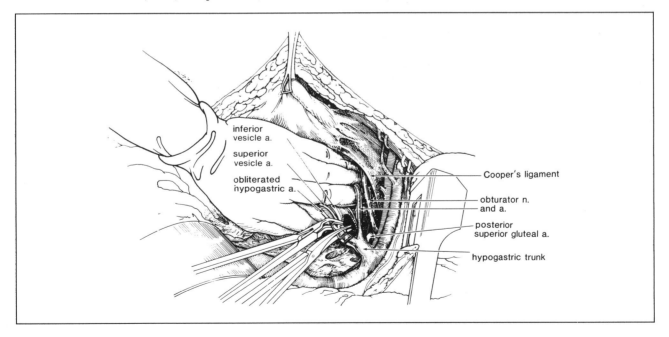

of fibrous tissue. Veins are similarly divided between 0 silk ligatures as encountered during dissection of the bladder pedicles. The inferior vesical arteries, which are at the inferior-most portion of the dissection of the pedicles, are generally left until later in the procedure.

The peritoneal reflection between the bladder and rectum can then be incised (Fig. 11-7). Care should be taken to maintain as much as possible of the peritoneum overlying the bladder. Once the rectovesical space has been entered, the posterior surface of the bladder (including Denonvillier's fascia overlying the seminal vesicles) can be freed bluntly from the underlying rectum as one proceeds caudad toward the perineum (Fig. 11-8). At this point, the entire bladder should be freed from the major portion of its fascial and vascular attachments in

Figure 11-7. *After the lateral pedicles of the bladder have been dissected inferiorly, the peritoneal reflection between the rectum and the posterior bladder wall should be incised to allow entry into the rectovesical space. (From Fair, WR, and Atlas, I, Radical cystectomy. In MJ Droller (ed),* Surgical Management of Urologic Disease: An Anatomic Approach. *St Louis: Mosby–Year Book, 1992, with permission.)*

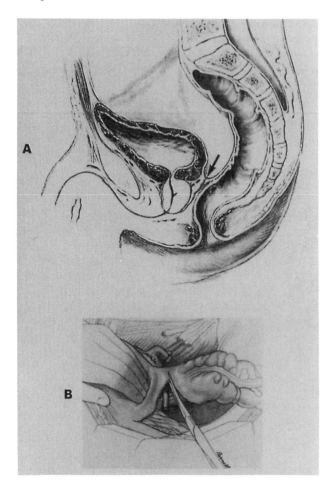

the pelvis. What remains are the inferior-most part of the bladder pedicles and the fascial layers on which the inferior portion of the bladder rests. Attention can now be focused on dissection of the prostate and urethra. The endopelvic fascia is incised laterally, extending anteriorly to the puboprostatic ligaments (Fig. 11-9). Adipose tissue in the retropubic space and superior to these ligaments is removed by blunt dissection and by suction. Any small vessels that may be encountered are cauterized. The puboprostatic ligaments are incised at their insertion in the periosteum of the pubic rami. This permits access to the dorsal vein complex.

A right-angle clamp is placed between the dorsal vein complex and the underlying urethra at the apex of the prostate, a 0 silk ligature is placed, and the dorsal vein complex is divided. If bleeding occurs, the ligature can be reinforced with a 0 chromic catgut suture ligature placed at the cut distal end of the dorsal vein (Fig. 11-10).

If the urethra is to be left behind, a right-angle clamp is placed around the urethra at the apex of the prostate and within the lateral fascial bundles that hug the urethra laterally. A tunnel is created posteriorly, and an umbilical tape can be placed. The urethra is then entered sharply on its anterior surface (Fig. 11-11). The indwelling catheter is grasped with a Kocher clamp and divided with the balloon kept inflated. The remainder of the urethra is then divided within the lateral fascia above the umbilical tape and a right-angle clamp.

The prostate can then be retracted cephalad using the indwelling catheter as an anchor. The rectourethralis muscle lying posteriorly is divided sharply and then dissected cephalad to the reflection of Denonvillier's fascia lying over the base of the seminal vesicles and ampullae of the ejaculatory duct (Fig. 11-12). This fascia is entered to expose the posterior surface of the seminal vesicles, and a tunnel can be created joining with the space that had been developed between the rectum and the bladder from above.

The endopelvic fascial reflection on the anterolateral surface of the prostate can be divided anteriorly to permit preservation of the nerve (neurovascular) bundles that maintain potency (Fig. 11-13). These bundles should fall away toward the rectum, permitting further dissection of the lateral pedicle of the prostate and of the inferior portion of the bladder (containing the inferior vesicle artery) on either side. Vessels are divided between clips or 00 chromic ligatures. In the setting of prior radiation therapy, thickened fibrous tissue in these areas may prevent a nerve-sparing procedure from being accomplished. In these instances, the remaining portions of lateral pedicle tissue and the inferior vesical

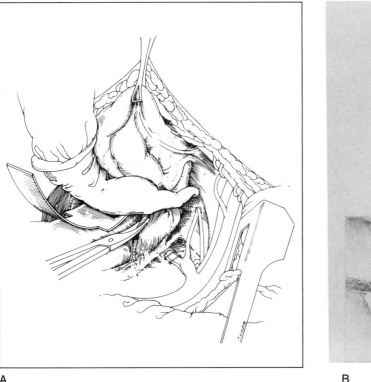

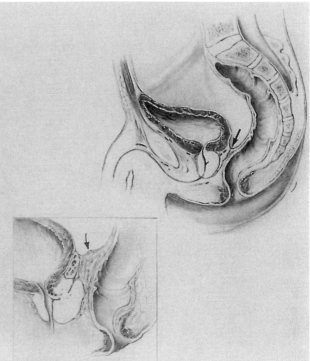

A   B

Figure 11-8. *Blunt dissection in the rectovesical space is used to elevate the bladder and seminal vesicles from the rectum (A) along Denonvillier's fascia (B). (Part A from Skinner, DG, Technique of radical cystectomy. Urol Clin North Am 8:353, 1981; and Part B from Skinner, DG, and Lieskovsky, G, Technique of radical cystectomy. In DG Skinner and G Lieskovsky (eds),* Diagnosis and Management of Genitourinary Cancer. *Philadelphia: Saunders, 1988, with permission.)*

Figure 11-9. *The endopelvic fascia is incised lateral to the prostate and extended anteriorly to the level of the puboprostatic ligaments. The ligaments are divided near their attachment to the pubic rami. (From Fair, WR, and Atlas, I, Radical cystectomy. In MJ Droller (ed),* Surgical Management of Urologic Disease: An Anatomic Approach. *St Louis: Mosby–Year Book, 1992, with permission.)*

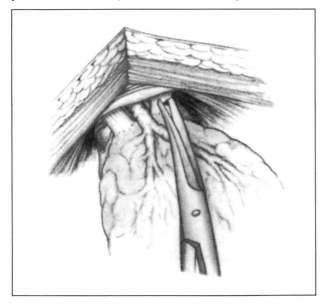

artery on either side can simply be divided between clamps and suture ligatures of 00 silk or chromic catgut and the specimen removed.

The distal stump of the urethra can be used for anastomosis to a segment of bowel that has been fashioned into a pouch if it is intended to preserve voiding capability. The external urethral sphincter mechanism will have been preserved if the urethra was divided just distal to the prostatic apex.

If the urethra is to be incorporated with the surgical specimen, dissection is continued both bluntly and sharply within the lateral fascia on either side of the urethra to mobilize it from the corporal bodies. Both corporal bodies and the penis are inverted during the course of retraction and dissection. Sharp dissection is needed to free the fossa navicularis from the glans penis (Fig. 11-14). The penis is then restored to its normal position by direct pressure on the corporal bodies to reevert them.

The urethra also may be dissected by making an incision in the perineum, circumscribing the bulbar urethra, and then proceeding with dissection of the remainder of the urethra as described above (Fig. 11-15).

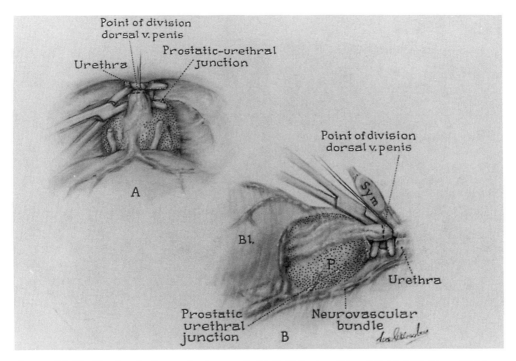

Figure 11-10. *The dorsal vein complex is secured with 0 silk ligature (A) and divided (B). (From Walsh, PC, Technique of radical retropubic prostatectomy with preservation of sexual function: An anatomic approach. In DG Skinner and G Lieskovsky (eds),* Diagnosis and Management of Genitourinary Cancer. *Philadelphia: Saunders, 1988, with permission.)*

Figure 11-11. *A. The urethra is entered sharply in the midline at the apex of the prostate. The indwelling urethral catheter is grasped with a Kocher clamp and divided distal to that clamp to maintain inflation of the catheter balloon. B. The remainder of the urethra is then divided distal to the apex of the prostate. (From Ring, KS, Olsson, CA, and Benson, MC, Surgery for prostate cancer. In MJ Droller (ed),* Surgical Management of Urologic Disease: An Anatomic Approach. *St. Louis: Mosby–Year Book, 1992, with permission.)*

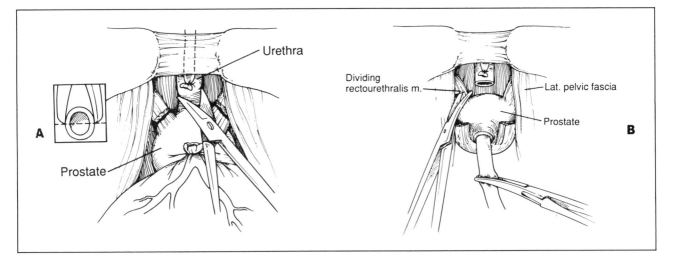

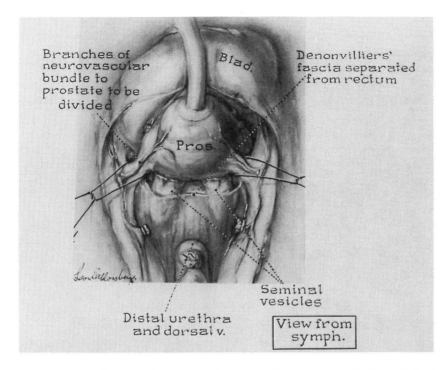

Figure 11-12. *The tissue plane between the rectum and the prostate can be dissected sharply and bluntly to permit cephalad retraction of the prostate and visualization of Denonvillier's fascia over the seminal vesicles. This can be divided to expose the posterior surface of the seminal vesicles. (From Walsh, PC, Technique of radical retropubic prostatectomy with preservation of sexual function: An anatomic approach. In DG Skinner and G Lieskovsky (eds),* Diagnosis and Management of Genitourinary Cancer. *Philadelphia: Saunders, 1988, with permission.)*

Figure 11-13. *The reflection of the endopelvic fascia on the lateral aspect of the prostate is divided to obtain exposure to the lateral prostatic pedicles. These can be divided between ligaclips or 00 chromic catgut ligatures. (From Walsh, PC, Technique of radical retropubic prostatectomy with preservation of sexual function: An anatomic approach. In DG Skinner and G Lieskovsky (eds),* Diagnosis and Management of Genitourinary Cancer. *Philadelphia: Saunders, 1988, with permission.)*

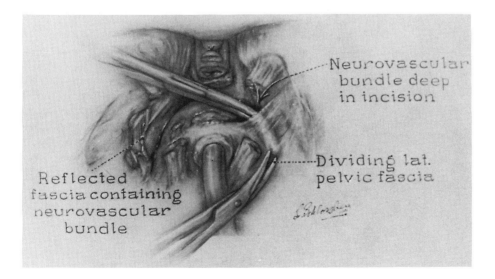

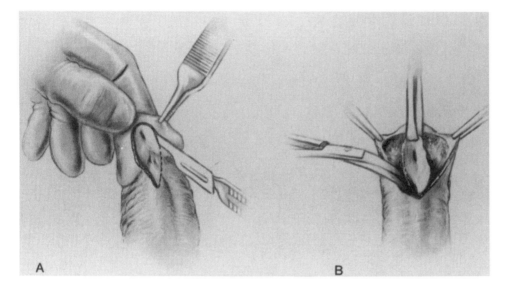

Figure 11-14. *When the urethra is to be incorporated into the surgical specimen, dissection should proceed along the course of the urethra distally using both blunt and sharp dissection with retraction on the urethra so as to evert the corporal bodies and the penis in approaching the fossa navicularis. This is generally excised by sharp dissection to the external meatus. (From Ahlerling, TE, and Lieskovsky, G, Surgical treatment of urethral cancer in the male patient. In DG Skinner and G Lieskovsky (eds), Diagnosis and Management of Genitourinary Cancer. Philadelphia: Saunders, 1988, with permission.)*

Figure 11-15. *The middle and distal urethra can be dissected perineally. A midline or inverted-U-shaped incision can be made and the bulbar urethra identified by palpation of the indwelling catheter. This is circumscribed, and the distal and proximal extents of the urethra are freed by blunt and sharp dissection. Urethral branches of the pudendal arteries are divided between small ligaclips. (From Ahlerling TE, and Lieskovsky, G, Surgical treatment of urethral cancer in the male patient. In DG Skinner and G Lieskovsky (eds), Diagnosis and Management of Genitourinary Cancer. Philadelphia: Saunders, 1988, with permission.)*

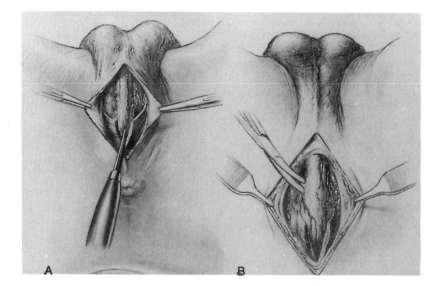
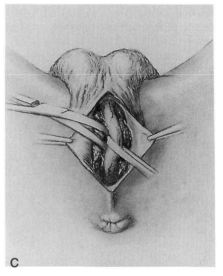

It is important in each of these dissections to ligate the pudendal arterial branches to the urethra to prevent troublesome bleeding.

In females, the uterus, cervix, and anterior vaginal wall are incorporated into the surgical specimen. The broad ligament on each side is divided along the course of the external iliac artery, the round ligament is divided between 2-0 chromic catgut ligatures, and the uterus and bladder are dissected together as described above, but with separate ligation of the uterine arteries on either side (Fig. 11-16). During this dissection, the uterus should be retracted anteriorly and the posterior wall of the vagina incised. The location of this incision can be identified by placement of a spongestick into the vaginal vault (Fig. 11-17). The incision should then be extended laterally toward the perineum such that the urethra in the anterior vaginal wall can be incorporated in the specimen. Although some have described incorporation of the posterior vaginal wall in the dissection, this generally is not necessary when one considers the pathway of disease extension from the bladder.

After the specimen has been removed, the vagina can be reconstructed by approximating the cephalad edge of the cut posterior wall to the anterior margin. This obliterates the perineal defect created by removal of the anterior vaginal wall and underlying urethra and permits maintenance of a vaginal vault for sexual function.

Radical Cystectomy After Radiation Therapy/Chemotherapy

When invasive bladder cancer has been treated with "definitive" radiation and/or chemotherapy rather than cystectomy, persistence or recurrence of disease, as documented by extensive transurethral resection, may prompt reconsideration of cystectomy to achieve possible cure or, when necessary, palliation. The procedure in this setting is similar to that described above. However, both chemotherapy and radiation therapy may have produced fibrotic changes that prevent or obscure identification of anatomic landmarks and normal fascial planes that would ordinarily facilitate dissection. In these situations, dissection should commence over the external iliac arteries as previously described and proceed by sweeping fibroadipose tissue and lymph nodes medially. The lateral bladder pedicles should then be divided with ligation of the vesical arteries and veins as they are encountered and division of the ureters as described above. If the fibrous reaction is too dense to permit this, the peritoneal reflection overlying the retrovesical space can be incised and the posterolateral pedicles clamped and suture ligated without identifying each individual vessel, proceeding in a caudad direction toward the perineum.

Further dissection along anatomic landmarks pro-

Figure 11-16. *A. Radical cystectomy in the female incorporates excision of the uterus, the adnexae, the cervix, and the anterior wall of the vagina. B. Access to the bladder pedicles involves division of the round ligaments between 00 chromic catgut ligatures and division of the broad ligament attachments as shown. (From Fair, WR, and Atlas, I, Radical cystectomy. In MJ Droller (ed),* Surgical Management of Urologic Disease: An Anatomic Approach. *St Louis: Mosby–Year Book, 1992, with permission.)*

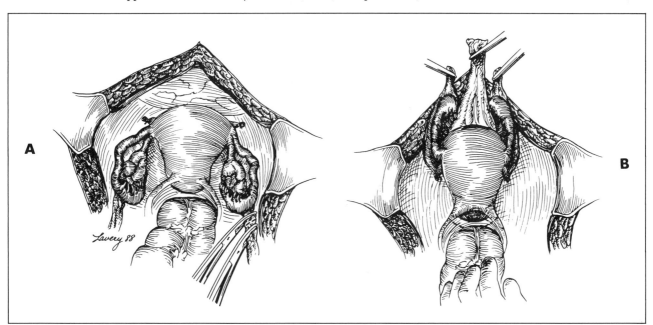

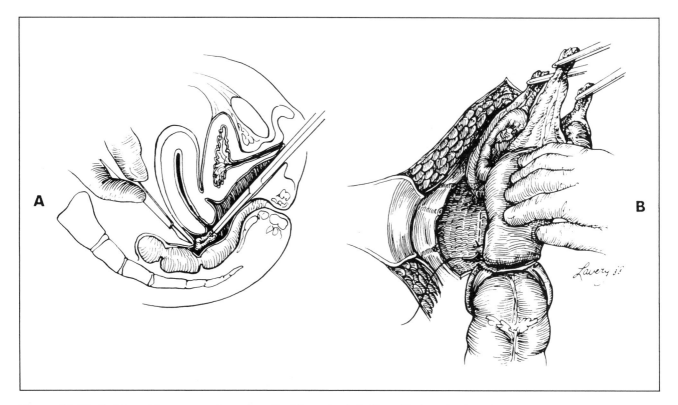

Figure 11-17. *Excision of the uterus and anterior wall of the vagina is facilitated by introduction of a sponge stick in the vaginal vault posterior to the cervix and incision of the vaginal wall over the instrument. Anterior exenteration is completed by incision of the lateral vaginal walls with circumscription around the urethral meatus. (From Fair, WR, and Atlas, I, Radical cystectomy. In MJ Droller (ed),* Surgical Management of Urologic Disease: An Anatomic Approach. *St Louis: Mosby–Year Book, 1992, with permission.)*

ceeds as visualization and palpation permit. When this is not possible, blunt and sharp dissection should be used in an attempt to outline the bladder and incorporate as much surrounding tissue as possible, always sweeping medially toward the bladder and then toward the perineum. It is often not possible in these instances to preserve the neurovascular bundles that permit retention of potency. Usually, the urethra is incorporated into the dissection, and forms of urinary diversion that do not include the urethra are chosen.

Complications

The major risks of transurethral resection, whether in an initial or reoperative setting, are hemorrhage and bladder perforation. Each of these can be avoided by adhering to the precautions and principles of resection described above.

The major risks involved in reoperative cystectomy include hemorrhage and rectal injury. The first can be avoided by careful dissection and knowledge of the location of vessels during the course of dissection. The second can be avoided by careful dissection of the plane between the bladder and the rectum. Generally, these tissues should separate easily. If they do not, the dissection should not be forced, since an incorrect plane may have been entered (either between the seminal vesicles and the bladder or into the serosa of the rectum). In these circumstances, the correct plane should be sought by redirecting the path of dissection.

If rectal injury is identified, the tear often can be closed in multiple layers and the anal sphincter then mechanically dilated to prevent retention of fecal material and to permit healing to occur. Intravenous and then oral hyperalimentation should be begun, and oral intake of other than fully absorbable foodstuff should not be permitted for 3 to 4 weeks and then only following testing of the repair by a barium study. In the setting of prior radiation therapy, the injury should be repaired, but a diverting colostomy also should be performed to permit sufficient time for healing. The colostomy can then be closed at a later time when the injury has been demonstrated to have healed fully.

Attempts to preserve potency by preservation of the neurovascular bundles should not compromise the extent of surgery. Those considerations which may prompt efforts in this regard in the performance of radical prostatectomy for prostate cancer may be similarly relevant in the case of bladder cancer. On the other hand, loss of potency should not be regarded as a complication of cystectomy.

Conclusions

Reoperation for bladder cancer encompasses a number of factors that reflect the various forms of bladder cancer that are seen and the various settings in which they appear. Thorough consideration of these factors and careful dissection or resection are critical if reoperation is to be performed in a safe and effective manner and if it is to achieve the desired result.

Bibliography

Abel, PD, Hall, RR, and Williams, G. Should T$_1$ transitional cell cancer of the bladder still be classified as superficial? Br J Urol 62:235, 1988.

Fair, WR, and Atlas, I. Radical cystectomy. In MJ Droller (ed), Surgical Management of Urologic Disease: An Anatomic Approach. St Louis: Mosby–Year Book, 1992, p 591.

Fitzpatrick, JM. The natural history of superficial bladder carcinoma. Semin Urol 11:127, 1993.

Heney, NM, et al. Superficial bladder cancer: Progression and recurrence. J Urol 130:1083, 1983.

Herr, HW. Progression of stage T$_1$ bladder tumor after intravesical bacillus Calmette-Gúerin. J Urol 145:40, 1991.

Herr, HW, and Laudone, VP. Intravesical therapy for superficial bladder cancer. AUA Update 8:90, 1989.

Loughlin, KR, and Richie, JP. Approaches in urinary tract replacement. In MJ Droller (ed), Surgical Management of Urologic Disease: An Anatomic Approach. St Louis: Mosby–Year Book, 1992, p 1145.

Reiner, WG, and Walsh, PC. An anatomical approach to the surgical management of the dorsal vein and Santorini's plexus during radical retropubic prostatectomy. J Urol 121:198, 1979.

Skinner, DG. Technique of radical cystectomy. Urol Clin North Am 8:353, 1981.

Walsh, PC. Technique of radical retropubic prostatectomy with preservation of sexual function: An anatomic approach. In DG Skinner and G Lieskovsky (eds), Diagnosis and Management of Genitourinary Cancer. Philadelphia: Saunders, 1988, p 753.

Walsh, PC, and Schlegel, PN. Radical pelvic surgery with preservation of sexual function. Ann Surg 208:391, 1988.

Whitmore, WF. Total cystectomy. In EH Cooper and RE Williams (eds), The Biology and Clinical Management of Bladder Cancer. Oxford: Blackwell Scientific Publishers, 1975.

Exstrophy of the Bladder

LOWELL R. KING

The modern techniques for managing exstrophy involve planned reoperations in boys. However, almost all affected babies seem to need more than one procedure. The reason is that, in a sense, the bladder exstrophy and epispadias, with missing sphincters, is only the most obvious part of the anomaly. The pelvic bones are widely separated, so the acetabula are turned out, and the children develop a waddling gait. The musculature of the lower abdominal wall and perineum lack normal central attachments, so inguinal hernia, rectal prolapse, and uterine prolapse are commonly associated. In males, epispadias repair results in a stubby penis that is tethered to the abdominal wall on erection unless extreme care has been taken to move lots of additional skin to the dorsum of the penis before the urethra is constructed. Formation of a "sphincter mechanism" by tubularizing the bladder base remains an uncertain way to provide continence. Even when a good result is achieved, the bladder may remain small, and augmentation may be required. Most children with exstrophy reflux after simple bladder closure. Abdominal skin flaps are required to rotate hair-bearing skin and soft tissue into the midline to restore the normal contour of the body wall and the escutcheon and to push the penis downward. No wonder the management of exstrophy has been termed the "ultimate challenge" in pediatric urology.

On the other hand, most children with exstrophy are otherwise normal, with normal kidneys and renal function. The most important aim in management is to keep the kidneys normal. If the bladder reconstruction goes awry, there is no shame in changing course and doing a urinary diversion to protect renal function. Sev-eral forms of continent diversion are reasonable alternatives to reoperations on the bladder outlet that have a diminishing chance of success. Diversion can be an advantage in boys in that all energies can be focused on reconstruction of the genitalia without concern about urethral continence.

Early Bladder Closure

Histologic studies of bladder exstrophy (Culp) revealed that the muscle is relatively sparse with the fibers separated by relatively acellular amorphous tissue and sometimes collagen. These observations were used to argue that the exstrophic bladder is inherently abnormal, a rationale for primary urinary diversion without an attempt at functional closure. However, Jeffs and others have shown that continence often can be achieved, even when the exstrophic bladder is initially very small. Almost all now agree that bladder closure should be carried out within a few days of birth before the bladder becomes inflamed.

Posterior pelvic osteotomies were introduced in 1958 as an adjunct to bladder closure. The osteotomies allow the bladder neck to be folded more posteriorly into the pelvis and relieve tension on the anterior abdominal wall closure. Babies still need to be placed in Bryant's traction or a spica cast postoperatively to prevent disruption. It was hoped initially that the displacement of the bladder neck would provide eventual continence by restoring a more "normal" urethrovesical angle, but this maneuver alone is rarely adequate.

Some advocate closure at a day or two after birth without osteotomies, relying on the effect of maternal relaxin to keep the joints pliable enough to permit healing of the anterior wall defect. I feel that posterior ileal osteotomies are safe and easy to perform and add a safety factor. Alternately, anterior osteotomies are safe in the hands of an experienced pediatric orthopedist. Dehiscence of the exstrophy closure is a serious complication, since inflammation and scar in the repair of the bladder neck reduce the chance of eventual continence after secondary reconstruction.

Posterior Ileal Osteotomies

The baby or child is placed prone. The sacroiliac joints and the sciatic notch are palpated. An incision is made about 1 cm lateral to the sacroiliac joint from the upper border of the ileum to the notch. Muscle fibers are divided or stripped laterally to expose the ileal bone. The upper border is cartilaginous and can be cut with a knife. The outer table of bone is then incised with a sharp osteotome and mallet. The inner table is divided in the same fashion, keeping a blunt osteotome inserted into the sciatic notch pressed against the bone. This protects the gluteal artery. The same procedure is then repeated on the other side. After the wounds are closed, the patient is turned supine for closure of the exstrophy.

In girls, the epispadias may be repaired at the time of exstrophy closure. In boys, it is virtually always mandatory to obtain more penile length prior to the epispadias repair. If the urethra is formed at the time of bladder closure, the penis will not be dependent when flaccid and will be tethered to the abdominal wall on erection.

Techniques of Exstrophy Closure

In general, no attempt is made to fabricate a continence mechanism at this stage. The bladder is circumscribed. The umbilicus may be excised or may be detached from skin and bladder and moved upward to the midabdominal wall (Fig. 12-1). Retaining the umbilicus in this way seems to carry little risk of wound infection, and most children seem to want an umbilicus rather badly. In girls, the incision is now carried down to the bladder base, outlining a bladder neck and urethra that are no. 12 to 16 French in caliber. The urethra should be detached completely from the pubic rami before it is tubularized. These incisions should be against the periosteum, retaining all soft tissues alongside the bladder neck and urethra for a second layer to buttress the closure. Also, when the bladder neck is detached com-

Figure 12-1. *A. The bladder is circumscribed. The umbilicus is excised or explanted superiorally on its pedicle. The periexstrophy skin flaps are based distally. B. The proximal corpora cavernosa are exposed and partially detached from the pubic rami. The corporal bodies are approximated with 3-0 chromic catgut. C. The paraexstrophy skin flaps are rotated onto the penile shaft and sewn to the divided edges of the urethral plate. D. The bladder is closed with two layers of heavy (2-0) chromic catgut. A Malecot catheter is employed, and ureteral stents are placed to keep the penis as dry as possible. These exit through the bladder neck. A Tegaderm dressing is placed on the penis.*

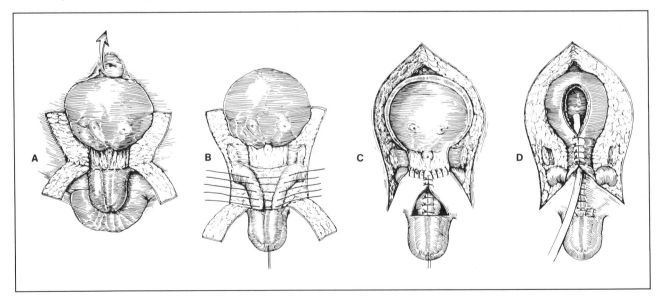

pletely, it can drop into the pelvis, away from the bone. Bladder closure is completed around a small Malecot or urethral catheter using two layers of absorbable sutures whenever possible. Ureteral stents are also placed and sewn to the bladder with 5-0 chromic catgut in an attempt to keep the wound as dry as possible. These stents exit by means of the urethra.

The pelvic bones are then approximated, at least partially, with heavy no. 1 nonabsorbable sutures placed through periosteum and bone. Approximation of the pubic bones relieves tension and makes the wound closure easier. Finger drains that can be put on gentle suction are placed in the pelvis alongside the bladder and exit through lateral stab wounds. The rectus muscles are approximated loosely with absorbable sutures, but the overlying fascia is closed with a 1-0 nonabsorbable monofilament suture. I like to invert the knots to minimize later erosion. After wound closure is complete, the baby is placed in a relatively tight spica cast or in traction.

Penile Lengthening

In males, "paraexstrophy" skin flaps are rotated onto the dorsum of the penis at the time of the exstrophy closure (Duckett). The thin skin just lateral to the exstrophic bladder and above the bladder neck is almost non-hair-bearing and is suitable to be incorporated eventually into the neourethra. Flaps about 1 cm in width and 1.5 to 2 cm in length are outlined, based on the most proximal portion of the urethra (see Fig. 12-1). After the flaps are raised and defatted, the urethral plate is divided about 1/2 cm distal to the verumontanum. The corpora cavernosa are exposed. The urethral plate is then dissected distally from the underlying corpora nearly to the coronal sulcus. The flaps are then rotated to cover the exposed corpora. They are sutured to adjacent skin edges, to each other, and to the edges of the urethral plate with 5-0 chromic sutures. The exstrophy closure is then completed as described above.

This is also a good time to position the eventual meatus more ventrally, at the tip of the penis. The glans is divided in the midline distal to the end of the urethral groove. Then 5-0 chromic sutures are used to advance the urethral plate more distally. This will result in a meatus that is centered on the glans after the epispadias is repaired.

The most feared complication after bladder closure is dehiscence, which occurs occasionally in spite of all the precautions described above. When this happens, the surgeon's instinct is to reclose the exstrophy. However, this usually should not be attempted until healing

has occurred, i.e., until 3 to 6 months have elapsed. Immediate reclosure generally results in wound infection and another dehiscence. Early secondary closure is complicated by a lack of tissue elasticity and the inability to approximate the tissues with precision. The exstrophic bladder is covered by plastic wrap or petrolatum gauze until closure can be achieved.

Reclosure of the Bladder

After healing is complete, the bladder is reclosed using essentially the same technique. Osteotomies may be repeated, or facial flaps may be raised to cover the lower midline defect in the abdominal wall. I usually prefer both maneuvers.

The skin and subcutaneous tissue above the reclosed exstrophy are incised in the midline to expose the rectus fascia above and lateral to the defect in the abdominal wall left by closing the bladder. Large fascial flaps are raised, using the medial edge of the rectus as the hinge. The fascial flaps should be slightly larger than the defect they are to cover. One flap is first turned and sutured in place with nonabsorbable sutures. The contralateral fascial flap buttresses this closure. If osteotomies also have been performed, a spica cast or Bryant's traction is employed again postoperatively.

Once the bladder has been closed and has healed, surveillance is maintained until 1½ to 2 years of age. Additional surgery to lengthen the penis by transposing more skin onto the dorsum can be performed during this interval if indicated. Sonography is used to be sure the bladder empties and that there is no emergent hydronephrosis. Cystography is performed to detect reflux and to estimate bladder capacity. Some bladder growth can be anticipated, even when there is little or no urethral resistance. The bladder needs to have about a 75 cc or greater capacity for the Young-Dees incontinence operation that follows. This is usually combined with ureteral reimplantation to correct reflux and to move the ureters above the trigone, which permits an increase in the length of the trigonal tube formed to serve as the sphincter (Leadbetter).

Incontinence Procedure

All agree that precision is required in performing a Young-Dees-Leadbetter type of incontinence procedure. The problem is that even when it is done in a standardized fashion, the results continue to be inconsistent. For this reason, many now recommend intraoperative manometrics as a guide in deciding how tight to make the bladder neck and the tubularized trigone.

The bladder is opened in the midline. The ureteral orifices are identified. The ureters are then mobilized extravesically and transected where they enter the bladder. The distal stumps are tied with chromic catgut.

Attention is then turned to the trigone. I outline a mucosal strip 1 cm wide and 3.5 cm long running from the bladder neck proximally to the rostral margin of the trigone (Fig. 12-2). The bladder mucosa on either side of this strip is excised, denuding the underlying lateral detrusor muscle. The strip of mucosa is then tubularized over a no. 8 French catheter using a running, locked, 3-0 or 4-0 chromic suture. Next, the denuded bladder muscle on either side is mobilized to buttress the closure of the neourethra. Three 0 sutures are preferred.

Using the cautery, I then detach one lateral triangle of denuded detrusor from the still open bladder. This muscle flap is drawn over the neourethra as a second layer to buttress the closure. The opposite muscle flap is detached from the distal two-thirds of the tube and drawn across the new bladder neck as a separate buttress placed superiorly over the new bladder neck (Monfort, Fig. 12-2). The effect of these maneuvers is to make a relatively narrow uniform tube from healthy trigonal muscle hopefully to serve as a sphincter. The closure is buttressed by whatever adjacent tissue is available. Since the trigonal tissue employed is not really sphincter muscle, it seems likely that continence depends on the muscle tone exerted along the length of the tube. The neo-

urethra is therefore suspended to the inside of the abdominal wall as the wound is closed using a nonabsorbable suture on either side above and below the new bladder neck.

The ureters are then reimplanted transversely into the back wall of the bladder above the trigone, taking care to form an adequate submucosal tunnel to prevent reflux. The ureteral reimplants are stented. After the bladder is closed around a suprapubic tube, manometrics—a leak-point profile—can be obtained. This test has not yet been well standardized. If fluid run into the suprapubic tube exits freely from the urethra, resistance is obviously inadequate. The upper portion of the repair must be taken down and tightened. I have found a leak point of 60 mmHg to result in subsequent hydronephrosis on occasion, so I prefer a reading in the 35- to 55-mm Hg range. Considerable manometric testing is now being done in exstrophy patients, and more precise guidelines are likely to be available in the near future. Jeffs has recently found much higher pressures to be safe and not to result in hydronephrosis, while increasing the chance of continence.

Epispadias Repair

In boys, the epispadias repair is performed in conjunction with the continence procedure described above. In concept, the epispadias repair is simple—a 12- to 14-mm strip of skin on the dorsal surface of the penis is simply

Figure 12-2. *The incontinence procedure. (Left) The ureters are reimplanted into the back wall of the bladder above the trigone. A strip of bladder mucosa 1 cm wide is tubularized around a no. 8 French catheter using a running locked 3-0 chromic suture. The bladder base lateral to this tube is deepithelialized. (Center) One flap of denuded bladder is drawn over the tube and sutured to the bladder muscle behind with interrupted sutures. (Right) The other bladder flap is rotated rostrally and is used to buttress the new bladder neck. The bladder is then closed in two layers around a Malecot catheter.*

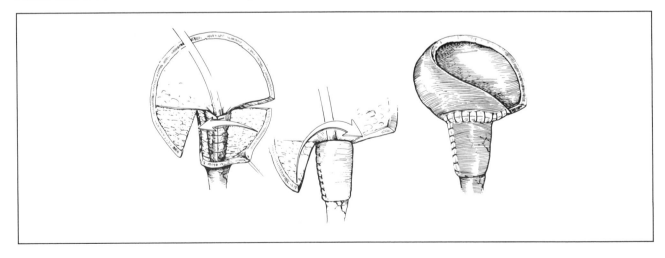

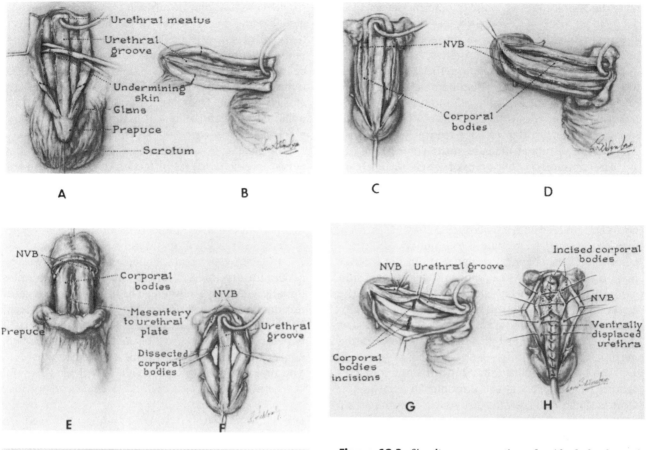

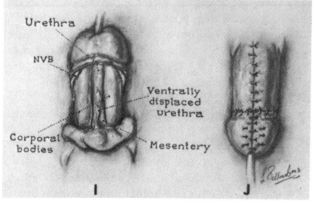

Figure 12-3. *Simultaneous correction of residual chordee and urethroplasty in an older patient. A. A strip of dorsal skin will serve as the neourethra. B. Adjacent penile skin is mobilized. C, D. The lateral neurovascular bundles are identified and mobilized. E. The corpora cavernosa are separated after the penis has been degloved. F. The dissection in continued dorsally. G. Incision into the corporal bodies, which will be reapproximated above the neourethra. H. The neourethra is formed to the tip of the glands, and the corpora cavernosa are approximated above. I. Ventral view. The urethra now lies more normally, in the groove between the corpora cavernosa. J. Completed repair. (Reprinted with permission: Gearhart, JP and Jeffs, RD, Exstrophy of the bladder, epispadias, and other bladder anomalies. In PC Walsh, et al (eds),* Campbell's Urology, *6th ed. Philadelphia: Saunders, 1992.)*

tubularized using running, locking, 4-0 sutures. In practice, care must be taken to maintain penile length and to form the penis into a cylinder that is cosmetically pleasing. After the skin strip that is to become the neourethra is outlined, the penis is degloved from an incision around the corona. Two or three 3-0 absorbable sutures are placed ventrally to approximate the denuded corporal bodies. These sutures correct the dorsal glandular tilt. Next, the incisions along the sides of the neourethra are deepened to the corpora. The neourethra is tubularized,

and 3-0 long-lasting absorbable sutures are again used to roll the corpora together over the neourethra dorsally. These give the penis the desired cylindrical shape and correct the outward rotation of the corpora, at least distally. The urethra also may be transposed ventrally, as depicted in Figure 12-3.

Skin coverage is obtained by unrolling the ventral hood and transposing it dorsally to the top of the penis to cover the distal penile shaft. Proximal skin coverage of the epispadias repair is more difficult to achieve. Skin is always in short supply. It may be possible to approximate the lateral edges of penile skin, in two layers, over the bladder neck area and proximal neourethra, but closure in this manner may again tend to tether the penis and angulate it upward. Alternatively, a skin flap or parts of flaps can be rotated from the abdominal wall to cover the base of the penis and proximal shaft. This may seem like an excessive addition to an already lengthy procedure, but the cosmetic result is superior. Also, use of such a flap or flaps reduces the risk of a troublesome fistula at the base of the penis.

The common complications of epispadias repair are a proximal fistula, a fistula at the corona, and a meatus that is on the dorsal aspect of the glans. In 6 months, after healing is complete, the fistula is closed in two layers and covered with a generous skin flap. The meatus may be centered by placing a tourniquet around the penis and incising the glans deeply from the inferior margin of the meatus to a point in the midline 3 mm beneath the center of the glans. The back wall of the neourethra is advanced to this point. The edges of the superior margin of the meatus are then excised, and the glans is approximated in two layers to advance the meatus.

The main complications of the incontinence procedure are obstruction and continued incontinence. Obstruction may be due to a stricture in the tubularized trigonal tube or penile urethra or even to complete obliteration of the trigonal tube. A retrograde urethrogram may clarify the situation. A cystoscopy is warranted, since discrete strictures may be managed successfully by "cold knife" or laser incision of a discrete stricture. Occasionally, a local skin flap also can be used to repair a discrete stricture, although this must be deferred until healing is complete.

Recurrent obstruction or obliteration of the trigonal tube is usually best managed by continent urinary diversion. Any of several standard techniques can be employed. Since children with exstrophy generally have normal anal sphincters and bowel control, I tend to like ileocecal ureterosigmoidostomy, described below, as a permanent means of continent diversion.

Incontinence on Obstruction after an Incontinence Repair

After a Young-Dees type of bladder tubularization, continued incontinence of some degree is the rule for several months. This may be due to overflow; a bladder sonogram just after the suprapubic tube has been removed may suggest this cause. An attempt may be made to institute intermittent catheterization, but con-

structed urethras may be difficult to catheterize. Incomplete bladder emptying can be tolerated and may even be a good prognostic sign if it does not result in infection or hydronephrosis. Should these occur, a Cystocath can be inserted and maintained for 2 to 4 additional weeks. If inability to empty persists, the child should be evaluated for stricture. If the trigonal tube is simply too tight, it should be overdilated at this time, usually to about no. 14 to 16 French.

In general, leaking from an empty bladder may persist for several weeks or months before healing and tightening of the trigonal tube begins to provide needed urethral resistance. These operations tend to take a lot of time to "come right." Parents need a lot of support in this period, but if the child is leaking from an empty bladder, instrumentation should be deferred.

In Jeffs' view, continence occurs gradually. The maximum dry interval, often only 10 to 15 minutes initially, gradually lengthens. The dry period is longer at rest than when the child is active. If this trend is seen, continued observation is best. The dry interval will hopefully increase to 1 to 2 hours within a year or two. Enuresis usually continues until a dry interval of 2 to 3 hours during the day is achieved. This may take several years. In short, successful incontinence surgery may take a long time before it is seen as successful by the family. A program of timed voiding may help in the interim.

When leaking from an empty bladder—total incontinence—persists for more than 6 months after trigonal tubularization, additional surgery usually will be required. Possibly about one-third of such boys may gain control at puberty as the prostate grows, increasing urethral resistance, but children generally should not be expected to tolerate incontinence throughout childhood. The risk of severe and persistent psychological damage is simply too high.

Patients are reevaluated about 6 months after surgery when total incontinence persists. Causes include a bladder that has remained very small, a noncompliant bladder, and of course, inadequate urethral resistance. A leak-point pressure is estimated at the time the cystometric study is performed.

A very small or noncompliant bladder is usually best treated by cystoplasty. Since voiding occurs with straining after this procedure, it is important to be sure that the parents can perform intermittent catheterization prior to the cystoplasty in case it should be needed postoperatively. Some children, especially those with sensate urethras, are terrorized by the catheter and need a good bit of counseling before intermittent catheterization can be instituted successfully (Gil).

If urethral resistance is nil, an additional incontinence procedure should be performed at the time of the cystoplasty. I narrow the tubularized trigone and new bladder-urethral junction, making the urethra tight around a no. 8 French catheter. In girls, I suspend the bladder neck with a facial sling out from the edge of the rectus fascia. Some form of urethral suspension is again important to maintain the length and configuration of the trigonal tube.

When the bladder is growing and is compliant, additional urethral resistance needs to be provided. This is done by tightening the trigonal tube, as described above, or by implanting an artificial sphincter or transplanting a muscle around the bladder neck. The neourethra should not be opened at the time an artificial sphincter is implanted because erosion of constructed urethras by the sphincter cuff is a serious problem and a relatively common complication.

Technique of Artificial Sphincter Implantation

The neourethra is mobilized circumferentially. If it is opened, the urethra is simply narrowed and the sphincter implantation is deferred. When the urethra is mobilized successfully, it is wrapped in omentum. The cuff of the artificial sphincter is placed over the omentum, reducing the risk of urethral erosion. Activation of the sphincter is deferred for several weeks postoperatively.

Formation of a Sphincter

Another approach to persistent incontinence is to transplant a somatic muscle, usually from the thigh or the palmaris longus, to serve as a sphincter. In the Gierup operation, a long muscle is first denervated to convert it to a more anaerobic type of metabolism. It is then transplanted around the bladder neck as a free graft—without reinnervation or revascularization. It may then regenerate with the characteristics of a sphincter. Good results have been reported.

A newer approach is to recreate the normal sphincter with a transplanted somatic muscle (King and Serafin). A segment of the sural nerve is anastomosed to the motor branch of the pudendal nerve that runs to the external urinary sphincter. The nerve fibers are allowed to grow into the graft, which takes 6 to 12 months. A long muscle is then harvested, wrapped around the bladder neck and proximal urethra, and revascularized.

The nerve to this muscle is then attached to the sural nerve graft. After healing and time for nerve growth, the new sphincter becomes normally innervated. This is a very promising approach, but none of my patients is really evaluable as yet.

Even with all these possibilities, some children remain incontinent. After two or a maximum of three operations on the bladder outlet, some form of continent diversion should be elected. Since patients with exstrophy generally have normal bowel control and a normal anal sphincter, I usually prefer ileocecal ureterosigmoidostomy. This is a form of intact ureterosigmoidostomy designed to avoid the late risk of colon carcinoma that occurs near the site that the ureters are implanted with the intact colon.

Technique of Ileocecal Ureterosigmoidostomy

The bowel is cleansed and sterilized prior to surgery. The ileocecal segment is taken from continuity with the bowel, detaching about 10 to 12 cm of cecum and about 14 cm of terminal ileum. The antireflux mechanism is a stabilized ileal intussusception through the ileocecal valve (Fig. 12-4). To facilitate this, the mesentery is detached from 6 cm of the distal-most ileum. An intussusception about 5 cm in length is then formed. The full thickness of outer posterior layer of the intussusception is then opened with the cautery. Mucosa is denuded from a facing disk of cecal wall. The muscular edges of the incision in the intussusception are then sewn to the exposed cecal muscle with 2-0 chromic sutures, keeping the intussusception slightly on the stretch. A row of 3-0 silk sutures between the cecum and the base of the intussusception completes the antireflux nipple.

A long ellipse is then removed from the medial aspect of the lower sigmoid. The cecum is rotated for anastomosis to the sigmoid using two layers of 2-0 or 3-0 gut. Before the bowel is closed, two stents are threaded through the sigmoid lumen and through the nipple valve. These will stent the ureters after their anastomosis to the ileal tail proximal to the intussusception. I usually spatulate and join the ureters and anastomose them end-to-end to the ileal stump, which is shortened or tailored to prevent redundancy or kinks.

In this way, the transitional epithelium of the ureters is removed from the bacteria in the fecal stream, at least theoretically obviating the increased risk of colonic malignancy seen after conventional ureterosigmoidostomy.

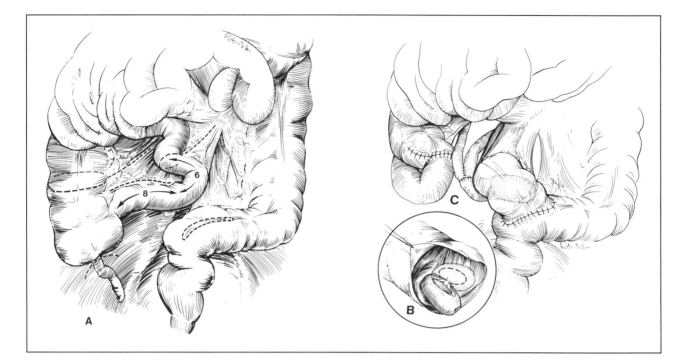

Figure 12-4. *Ileocecal ureterosigmoidostomy. This is a method of performing intact ureterosigmoidostomy that probably does not carry the increased risk of bowel malignancy in later life. A. The ileocecal segment is employed, as in ileocecal cystoplasty. About 14 cm of terminal ileum and 10 cm of cecum are removed from the intestinal tract. B. An intussusception 5 cm long forms the antireflux mechanism. The muscle of the outer wall of the intussusception is sewn to adjacent cecal muscle from which the mucosa has been removed. C. The cecum is anastomosed to the sigmoid in two layers. The ureters are then attached to the ileal "tail" proximal to the intussusception.*

Late Complications of Bladder Exstrophy

At adolescence, several other problems may become apparent. The penis may be involved in torsion or twisted. One corpora cavernosa may be longer or wider than the other, resulting in an asymmetrical erection. This problem needs to be individualized. If angulation of the penis interferes with vaginal penetration, treatment is obviously mandatory. The penis is degloved, and an artificial erection is performed. Angulation is corrected by removing one or two wedges of corpora cavernosa. A slight overcorrection is desirable at the time of surgery to completely correct the bend. Torsion or twisting of the corpora is treated by separating the corpora and realigning them, using heavy 2-0 or 3-0 absorbable sutures. Additional skin flaps may be needed to resurface the penis adequately on the short side to prevent reangulation.

The common serious late complication is dorsal tethering of the penis due to a short urethra. The urethra must then be divided and dissected free of the corpora until the penis becomes dependent. The resulting defect

in the urethra is bridged with a free graft, since there is not usually enough penile skin for a vascularized island flap. When there is no penile skin for the urethral graft, bladder mucosa, a buccal graft, or thin skin harvested from the neck below the beard line are the best alternatives.

A stent is again employed, and supravesical urinary diversion is maintained for 10 to 12 days. Generous rotational skin flaps are employed to help in covering the graft without tension.

Finally, the escutcheon is usually separated in the midline by non-hair-bearing skin. This does not become apparent until the hair starts to grow at puberty. The non-hair-bearing midline skin is detached in an inverted V and slides inferiorly to the junction of the penis with the abdominal wall. Rotation flaps of lateral hair-bearing skin, with fat attached, are interdigitalized across the midline. The fat is left attached to avoid a depression in the abdominal wall at the exstrophy site. Small suction drains are left under the skin flaps for a few days, and a compression dressing is employed postoperatively.

Summary

There are no shortcuts in the management of exstrophy. Preservation of normal renal function should be the overriding concern. Almost all patients can now be made continent by some maneuver, but multiple operations are usually required. In males, great care should be taken to obtain adequate penile length before the urethroplasty is performed.

The payoff is a happy, dry, well-adjusted patient who can function well sexually in the gender assigned. Currently, such results are still noteworthy but will hopefully become routine. The disease is stressful to family, patient, and surgeon alike, but the rewards are great.

Bibliography

Crissey, MM, Steel, GD, Gittes, RR. Rat model for carcinogenesis in ureterosigmoidostomy. Science 207:1079, 1980.

Culp, DA. The histology of the exstrophied bladder. J Urol 91:538, 1964.

Diamond, DA, and Ransley, PG. Bladder neck reconstruction with omentum, silicone and augmentation cystoplasty. J Urol 136:252, 1986.

Duckett, JW. Use of paraexstrophy skin pedicle grafts for correction of exstrophy and epispadias repair. Birth Defects 13:175, 1977.

Gearhart, JP, and Jeffs, RD. Management of failed exstrophy closure. J Urol 146:610, 1991.

Gearhart, JP, and Jeffs, RD. Augmentation cystoplasty in failed exstrophy reconstruction. J Urol 139:790, 1988.

Husmann, DA, McLori, GA, and Churchill, BM. Closure of the exstrophic bladder: An evaluation of the factors leading to its success and its importance in urinary continence. J Urol 142:522, 1989.

Jeffs, RD, Guice, SL, and Oesch, I. The factors in successful exstrophy closure. J Urol 127:974, 1982.

Kass, EJ. Dorsal corporeal plication: An alternative technique for the management of severe chordee. J Urol 150:635, 1993.

Kelley, JH, and Eraklis, AJ. The procedure for lengthening the phallus in boys with exstrophy of the bladder. J Pediatr Surg 6:645, 1971.

Koff, SA. A technique for bladder neck reconstruction in exstrophy: The cinch. J Urol 144:546, 1990.

Koff, SA, and Eakins, M. The treatment of penile chordee using corporeal rotation. J Urol 131:931, 1984.

Mesrobian, HGJ, Kelalis, PP, and Kramer, SA. Long-term followup of cosmetic appearance and genital function in boys with exstrophy: Review of 53 patients. J Urol 136:256, 1986.

Montfort, G, et al. Transverse island flap and double flap procedure in the treatment of congenital epispadias in 32 patients. J Urol 138:1069, 1987.

Nill, TG, Peller, PA, and Kropp, KA. Management of urinary incontinence by bladder tube urethral lengthening and submucosal reimplantation. J Urol 144:559, 1990.

Perlmutter, AD, Weinstein, MD, and Reitelman, C. Vesical neck reconstruction in patients with epispadias-exstrophy complex. J Urol 146:613, 1991.

Schultz, WG. Plastic repair of exstrophy of the bladder combined with bilateral osteotomy of the ilia. J Urol 92:659, 1964.

Skef, Z, et al. Use of inferior rectus myocutaneous flap for coverage of bladder exstrophy defect. J Pediatr Surg 17:718, 1982.

Winslow, BH, et al. Epispadias and exstrophy of the bladder. In JC Mustarde and IT Jackson (eds), Plastic Surgery in Infancy and Childhood, 3rd ed. New York: Churchill Livingstone, 1988, pp 511–527.

Woodhouse, CRJ. Reconstruction of the epispadias penis in adolescence. Progr Pediatr Surg 23:165, 1989.

Woodhouse, CRJ, and Kellett, MJ. Anatomy of the penis and its deformities in exstrophy and epispadias. J Urol 132:1122, 1984.

Vesicovaginal Fistulas

ELROY D. KURSH

Reoperation for vesicovaginal fistulas is one of the most perplexing urologic problems to manage. The patient and surgeon usually experience a tremendous sense of frustration. Often the patient enters the hospital to undergo a straightforward hysterectomy. When a vesicovaginal fistula (VVF) develops, she not only has to contend with the urinary incontinence, but she also faces a second surgical procedure. It is easy to envision why the anger and frustration mount if the incontinence and fistula persist after an attempted surgical repair.

Recurrence of a VVF after use of a particular technique of repair is an unfortunate complication that demands careful attention to detail. Understandably, patients require a considerable amount of emotional support. Coping with yet another failure is almost too much to ask of any individual. Therefore, it is essential for the urologist to employ a technique that maximizes the chance for a successful outcome, which requires the interposition of fresh, well-vascularized tissue between the bladder and vagina.

Vesicovaginal fistulas that develop after radiation therapy constitute yet another complex surgical problem. Most of these fistulas occur following radiation therapy for carcinoma of the cervix and develop within 6 to 12 months after cessation of radiation therapy. However, there is evidence that urinary and rectosigmoid complications are increasing in incidence 5 years after treatment has been completed and may be noted even 30 years later. Not only does the radiation therapy cause significant tissue injury, but necrosis may be enhanced by progressive arteriosclerotic vascular disease that is frequently associated with aging. Failure to surgically correct radiation-induced VVFs is not uncommon. Another attempt at repairing a recurrent radiation fistula may be considered, but it is even more critical to interpose well-vascularized tissue between the bladder and vagina.

Clinical Presentation

Patients present with varying degrees of urinary incontinence that usually develops shortly after the initial attempt to surgically correct the VVF. A small fistula may be associated with small amounts of persistent incontinence with intermittent normal voiding from the urethra. On the other hand, a woman with a large fistula usually has continued urine leakage from the vagina with little or no normal voiding. It is important to consider that the patient may have a ureterovaginal fistula that has been overlooked. Unless the ureterovaginal fistulas are bilateral, these patients note persistent leakage from the vagina as well as intermittent normal voiding from the urethra.

Evaluation

Even after a patient has undergone an attempt to repair a VVF, it is essential to do several diagnostic studies to be certain of the etiology of the urinary incontinence. This is especially true if the patient underwent the initial VVF repair elsewhere and was referred for continued management of a recurrent fistula. I have managed patients who were referred for secondary VVF repairs who did not have VVFs at all but instead had ureterovaginal fistulas. Therefore, it is emphasized that a definite diagnosis must be established before planning and undertaking surgery.

A bladder filling test confirms the diagnosis of a VVF by noting drainage of fluid from the fistula site in the vagina, which is inspected with the use of a speculum as the fluid is injected into the bladder by means of a catheter or cystoscope. If necessary, various dye solutions such as indigo carmine or methylene blue may be used to fill the bladder as the possible fistula site in the vagina is observed for leakage of the dye.

It is important that the urologist have a knowledge of the status of the upper urinary tracts to be certain that the patient does not have a ureterovaginal fistula. This is especially true because it is not uncommon for a ureterovaginal fistula to be associated with a VVF. Therefore, if the presence of a ureterovaginal fistula has not been adequately assessed, an intravenous pyelogram (IVP) should be performed. If a ureterovaginal fistula is present, a varying degree of hydroureteronephrosis is usually noted, since obstruction almost always coexists with this type of fistula. An abnormal course of the ureter may be visualized along with urine exiting into the vagina. Often, a retrograde pyelogram may even be superior in demonstrating the site of the ureterovaginal fistula and the passage of contrast material from the ureter into the vagina.

Another essential part of the assessment is to perform a cystoscopic examination. I have not usually found it necessary to employ general anesthesia to perform the examination, which has been the traditional approach, and generally use topical or no anesthetic. Cystoscopy helps identify the presence of a VVF and the degree of associated inflammation. It is also important to evaluate the number, size, and location of single or multiple fistulas.

Other studies such as a cystogram are not usually required. A number of other dye studies also can be performed, such as inserting a vaginal tampon followed by filling the bladder with a dye solution. Staining of the uppermost part of the tampon is indicative of a VVF, while staining of the outermost part of the tampon may represent urinary incontinence or a urethrovaginal fistula.

If the patient has a recurrent VVF following radiation therapy, it is imperative to be certain that recurrent cancer is not responsible for the fistula. Multiple biopsies of the fistula margin should be performed. Computed tomography (CT) of the abdomen and pelvis may reveal evidence of recurrent cancer. Likewise, obstruction of the upper urinary tracts must be viewed as evidence of recurrent cancer until this possibility has been excluded. If there is any doubt about the possibility of recurrent cancer, a short period of observation is worthwhile to help clarify the situation.

Timing of Surgery

When contemplating surgery, the urologist should time the repair to maximize the likelihood of a successful outcome, especially for a recurrent VVF. If a recurrent VVF is evident several days after an attempted initial repair, it is reasonable to consider repairing the fistula immediately before much inflammation ensues. After a week or 10 days, inflammation is usually maximum, and it is considerably more difficult to establish precise surgical planes.

Over the years, the standard management of a VVF was to delay surgery for 3 to 6 months to allow the edema and inflammation to resolve beforehand. A delay in repair provides a better-healed operative site with less inflammation, usually making it easier to establish proper surgical planes and increasing the likelihood of a successful surgical outcome. The social inconvenience and psychological impact imposed by delayed repair have led some to attempt to repair a VVF shortly after it is diagnosed. Persky and associates reported 6 successful repairs in 7 patients performed 7 days to 10 weeks after the initial surgery. The only failure in their series occurred in a patient with a combined vesicoureterovaginal fistula. Fourie reported 5 successful repairs in 6 patients employing an early suprapubic approach. Cruikshank reported successful early repairs in all 9 patients 13 to 19 days after hysterectomy using a vaginal approach. Wang and Hadley also reported a 100 percent success rate using a transvaginal approach for simple nonradiated VVFs in patients repaired before a 3-month waiting period elapsed. Badenoch and associates reported primary healing in all 19 patients using an abdominal approach whether or not the surgery was done in less than 6 weeks (7 women) or more than 6 weeks (12 women) after hysterectomy.

Likewise, the urologist managing a recurrent VVF is faced with the same difficult decision of when to optimally repair it. My own preference is to time the repair on the basis of the amount of visible associated inflammation. Patients are examined at regular intervals, with particular attention being placed on the vaginal side of the fistula, which is examined with a speculum. If the vagina appears uninflamed, well epithelialized, and free of granulation, cystoscopy is performed with topical or no anesthesia. If similar findings are noted in the bladder and pelvic examination reveals a pliable vagina without induration, surgery is undertaken. Several studies have supported this approach. Robertson noted a 97 percent cure rate in 100 patients when endoscopic timing of the repair was employed. It also has been noted in 20 patients that endoscopic timing led to repair an average of 2.4 months earlier as compared with an empirical delay with no decrease in the success rate.

A similar problem exists when dealing with recurrent radiation fistulas, which are often associated with varying degrees of acute necrosis and inflammation. It is preferable to allow the necrosis to demarcate before undertaking surgical repair, particularly for relatively acute radiation-induced fistulas occurring 6 to 12 months after cessation of radiation therapy.

Preoperative Management

A major problem for the patient is the management of urinary leakage while awaiting surgical repair. The continued odor and discomfort present a difficult social problem. Leakage may be minimized if the fistula is small by using a vaginal tampon and frequent voiding. Unfortunately, most fistulas are in the dependent portion of the bladder base and tend to cause considerable leakage. In general, incontinence underpants with various urine collection pads are necessary. Silica-impregnated pads are preferable because they trap the urine and help prevent extensive contact with the perineum. Today, there are many satisfactory urine collection pads that serve this purpose.

Another alternative is the use of the contraceptive diaphragm to attempt to trap enough urine to reduce urinary leakage. The diaphragm must completely cover the fistula and should be fitted properly to ensure good contact between its rim and the vaginal muscosa. Even a well-fitted diaphragm will not provide a watertight seal, making the addition of absorbent collection devices necessary.

Although some patients may require an indwelling Foley catheter for hygienic and psychological reasons, they are best avoided because of the risk of associated infection and the inflammation that they cause. For the same reason, use of an indwelling catheter may increase the delay period of when to optimally proceed with surgery. Additionally, indwelling catheters may not adequately vent urine leakage when the fistula is large and in a dependent position.

Before undertaking surgery, care is taken to ensure sterilization of the urine, and broad-spectrum parenteral antibiotic coverage is started. Preoperative preparation also includes mechanical and antibiotic bowel preparation, since it may be necessary to lyse a significant number of adhesions or resect bowel to gain adequate access to the pelvis. A povidone-iodine douch is administered the night before surgery.

Surgical Therapy

In order to strengthen the repair and maximize the chance of a successful outcome in a patient with a recurrent VVF, an alternative approach should be employed that incorporates the use of well-vascularized tissue interposed between the bladder and vagina. A number of tissues have been used for this purpose, including peritoneum, omentum, rectus abdominis muscle, gracilis muscle, bulbocavernosis muscle and fat pad, and a variety of other muscles.

Fulguration

A relatively simple approach that has a reasonable chance of success for the minute recurrent VVF is the use of fulguration to destroy the epithelial lining of the fistula tract. I recently reviewed my experience with endoscopic fulguration of VVFs in 14 women. Three women in this review were patients with recurrent fistulas after formal open abdominal or vaginal fistula repairs. In 2 of the 3 patients, fulguration resulted in resolution of the fistula. A Bugby electrode is inserted into the fistula either cystoscopically from the bladder or from the vagina. Following the procedure, the bladder is decompressed by means of a large indwelling catheter for 2 to 4 weeks. The theory behind the use of fulguration is that destruction of the epithelial lining of the fistula tract allows the bladder and vagina and their respective mucosal surfaces to heal from side to side. The fistula tract must be a few millimeters in size or less for the technique to be successful, and it is futile to attempt electrocoagulation of fistulas larger than 2 to 3 mm. It is recommended that a relatively low current be applied to attempt to confine the destruction to the epithelial lining of the fistula and avoid injuring the surrounding tissues. A pediatric Bugby electrode is often preferred to the larger adult size.

Martius Technique

Use of the bulbocavernosus muscle and fat pad was described by Martius in the late 1920s, but this technique was not introduced to the United States until the American translation of *Martius' Operative Gynecology*, edited by McCall and Bolton, became available in 1957. Today, most surgeons use the labial fat pad alone without going to the extent of dissecting out the bulbocavernosus muscle as initially described. Recent anatomic studies in a cadaver demonstrated that the standard Martius graft is composed of fibroadipose tissue from the labia majora and not from the bulbocavernosus muscle.

A number of vaginal incisions can be employed when performing the Martius' technique, although today most prefer a vaginal flap that is advanced later during the closure. A mediolateral episiotomy is often made to assist exposure. After the vaginal mucosa is dissected off the bladder side of the fistula, the bladder is closed by turning in the fistula in one or two layers. A separate labial incision is made on either side. The labial fat pad is mobilized with its pedicle, which is usually based posteriorly and is rotated under a subcutaneous tunnel and the vaginal muscosa to cover the bladder closure (Fig. 13-1).

The bulbocavernosus fat pad has a rich blood supply coming from several directions. Posteriorly and inferiorly, the graft is supplied by the posterior labial branches of the internal pudendal artery and vein. Anteriorly and superiorly, branches of the external pudendal

Figure 13-1. *The bulbocavernosus fat pad, which is based posteriorly, is mobilized and rotated medially beneath the labia and vaginal mucosa to overlay the closed fistula site. (Reprinted with permission from the American College of Obstetricians and Gynecologists. From Elkins TC, Delancey JOL, and McGuire EJ, The use of modified Martius graft as an adjunctive technique in vesicovaginal and rectovaginal fistula repair.* Obstet Gynecol *75:727, 1990.)*

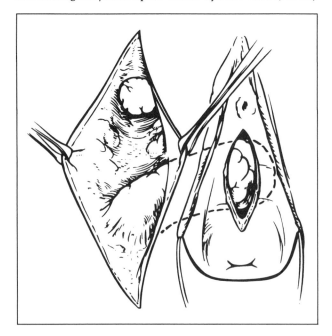

vessels proceed medially from its origin at the femoral vessels to enter the anterolateral aspect of the graft. This dual blood supply allows the surgeon the prerogative of basing the graft either anteriorly or posteriorly depending on the individual patient's anatomy and the site of the fistula.

Most descriptions today differ from Martius' original one, in which he employed the bulbocavernosus muscle itself. Use of the muscle requires a deeper dissection and is more likely to cause hemorrhage, which at times may be severe. The described technique is not only simpler and associated with less bleeding but also appears to be equally effective in bringing well-vascularized tissue over the fistula site. The blood supply of the graft is good, and the prominence of fibrous septa from the round ligament within the graft adds sufficient strength to afford rotation.

The vaginal muscosa is closed by a variety of techniques, completing this procedure. A myocutaneous flap based on the bulbocavernosus muscle and fat pad also can be used.

Abdominal Approach

I prefer to employ a suprapubic transvesical, transperitoneal approach for correction of complex recurrent VVFs. This approach has the advantage of providing excellent exposure of both the bladder and vaginal sides of the fistula and the ability to interpose a variety of well-vascularized tissues in order to maximize a successful outcome.

After induction of anesthesia, the patient is placed in the standard supine postion with the lower extremities spread slightly apart, or for more complex fistulas, it may be an advantage to place the patient in a lithotomy position with the lower extremities strapped in foot restraints to permit access to both the abdomen and vagina. Because of their ease of manipulation, the Allen universal stirrups are excellent for this purpose. Sequential compression devices are placed on the lower extremities. The vagina, perivaginal area, and entire abdomen are prepared with povidone-iodine, and the patient is draped to expose the abdomen. It is often helpful to pack the vagina with a packing soaked with povidone-iodine prior to preparing and draping the abdomen, since this greatly assists in localization of the vagina intraabdominally later in the procedure.

A lower abdominal midline incision is made. A transverse incision is avoided because it may be necessary to extend this incision to gain adequate access to the upper abdomen if mobilization of the omentum is required later in the procedure, and a longitudinal incision is required when employing the rectus abdominis muscle for interpositional pedicle material. Generally, it is necessary to lyse a number of adhesions to gain mobility of the small bowel, which is packed out of the way to allow clear exposure of the pelvis. The bladder is opened longitudinally in the midline, and ureteral catheters are usually passed to 25 cm bilaterally (Fig. 13-2). Bivalving the bladder is avoided in order to prevent a large posterior bladder closure later in the procedure. Avoidance of bivalving the bladder also may help preserve the bladder that is compromised from radiation injury and may facilitate maintenance of bladder capacity. Without attempting to separate the peritoneal reflection, a plane is established between the vagina and bladder. The previously packed vagina facilitates intraabdominal palpation of the vagina in order to locate the correct site of this plane. The peritoneum overlying the site is incised (Fig. 13-3*A*). Dissection between the bladder and vagina proceeds both bluntly and sharply, but usually sharp dissection is required (see Fig. 13-3*B*). Establishing the correct plane is greatly facilitated by dissecting along the taut anterior vaginal wall, which is readily palpable due to the previously placed vaginal pack. According to the judgment of the surgeon, it may be easier to begin this dissection before opening the bladder. After opening the bladder, it is helpful to insert a small Foley catheter or Fogarty catheter through the fistula from the open bladder in order to determine the exact location of the fistula as the dissection progresses. The dissection behind the bladder and in front of the vagina is done until the fistula is entirely defined and

Figure 13-2. *A. The bladder is opened longitudinally. B. A Foley catheter is inserted into the vagina via the fistula and ureteral catheters are usually inserted. (From Kursh, ED, Transabdominal vesicovaginal fistula repair. In ED Kursh and E McGuire (eds),* Female Urology. *Philadelphia: Lippincott, 1994.)*

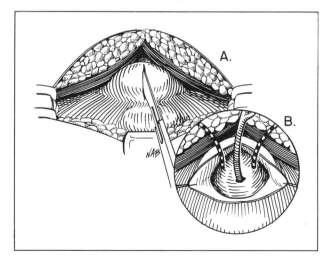

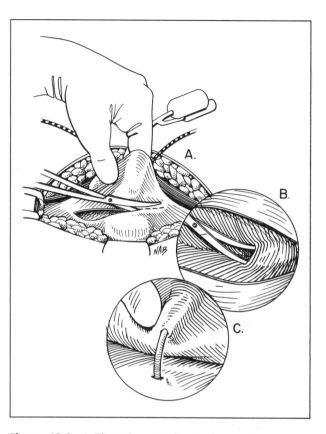

Figure 13-3. *A. The peritoneum that overlies the plane between the bladder and vagina is incised. B. Blunt and sharp dissection is used to dissect the anterior vagina off the posterior bladder wall. C. The dissection between the bladder and vagina is completed well below the fistula, which is defined by the catheter previously placed through it. (From Kursh, ED, and McGuire, E, Transabdominal vesicovaginal fistula repair. In ED Kursh and E McGuire (eds),* Female Urology. *Philadelphia: Lippincott, 1994.)*

the plane of at least a centimeter or two caudal to the fistula is established (see Fig. 13-3*C*).

The traditional approach for a repair of any fistula usually has included wide excision of the fistulous tract in order to freshen the margins and remove all the inflammatory and granulation tissue. It is my preference to sharply debride any inflammatory tissue and epithelium at the rim of the fistula, but no attempt is made to excise the entire vesical or vaginal sides of the fistulous tract for a particular distance (Fig. 13-4*A*). It is surprising how excision of a small fistulous tract can result in large openings in the bladder and vagina. Therefore, the major advantage of avoiding wide excision is diminishing the size of the defects in each component of the fistula. Other advantages include minimizing excessive bleeding from the freshly excised margins and possibly avoiding the need for ureteral reimplantation. In my experience, this method of handling the fistula margin has not

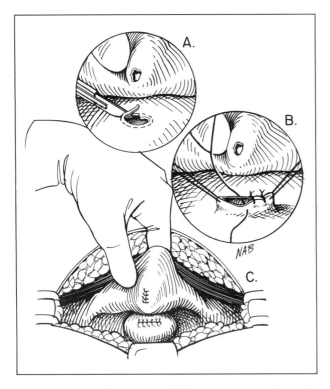

Figure 13-4. *A. The indurated inflammatory or granulation tissue at the rim of the fistula is sharply debrided for a short distance. B. The vaginal component of the fistula is closed transversely. C. Both the bladder and vaginal components of the fistula are completely closed in opposite directions. (From Kursh, ED, Transabdominal vesicovaginal fistula repair. In ED Kursh and E McGuire (eds),* Female Urology. *Philadelphia: Lippincott, 1994.)*

compromised the outcome. For a recurrent radiation fistula, it may be necessary to excise a larger amount of necrotic and fibrotic tissue in order to reach healthier, better-vascularized tissue.

The serosa and muscularis of the bladder are closed longitudinally with interrupted 2-0 absorbable suture material. The bladder mucosa is closed with a running 4-0 chromic catgut sutures. In order to avoid apposing sutures lines, the vagina is closed in an opposite transverse direction using interrupted 2-0 or 0 absorbable sutures after the vaginal pack is removed (see Fig. 13-4B). If the vagina is pliable enough, it may be feasible to invert the initial layer of closed vagina with a second layer using interrupted Lembert-type sutures of absorbable suture material. It is by no means necessary to always close the bladder and vagina in any particular direction. Each component of the fistula is closed in the manner that the surgeon deems is easiest based on the size and location of the fistula or multiple fistulas, the proximity of the ureteral orifices, and the patient's individual anatomy (see Fig. 13-4C).

A decision is made regarding the adequacy of repair that has already been completed and the degree of associated inflammation. If there is any concern about the risk of recurrence, I do not hesitate to use a rectus abdominis muscle flap interposed between the vagina and bladder. Otherwise, an omental pedicled graft is employed. After the fistula repair has been completed, the ureteral stents are removed. A large Foley catheter is employed as a cystotomy tube, which is brought through a separate stab incision, and a urethral Foley catheter is also inserted. Generally, a closed suction drain such as a Jackson-Pratt drain is placed in the space of Retzius and brought out through a separate stab incision.

Omental Flap

Pending the anatomy of the omentum, a number of omental flaps can be mobilized to gain adequate access to the pelvis. The arterial supply of the omentum comes from the right gastroepiploic artery, which is a branch of the gastroduodenal artery, and the left gastroepiploic artery, which is a branch of the splenic artery. The right and left omental arteries extend down their corresponding sides of the omentum, and there is a variable middle omental artery. If the patient has a long omentum, an L-shaped incision can be made in the omentum close to the transverse colon, basing the omental flap on either the right or left omental arteries (Fig. 13-5). If the omentum is short, it is necessary to mobilize it from the transverse colon and make the inverted-L-shaped incision close to the stomach in order to gain sufficient length of omentum to reach the pelvis. The latter maneuver invariably requires extending the abdominal incision.

Rectus Abdominis Muscle Flap

A rectus abdominis muscle is an excellent choice of tissue for repairing a number of pelvic defects, and it may be the premiere pedicle material when dealing with difficult VVFs. The muscle is well vascularized and its wide, relatively thin configuration makes it ideal for interposition between the bladder and vagina. There is minimal donor-site morbidity, and the tissue is readily available. Not only is the muscle in close proximity to the repair site, but gravity tends to keep the tissue well down in the lower portion of the pelvis, since the muscle is delivered from above.

Substantial scar tissue may be present in VVFs owing to the patient's propensity to form scar tissue

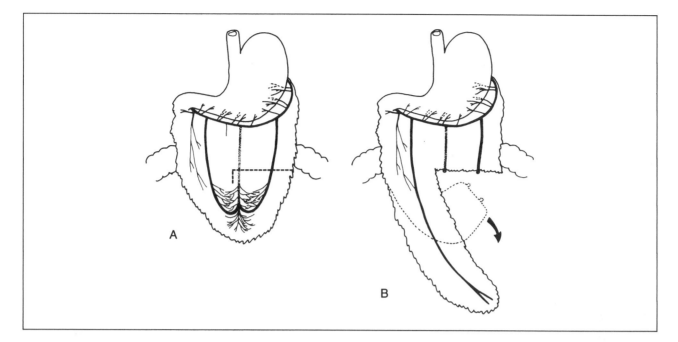

Figure 13-5. *Omental flap. A. If the patient has a normal-length omentum, the omental flap is fashioned by making an L-shaped incision below the transverse colon. It is usually preferable to base the flap on the right omental artery, as depicted here, since it is thought to be larger. B. The mobilized flap is rotated into the pelvis. (From Petty, WM, Lowy, RO, and Oyama, AA, Total abdominal hysterectomy after radiation therapy for cervical cancer: Use of omental graft for fistural prevention. Am J Obstet Gynecol 154:1222, 1986.)*

around deformities of this nature, and multiple repairs and radiation increase the likelihood of scar tissue. This scar tissue is associated with a general lack of stem cells that help promote good healing. Not only does fresh, well-vascularized tissue provide stem cells, but it also improves the blood supply of the poorly vascularized scar tissue. The increased vascularity of these tissues allows delivery of antibiotics and the components required for biologic debridement of the area.

The rectus muscles are generally regarded as the abdominal flexors as well as the anterior stabilizers of the spine. The origin of each muscle extends from the apex of the costal margin laterally across the fifth, sixth, and seventh costal cartilages and arises just below the origin of the pectoralis muscle. The anterior fascia of the two muscles, the pectoralis and the rectus, are, in essence, contiguous. The tendinous insertion of the muscle is the medial aspect of the pubic rim. The rectus abdominis muscle is encased in a sheath consisting of the anterior and posterior rectus fascia. This fascia unites in the midline to form the linea alba and laterally, where it divides again, to form the aponeurosis of the external oblique, internal oblique, and transverse abdominis muscles. There are three to four tendinous inscriptions within the muscle that result in segmentation of this

long, straplike muscle. The inferior blood supply of the rectus abdominis muscle comes from the inferior epigastric artery, which originates from the external iliac artery and then passes medially through the transversalis fascia into the rectus sheath. Encased in a fat pad, the artery proceeds medially and superiorly just above the posterior rectus sheath, entering the muscle from behind the middle of the lower third of the muscle. The venous drainage of the rectus abdominis muscle is by way of large venae comitantes (paired veins on either side of the artery) that run with the superior and inferior epigastric arteries.

The rectus abdominis muscle can easily be dissected free from its bed and transected at its insertion on the symphysis. It can then be divided at any point at or above the umbilicus, leaving it attached to its lower pedicle, the inferior epigastric artery and veins. From its branching point off the iliac vessels, the muscle and its pedicle have a 360-degree arc of rotation that allows the muscle to reach any point in the pelvis.

After the midline incision has been made, access to the rectus abdominis muscle is accomplished by dissecting through the medial border of the rectus fascia. The anterior rectus fascia is elevated off the muscle, usually for about the lower two thirds of the length of the muscle (from above the umbilicus down to the symphysis). A similar dissection is carried out at the level of the posterior rectus sheath. In the area of the tendinous inscriptions, the dissection needs to be meticulous because the muscle is especially adherent to the anterior rectus sheath in these areas. Damage to this area can result in devascularization of distant muscle segments. Leaving the entire anterior rectus sheath intact and in continuity with overlying subcutaneous tissue and skin aids in both closure of the midline wound and preservation of the blood supply to the overlying tissue. Once the dissection of the rectus muscle has been completed to the lateral border, it can be divided superiorly and at the tendinous insertion on the pubic rim inferiorly (Fig. 13-6). By lifting the muscle up, the inferior epigastric artery and associated veins are readily apparent. These vessels represent the vascular pedicle, which can be dissected out all the way to the external iliac vessels. Care should be taken to ligate the small branches that come off the pedicle as dissection progresses to the iliac vessels. Laterally, along the course of the muscle, the segmental arteries and nerves should be divided. This completely frees up the muscle, and a complete vascular island flap based on one vascular pedicle, the interior

Figure 13-6. *Rectus abdominis muscle flap. A rectus muscle flap is mobilized on its blood supply, the inferior epigastric artery. The muscle flap is completely detached both superiorly and inferiorly at its attachment to the symphysis pubis to allow sufficient mobility to swing it into the pelvis on its pedicle through an opening in the linea semilunaris. Inset shows the muscle flap sutured in place to cover the repaired bladder component of the fistula. (From Kursh, ED, Transabdominal vesicovaginal fistula repair. In ED Kursh and E McGuire (eds), Female Urology. Philadelphia: Lippincott, 1994.)*

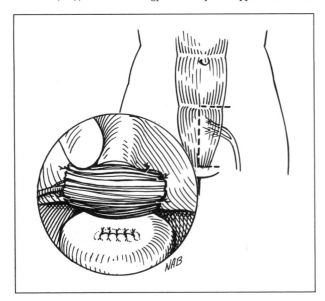

epigastric, is established. A vertical 5- to 6-cm incision is made in the most lateral aspect of the posterior rectus sheath in the area where the inferior epigastric artery takes off from the iliac artery. This incision is carried through the peritoneum, and the muscle is passed through it into the abdominal cavity. The posterior rectus fascia is then repaired, leaving a small 1-cm opening for the pedicle. This hole should not be made so small that it will constrict the pedicle but also not so large that there is a possibility for a hernia. The well-vascularized muscle flap is now passed down behind the bladder and sutured in between the repaired vagina and bladder with several tacking sutures of 2-0 or 0 absorbable suture material (see Fig. 13-6). Closure of the incision in the rectus fascia either can be performed separately or it can be incorporated into the midline abdominal wound closure.

It is not uncommon to employ both a rectus abdominis flap and an omental flap or a gracilis muscle flap and omental flap interposed between the bladder and vagina. Use of the omentum has the added advantage of helping absorb adjacent fluid collections that might accumulate in the pelvis.

Gracilis Flap

In the past, a gracilis muscle flap often was employed using a vaginal approach when dealing with complex or recurrent VVFs to increase the likelihood of a successful surgical outcome. Fleischmann and Picha described an abdominal method of using a gracilis muscle flap. The patient is placed in a lithotomy position and prepared and draped to allow access to each thigh. The initial portion of the procedure is performed as already described. Dissection between the bladder and vagina preceeds inferior to the fistula under either ureter in the direction of the thigh of the donor gracilis muscle. It is helpful for the examiner to keep the examining fingers of his or her free hand or the hand of an assistant in the vagina in order to help define the anterior edge of the vagina. The dissection terminates near the bladder neck in a plane beneath the endopelvic fascia in the prevesical space. An incision is made anteriorly in the endopelvic fascia extending for several centimeters on the side of the donor thigh to admit the belly of the gracilis muscle. This incision in the endopelvic fasica connects to the already established plane between the bladder and vagina where the gracilis muscle will be located (Fig. 13-7).

The gracilis muscle flap is usually prepared by a second surgical team, often headed by a plastic surgeon, although the primary surgeon also can perform this

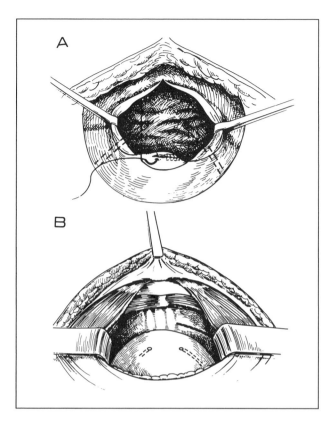

Figure 13-7. *A. The vaginal component of the fistula is closed, and dissection proceeds by creating a subvesical tunnel caudal to the fistula. B. A tunnel is established between the bladder and vagina extending to the prevesicle space through an incision in the endopelvic fascia. A parallel opening is made in the urogenital diaphragm to allow the gracilis muscle to be delivered into the pelvis. (From Fleischmann, J, and Picha, G, Abdominal approach for gracilis muscle interposition and repair of recurrent vesicovaginal fistulas. J Urol 140:553, 1987.)*

portion of the procedure. If a second surgical team is used, the gracilis muscle can be mobilized while the initial team is operating in the pelvis. Either a long skin incision extending over the course of the muscle on the medial thigh or three smaller skin incisions are made to permit mobilization and rotation of the muscle into the pelvis. The gracilis muscle is a relatively small adductor originating on the pubic arch that inserts into the proximal tibia. The muscle can be sacrificed without alteration in gait or use of the lower extremities. The distal tendinous insertion of the muscle is incised but is usually discarded later once the distal muscle belly is properly positioned and fixed in place. Two branches of the profunda femoris artery usually supply the muscle from a lateral position in the proximal third of the muscle. If there is any difficulty in localizing the arterial supply of the muscle, it is helpful to use a Doppler ultrasound

probe. In order to gain sufficient length, it may be necessary to sacrifice the distal artery, which usually can be done without altering viability of the muscle flap. The origin of the muscle on the pubic arch is not disturbed. A tunnel is created between the upper thigh and urogenital diaphragm using blunt and sharp dissection from both above and below. When establishing the tunnel, it may be helpful to make an additional incision in the ipsilateral labia majora. The muscle is rotated medially underneath the inferior pubic ramus to enter this space. If necessary, additional length may be gained by adducting the lower extremity. The muscle is brought through the openings in the urogenital diaphragm and the endopelvic fascia to enter the space posterior to the bladder (Fig. 13-8). After it is properly positioned, the muscle is fixed in place to the adjacent endopelvic fascia with interrupted 2-0 chromic catgut sutures. The distal end of the muscle is usually sutured in place on the bladder over the previously closed bladder side of the fistula (Fig. 13-9), but it also can be sutured over the vagina. Alternatively, the muscle can be brought through the obturator foramen to enter the pelvis rather than the urogenital diaphragm depending on the individual anatomy of the patient. Closed suction drainage is employed to drain the medial thigh.

Postoperative Management

Careful attention to fluid and electrolyte balance is maintained. Patients often have an associated paralytic ileus that requires nasogastric suction for several days until ample evidence of normal bowel activity resumes. Parenteral antibiotics are continued for several days, and oral antibiotics are administered when the patient resumes a normal diet.

Sequential compression devices are used until the patient is ambulating well. For a standard uncomplicated VVF repair, early ambulation is encouraged. On the other hand, if the gracilis flap is employed, the lower extremity of the donor gracilis muscle is kept relatively adducted and the bed is adjusted so that the lower extremity is elevated with the hips flexed. The patient is allowed to ambulate after a few days, but sitting in a chair is avoided to minimize the risk of venous stasis and possible venous thrombosis.

Drains are left in place until drainage is minimal. The urethral catheter is usually removed 5 to 7 days postoperatively. The patient is often discharged with the suprapubic cystostomy tube in place. For complex fistulas or following surgical correction of radiation-

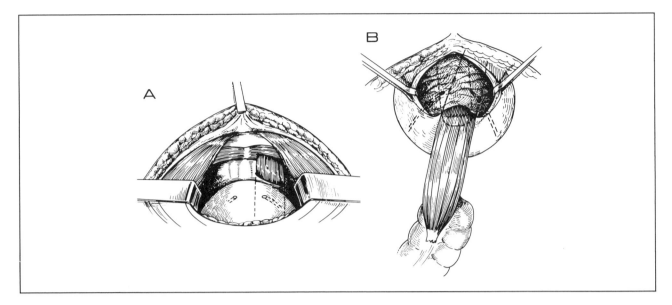

Figure 13-8. *A. The gracilis muscle is delivered to a position behind the bladder by passing it through the openings in the urogenital diaphragm and endopelvic fascia. B. The muscle flap is in position behind the bladder interposed between the bladder and vaginal components of the fistula. (From Fleischmann, J, and Picha, G, Abdominal approach for gracilis muscle interposition and repair of recurrent vesicovaginal fistulas. J Urol 140:553, 1987.)*

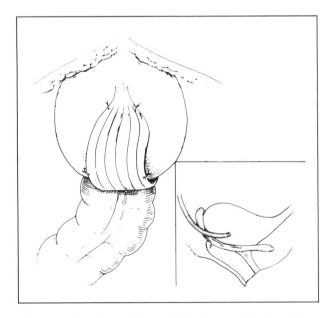

Figure 13-9. *The gracilis muscle flap is sutured in place. (From Fleischmann, J, and Picha, G, Abdominal approach for gracilis muscle interposition and repair of recurrent vesicovaginal fistulas. J Urol 140:554, 1987.)*

induced fistulas, the cystotomy tube is left in place for approximately 3 weeks. Often, a cystogram is obtained prior to removal of the cystostomy tube to verify the adequacy of repair.

Summary

Whatever approach the surgeon employs, fastidious attention to detail and proper surgical technique are mandatory. The planes between the bladder and vagina must be carefully dissected and defined, and the blood supply to pelvic structures must be maintained. Apposition of suture lines should be avoided. I feel that the repair described in this chapter has the distinct advantages of providing excellent visualization of both the bladder and vaginal edges of the fistula to maximize the strength of closure of each and the interposition of well-vascularized tissue between the vagina and bladder consisting of either omentum, rectus abdominis muscle, gracilis muscle, or both the omentum and one of these muscle flaps.

Bibliography

Badenoch, DF, et al. Early repair of accidental injury to the ureter or bladder following gynaecological surgery. Br J Urol 59:516, 1987.

Boronow, RC. Repair of radiation-induced vaginal fistula utilizing the Martius technique. World J Surg 10:237, 1986.

Cruikshank, SE. Early closure of post-hysterectomy vesicovaginal fistulas. South Med J 81:1525, 1988.

Elkins, TE, DeLancey, JOL, and McGuire, EJ. The use of modified Martius graft as an adjunctive technique in vesicovaginal rectovaginal fistula repair. Obstet Gynecol 75:727, 1990.

Fearl, CL, and Keizur, LWA. Optimum time interval from occurrence to repair of vesicovaginal fistula. Am J Obstet Gynecol 104:205, 1969.

Fleischmann, J, and Picha, G. Abdominal approach for gracilis muscle interposition and repair of recurrent vesicovaginal fistulas. J Urol 140:552, 1987.

Fourie, T. Early surgical repair of post-hysterectomy vesicovaginal fistula. S Afr Med J 63:889, 1983.

Hoskins, WJ, et al. Repair of urinary tract fistulas with bulbocavernosis myocutaneous flaps. Obstet Gynecol 63:588, 1984.

Ingleman-Sundberg, A. Pathogenesis and operative treatment of urinary fistulae in irradiated tissue. In AF Youssef (ed), Gynecologic Urology. Springfield, Ill: Charles C Thomas, 1960.

Kursh, ED, et al. Use of fulguration in the treatment of vesicovaginal fistulas. J Urol 149:292A, 1993.

Leach, GE, and Raz, S. Vaginal flap technique: A method of transvaginal vesicovaginal fistula repair. In S Raz (ed), Female Urology. Philadelphia: Saunders, 1983, pp 372–377.

McCall, ML, and Bolton, KA (eds). Martius' Gynecological Operations: With Emphasis on Topographic Anatomy. Boston: Little, Brown, 1957, pp. 322–333.

McCraw, JB, and Arnold, PG. McCraw and Arnold's Atlas of Muscle and Myocutaneous Flaps. Norfolk, Va: Hampton Press, 1986, pp 65–67, 297–299, and 389–392.

Obrink, A, and Bunne, G. Gracilis interposition in fistulas following radiotherapy for cervical cancer. Urol Int 33:370, 1978.

Orford, HJL, and Theron, JLL. The repair of vesicovaginal fistulas with omentum. S Afr Med J 67:143, 1985.

Perez, CA, et al. Radiation therapy alone in the treatment of carcinoma of the uterine cervix: II. Analysis of complications. Cancer 54:235, 1984.

Persky, L, Herman, G, and Guerrier, K. Non-delay in vesicovaginal fistula repair. Urology 13:273, 1979.

Petty, WM, Lowy, RO, and Oyama, AA. Total abdominal hysterectomy after radiation therapy for cervical cancer: Use of omental graft for fistula prevention. Am J Obstet Gynecol 154:1222, 1986.

Robertson, JR. Vesicovaginal fistulas. In WG Slate (ed), Disorders of the Female Urethra and Urinary Incontinence. Baltimore: Williams & Wilkins, 1982, pp 242–249.

Ryan, JA, Gibbons, RP, and Correa, RJ, Jr. Urologic use of gracilis muscle flap for non healing perineal wounds and fistulas. Urology 26:456, 1985.

Taylor, GI, and Corlett, RJ. The vascular territories of the body and their relation to tissue transfer. Plast Surg Forum 4:113, 1981.

Wang, W, and Hadley, HR. Non delayed transvaginal repair of high lying vesicovaginal fistula. J Urol 144:34, 1990.

Zoubek, J, et al. The late occurrence of urinary tract drainage in patients successfully treated by radiotherapy for cervical carcinoma. J Urol 141:1347, 1989.

14

Urethral Stricture

RICHARD TURNER-WARWICK
CHRISTOPHER CHAPPLE

The surgical restoration of a stable urethral lumen of even caliber is neither simple nor easy—unfortunately, therefore, the need for reoperation for urethral stricture is not uncommon. This is partly because some operative procedures are less reliable than others and partly because the potential reliability of the more appropriate definitive reconstructive procedures is sometimes underachieved.

The treatment of anterior bulbopenile strictures by internal urethrotomy alone, even when it is optically controlled, has proved unreliable in the long term. Repetition is commonly necessary so that, in reality, it is a general urologic procedure for their **management** rather than a "cure." However, developments in stricture surgery now enable us to offer restoration of efficient voiding and freedom from repeated instrumentation to the great majority of patients with anterior urethral stenosis.

The results of definitive procedures for urethral repair and reconstruction have improved greatly during the last two decades. Whereas a long-term stricture-free success rate of 70 to 80 percent used to be regarded as reasonably satisfactory, **a failure rate of more than about 5 percent in the first 5 years after a substitution reconstruction—and almost any restenosis in the long term after a one-stage anastomotic restoration of urethral continuity**—should cause aspiring reconstructive surgeons to reflect on ways to improve their results. Unfortunately, the expectations of long-term success with some of the less satisfactory substitution procedures are still overestimated by some surgeons—and the highly successful potential of anastomotic procedures, when used for appropriate cases, are not always realized.

This chapter is based on a review of a personal series of several thousand anterior urethral strictures and more than 600 restorations of pelvic fracture urethral distraction-defects. Owing to the predominant secondary specialist referral pattern in our series, the majority of our patients have required a reoperative procedure after one or more (sometimes very many) previous surgical endeavours.

Urethral Stricture Surgery

It is fundamentally important to recognize that reconstructions of glans-meatus bulbopenile spongy urethral strictures, sphincter-strictures, and pelvic fracture urethral distraction-defects are four quite distinct entities, each of which presents entirely different surgical problems that require quite separate consideration.

Furthermore, there are three basic procedure principles for urethral reconstruction:

1. **Regeneration**. Regeneration procedures depend on completion of part of the circumference of the neo-urethral lining by uroepithelial regeneration.
   a. *Natural regeneration*. The long-term success of urethral dilatation and internal urethrotomy is entirely dependent on whether the bare areas that they created can reepithelialize before the spongiofibrotic or hematofibrotic stenosis recurs—usually they do not.
   b. *Induced regeneration*. Reepithelialization can be induced by preventing approximation of the margins of the epithelial defects. The Hamilton-Russell (1914) procedure, later adopted by Dennis

Brown, was designed to induce epithelial regeneration of half the circumference of the neourethra by burying a "fixed, flat" urethral roof strip. Although this is not reliable as an isolated procedure for urethral reconstruction, it is an important principle in reconstructive surgery, and it is a component of our "combination" urethroplasty. Reepithelialization of the urethrotomized caliber also can be induced by the Wallmesh indwelling stent.

2. **Excision and reanastomosis.** Excision and spatulated overlap circumferential anastomosis provide the only stricture-resolving procedure that has the potential for 100 percent success in the long term (Turner-Warwick, 1973, 1989a). Unfortunately, this is only appropriate when the total length of a urethral abnormality is sufficiently short—thus few strictures, other than those resulting from external trauma and the relatively rare congenital variety, are truly suitable for it.

3. **Substitution.** No substitute for the urethra is as good as the urethra itself; although some are much better than others, all have inherent shortcomings. Consequently, there is a considerable incidence of early complications and a significant ongoing incidence of restenosis. "Combination" procedures can reduce the shortcomings of substitution procedures by confining their extent to the augmentation of a urethral roof strip that is fixed flat to prevent it from contracting; this reduces the circumferential proportion of a neourethral substitution to about 50 percent (Turner-Warwick 1968, 1972, 1989a, 1993a)

Each one of these three procedure principles has specific advantages and disadvantages that make it more appropriate or less inappropriate, in varying degrees, for any particular reconstructive problem. Thus, in general, the small but inevitable incidence of **complications resulting from urethral substitution procedures should never be introduced unnecessarily** for the resolution of strictures that are appropriate for repair by excision and spatulated circumferential anastomosis; on the other hand, **overextending the criteria that are critical to the success of an anastomotic procedure results in an escalating incidence of restenosis.** Adherence to these two simple principles can greatly reduce the need for reoperative procedures.

However well intended—and however well performed—any stricture operation that fails almost inevitably complicates the subsequent reoperative procedure—some only slightly, some critically, and some quite disastrously. Thus reoperative procedures range

from a relatively simple retrievoplasty to a complex "disaster plasty"—and worse. However, the actual procedures used for reoperation are rarely specifically designed for this purpose—they are generally an appropriate selection from the variety of reconstructive procedures that has been developed for the various complexities that also can result from other nonsurgical injuries.

Above all, the essence of successful reconstructive surgery, initial or reoperative, is to adapt the procedure according to the actual findings at operation. Thus reconstructive surgeons who are appropriately experienced in the range of surgical options generally use the TITBAPIT ("take it to bits and put it together") principle and are disinclined to decide, preoperatively, on the most appropriate procedure for a particular case—especially when it involves reoperation.

The Anterior Bulbo-penile Spongy Urethra

In this chapter, consideration of reoperative anterior urethral procedures is confined to the bulbomembranous urethra because a separate chapter is devoted to penile and glans-meatal hypospadiac retrievoplasty.

Some Basic Considerations of Surgical Anatomy

The Structure of the Anterior Urethra

An understanding of the surgical anatomy of the urethra—and its healing response to injury of any kind—is fundamental to its reconstruction and re-reconstruction. The wall of the bulbopenile urethra is formed by a layer of uroepithelium applied, almost directly, to the vascular spaces of the erectile tissue. It is the natural thrombotic healing response of this delicate underlying spongy tissue—and the extent of the consequent **spongiofibrosis**—that largely determines the nature of a stricture of the spongy urethra and its tendency to restenosis after surgery.

The Distribution of the Spongy Tissue

Throughout the length of both the penile and bulbar urethra, **the dorsal spongy tissue that forms its roof in the 12 o'clock position is only 3 to 4 mm thick** (Fig. 14-1). In the penile area, the lumen of the urethra is **concentric** within the erectile spongy tissue so that, circumferentially, this is only 3 to 4 mm thick. However, in the bulbar area, the lumen is **dorsally eccentric** within the bulk of the bulbospongy expansion so that while only 3 to 4 mm separate it from a penile corpora dorsally, inferolaterally, it is 10 to 15 mm thick.

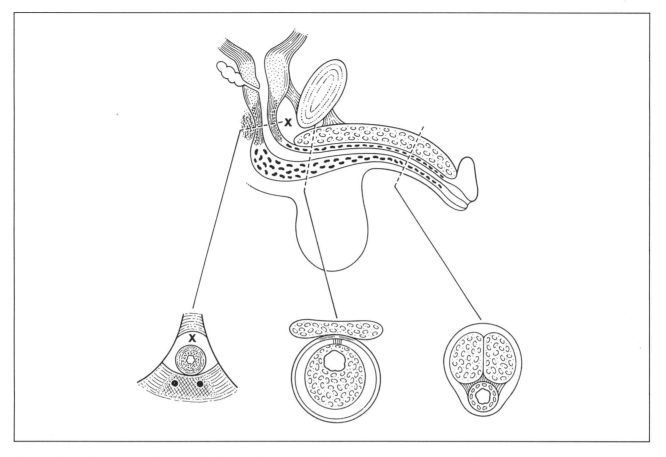

Figure 14-1. *Anatomic relationships. The lumen of the penile urethra is concentrically arranged within the spongy tissue, but in the bulbar area it is dorsally eccentric; thus throughout the whole length of the anterior bulbopenile urethra, the thickness of the spongy tissue on the dorsal (12 o'clock) roof aspect is only 3 to 4 mm. The subprostatic membranous urethra relates anterolaterally to the "pubourethral" space (X), and posteriorly, it is densely adherent to the perineal body. Posterolaterally (4–8 o'clock), it relates to the nervi erigentes. (Copyright 1987 by the Institute of Urology.)*

This grossly eccentric disposition of the spongy tissue in the bulbar area is not only relevant to the selection of the optimal site for internal urethrotomy but also commonly dictates the need for a definitive **spongioplasty**—to redeploy its bulk—in the course of definitive bulbar and bulboprostatic urethral reconstructions.

The Surgical Significance of "Spongiofibrosis" and the "Gray Urethra"

The natural spongiothrombotic healing response of the urethral spongy tissue and the consequent spongiofibrosis (Fig. 14-2) are fundamental factors that predispose the bulbopenile urethra to stricture formation and to postoperative restenosis. Thus proximal and distal to almost every stricture, with the exception of the rare congenital variety, the urethral lumen is surrounded by a subepithelial layer of spongiofibrosis, and it is the

extent of this that determines not only the nature of the stricture but also the most appropriate surgical procedure for its resolution (Turner-Warwick, 1989a).

The longitudinal extent of the spongiofibrosis associated with a stricture is the most important factor that determines both the type and extent of a definitive surgical reconstruction (Fig. 14-3). Surgery involving a residually spongiofibrotic urethra has a high stricture recurrence potential unless special precautions are taken to prevent this.

Unfortunately, failure to appreciate the surgical significance of spongiofibrosis is still a common cause of recurrent stenosis after stricture surgery (Turner-Warwick, 1968, 1973, 1989b). It is fundamentally important to appreciate that a surgically significant spongiofibrosis associated with a stricture often extends into a segment of the adjacent urethra, **the caliber and radio-**

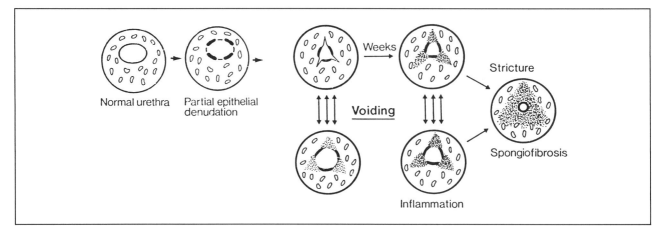

Figure 14-2. *Urethral healing. After partial denudation of its lining, the natural closing pressure that evacuates the bulbopenile urethra approximates the margins of the uroepithelium; the intervening clefts are intermittently opened by the voiding stream, and the spongy tissue thus exposed gradually becomes spongiofibrotic and the lumen stenotic. (Copyright 1987 by the Institute of Urology.)*

graphic appearance of which may be quite normal; to emphasize the surgical importance of this unstrictured segment of urethral abnormality, we sometimes refer to it as the "gray urethra." Often the true extent of the spongiofibrosis associated with a stricture is not apparent until the urethra is opened at the time of operation.

Thus, to avoid an incidence of predictable restenosis, both anastomotic and substitution procedures should extend 2 cm into macroscopically normal "pink" urethra—both proximal and distal to the urethral abnormality—whenever possible and not be limited merely to the relatively short segment that is actually strictured (Turner-Warwick, 1968, 1973, 1989a).

The Treatment Options

Internal Stricturoplasty

The basic principle of stricturotomy is to enlarge the urethral lumen by a urethrotomy incision that extends through the layer of suburoepithelial spongiofibrosis associated with the stricture. When the incision reaches a layer of "supple" surrounding tissue, the neolumen can expand—this supple layer may be either the relatively normal spongy tissue surrounding the spongiofibrosis or the adjacent adventitial tissue outside it.

The traditional sector for a urethrotomy incision is in the 12 o'clock position; however, in the bulbar area, this is questionable, because the urethral lumen is grossly eccentric within its surrounding spongy tissue, so incisions in the 4 to 8 o'clock position are more likely to extend through the layer of spongiofibrosis into a supple layer (Turner Warwick, 1989a) (Fig. 14-4). Cer-

tainly the 12 o'clock position is inappropriate at the meatus because any incision there—other than at precisely 6 o'clock—risks a distortion that can create a troublesome spraying of the stream.

In recent years, urologic enthusiasm for the Sachse optical urethrotomy procedure has tended to overshadow the equally valuable Otis urethrotome—in fact, they are complementary instruments. The endoscopic appearances of the urethrotomy incisions created by the two instruments are generally indistinguishable immediately thereafter, and it is questionable whether there is any significant difference in their healing.

The long-term success of an internal urethrotomy depends on whether the incisional clefts reepithelialize before they close—commonly they do not—so in the majority of cases it has to be repeated, and the incidence of long-term stricture-free success diminishes quite rapidly with this repetition.

The major potential disaster of the treatment of a bulbomembranous stricture by urethrotomy is a posterior extension of this into the distal sphincter mechanism—this is potentially disastrous because of the risk that a sphincterotomy over the 3 to 4 mm thickness of the intramural distal sphincter of the membranous urethra renders it incompetent (Fig. 14-5). Such an indiscriminate extension of its use into the sphincter—active posterior urethra—can result in complications that compromise or even preclude a definitive reconstruction that is successful in the long term.

Although the urethrotomy of a bulbar urethral stricture is likely to marginally increase the extent of its associated abnormal spongiofibrotic segment, this does

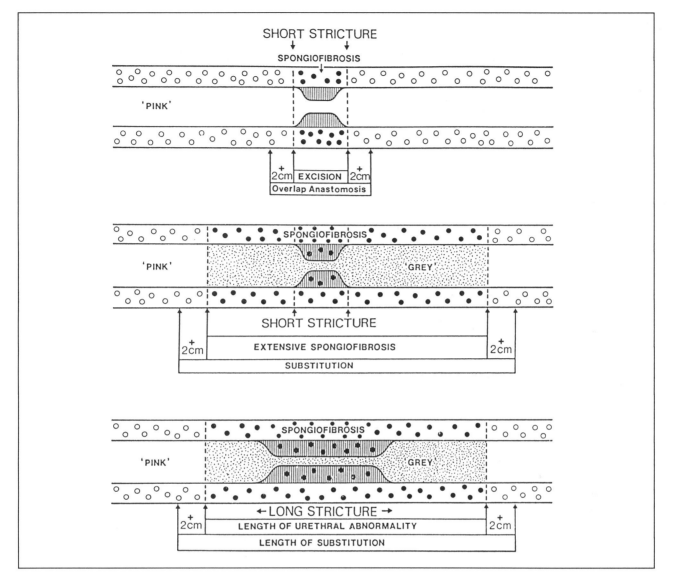

Figure 14-3. *Spongiofibrosis. It is the extent of the urethral abnormality, not the stricture itself, that determines whether an anastomotic or a substitution repair procedure is appropriate. The lumen of "gray" spongiofibrotic urethra proximal and distal to a stricture is not stenosed, but nevertheless, it has a stricture potential that is exacerbated by surgical procedures; a surgical repair should therefore extend into the normal "pink" urethra. (Copyright 1987 by the Institute of Urology.)*

not significantly complicate any subsequent **substitution** procedure that may be required—nor does it significantly reduce the expectation of stricture-free success that this procedure can offer. However, the urethrotomy of a short stricture that is eminently suitable for anastomotic repair may critically compromise this much superior option. Thus, **provided the length of a stricture is not sufficiently short to be otherwise suitable for an anastomotic repair**, and **provided the incision is not extended into the distal sphincter mechanism and**

thus compromise its competence, there is rarely a contraindication to the trial of a urethrotomy.

When a proven stricture obstruction recurs after urethrotomy, there are several conservative treatment options:

1. Simple dilation to maintain the normal posture-throtomy urethral caliber. After appropriate instruction, many patients can manage self-dilation by the passage of a soft plastic dilator or catheter, repeated as

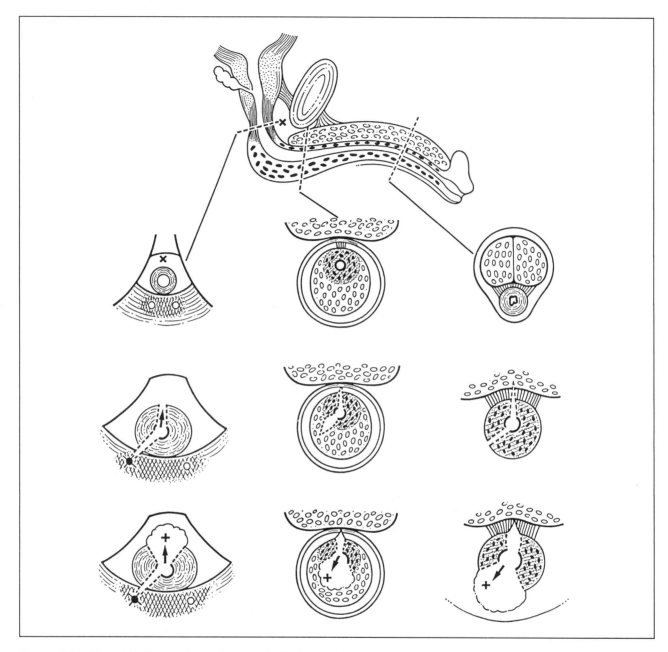

Figure 14-4. *The optimal sector for urethrotomy. In the bulbopenile spongy urethra, stricturotomy incisions in the 4 to 8 o'clock sector are more likely to extend into a supple tissue plane than in the traditional 12 o'clock site, where the spongy tissue is only 3 to 4 mm thick and is commonly obliterated by spongiofibrosis. A urethrotomy that transects the 3- to 4-mm thickness of the distal sphincter in the membranous urethra commonly impairs its functional occlusion. (Copyright 1987 by the Institute of Urology.)*

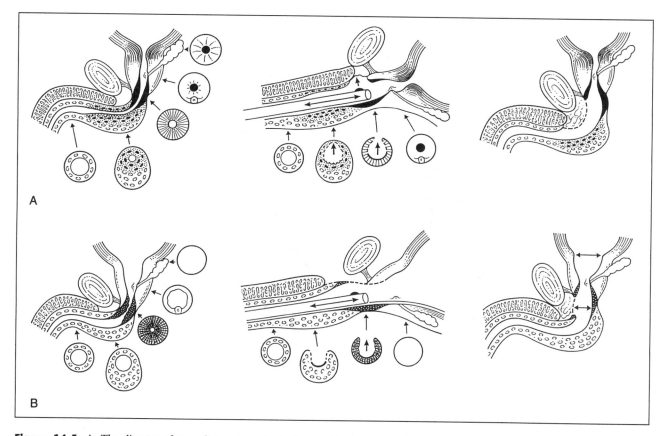

Figure 14-5. *A. The disaster of extending a posterior bulbar urethrotomy into the sphincter-active membranous urethra. Incompetence of the distal sphincter mechanism resulting from such an incision does not become clinically apparent if the bladder-neck sphincter is competent, but incontinence is likely to develop after a routine bladder-neck–ablating prostatectomy. B. Urethrotomy of a sphincter stricture after prostatectomy commonly results in the disastrous complication of incontinence. The essence of the treatment of sphincter strictures is preservation of the residual functional occlusion of the damaged remnants of the mechanisms. (Copyright 1987 by the Institute of Urology.)*

often as necessary (usually every week or so), to ensure its easy passage.

2. Repeated stricturotomy—as frequently as necessary to relieve recurrent stricture obstruction—often at decreasing intervals. This is generally inadvisable over an extended period because it tends to increase the local fibrotic scarring

3. Induced reepithelialization by an indwelling stent—such as the self-expanding Wallmesh stent (Milroy et al., 1989)—which maintains the urethrotomized caliber of the spongy urethra. The early results of this technique are encouraging, but it is much less successful for the resolution of distraction-defects after traumatic injuries. However, mesh-stent failures present complex reoperative problems because they generally require a block resection of the whole length of the stented segment of the urethra and a circumferential substitution procedure (Fig. 14-6).

The alternative to conservative treatment is a definitive retrieval reconstruction—usually a substitution procedure.

Definitive Urethral Reconstruction

The Principles of Anastomotic Bulbar Elongation Urethroplasty. To achieve a reliable stricture-free restoration of urethral continuity by anastomosis after the excision of a urethral stricture or distraction-defect, the basic essential is a tension-free, 2-cm spatulated overlap of normal, spongiofibrosis-free urethral ends—appropriate mobilization and lengthening of the urethra are naturally required to achieve this if chordee-creating tension is to be avoided.

The bulbar segment is the only part of the urethra that can be mobilized to provide surgically useful elastic lengthening. This is so because the available longitudinal elasticity of the penile urethra is nearly fully

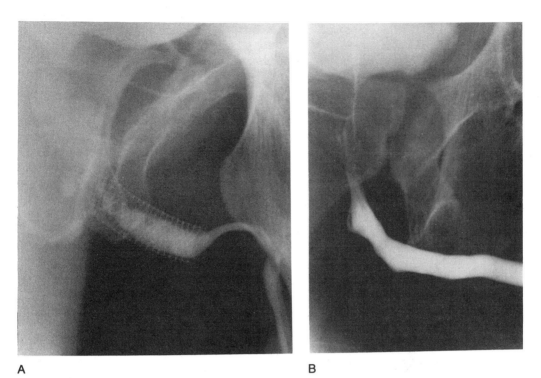

A   B

Figure 14-6. *An apparently short stricture treated by recalibration and insertion of a Wallmesh stent. A distal recurrence of the stricture was treated by insertion of a second "piggy-back" stent. The proliferative endostent fibrosis could not be controlled endoscopically because of the angulation of the stents, so a block resection removal was required. A. Although it was anticipated that the PIPS plasty substitution would probably need to be circumferential, in the event it was hemicircumferential because it was possible to create an anastomotic fixed flat roof strip after mobilization of the remnants of the bulbar urethra. B. (Copyright 1992 by the Institute of Urology.)*

stretched during an erection, so any attempt to gain additional urethral length by mobilizing and stretching it results in curvature-chordee of the penile shaft (Turner-Warwick, 1973, 1983a, 1989a).

Mobilization of a normal bulbar urethra between its membranous and penile junctions generally achieves 4 to 5 cm of elastic lengthening in the adult (proportionally less in children). This is the basis of bulbar elongation advancement urethroplasty (BEAU) procedures (Turner-Warwick, 1973, 1989a, 1991). This lengthening of the bulbar urethra can be used to resolve either a prostatobulbar pelvic fracture urethral distraction-defect proximally or a short bulbopenile stricture distally. The BEAU procedure also can be used for the anastomotic meatoplasty BEAM correction of a hypospadiac urethral foreshortening and retrievoplasty (Turner-Warwick, 1993b).

However, when the bulbar urethra itself is damaged, as in a fall astride injury, the local abnormality naturally reduces its elongation potential, so a tension-distortion base-angle chordee tends to result if a spatulated anastomotic repair is attempted when total length

of the bulbourethral abnormality exceeds about 1 cm. Thus suitability for an anastomotic restoration of bulbourethral continuity is virtually confined to short strictures resulting from external trauma, such as straddle injuries and the occasional congenitally based "Cobbs ring" stricture, when the length of the spongiofibrosis has not been increased by a previous urethrotomy (Turner-Warwick, 1973, 1989a). Thus an anastomotic procedure is rarely suitable for a retrievoplasty.

Substitution Urethroplasty. Substitution procedures are commonly required for anterior urethral reoperative reconstruction because of the length of the spongiofibrotic abnormality associated with the great majority of surgical failures. Unfortunately, there is no perfect substitute for the urethra—some are much better than others, but all have inherent shortcomings and, consequently, a commensurate incidence of complications and restenosis.

"Wet" or "Dry" Skin? "Wet" epidermal surfaces, such as those of the urethra, the foreskin, the mouth, the vagina, and the labia, are specially adapted to their moist

environment, whereas "dry surface" skin, such as that of the scrotum, the thigh, and the abdomen, tends to become inflamed and eczematous when constantly urine sodden. Thus some donor skin areas are relatively **inappropriate**. However, penile skin can be regarded as "semidry" skin; it is distinctly moisture resistant and almost hairless—consequently, it is much more appropriate for urethral substitution than scrotal skin. This is quite evident from the relatively satisfactory long-term results of penile skin substitution for the resolution of hypospadiac deformities over many decades.

Pedicled or Free Grafts? The survival of pedicled skin, with an efficient blood supply, is naturally more reliable than a free graft, which depends on gaseous and nutrient diffusion from the graft bed. Furthermore, the ultimate success of a one-stage free-graft procedure naturally depends on its 100 percent survival because a partial loss involving any proportion of its circumference results in a commensurate reduction of the caliber of the reconstructed lumen in that area and, consequently, restenosis. Furthermore, unlike a pedicled graft, if the length of a free graft is doubled, the stricture risk resulting from a partial "failure of take" also must be doubled.

When appropriate skin is available on a pedicled basis, it is generally preferable to a free graft. However, when a pedicled graft of suitable skin cannot be mobilized sufficiently, or when previous surgery has critically impaired its blood supply, free grafts enable appropriate "wet" or "moist" donor skin to be used, and this may be preferable to an easily available pedicled graft of relatively inappropriate scrotal skin.

Terminological Inexactitudes

Use of the word *flap* specifically to identify the transposition of skin that has a vascularized pedicle has become less accurately descriptive with the development of the microvascular transposition; thus, in this terminology, a microvascularized pedicled graft now has to be described, paradoxically, as a "free flap" when, in reality, it is not. There is much to commend the simple traditional terminology—*free grafts, pedicled grafts,* and *revascularized grafts.*

Similarly, for two reasons it is inaccurate to describe a pedicled graft of scrotal skin (and even less the penile skin) as "based on dartos fascia." In reality, its vascularization is based on the vessels within its remarkably mobile subcutaneous tissue—not on "fascia," which is generally a relatively avascular structure. Furthermore, the greek word *dartos* relates the subdermal corrugating muscle of the scrotal skin—the contraction of which retracts it—it does not appropriately describe the scrotal

skin itself, its subcutaneous tissue, or the blood supply of the scrotum as a whole—and still less that of the penile skin.

Pedicled-Skin Substitution

Scrotal Skin. The mobility of the scrotal skin facilitates its surgical use on a subcutaneous pedicle (sometimes erroneously described as a "dartos pedicle"). However, scrotal skin has two serious shortcomings which greatly compromise its value as a urethral substitute:

1. It is a "dry surface" skin that is particularly prone to develop eczematous and inflammatory reactions ("stenosing scrotitis") when urine sodden.
2. It is hair-bearing. Occasional hairs growing in the lumen of a urethral substitution reconstruction rarely cause problems if its caliber is normal; however, scrotal skin substitutions in the bulbar area often become sacculated, and hairs growing in pockets of stagnant urine tend to become encrusted, resulting in stone formation and infection.

The two-stage Turner-Warwick (1968) drop-back scrotourethral inlay procedure was developed specifically to provide an access for procedures to overcome these well-recognized shortcomings during the interval. However, when possible, the use of scrotal skin is generally best avoided, particularly for *circumferential* substitution, and certainly, we do not advocate its use on a one-stage PISS graft basis because this does not allow the adjustments and epilation necessary to reduce the incidence of its inherent complications. In our series, the complications of PISS-plasty have been a common indication for a retrieval PIPS plasty.

However, scrotal skin remains an invaluable component of a "combination" procedure when a two-stage observational scrotourethral inlay is required for a particularly complex bulbar reconstruction—as it sometimes is for reoperative procedures—and also as a permanent scrotourethral inlay after urethrectomy for gross chronic inflammation (the classic fistulous "water-can" perineum), for urethral tumors, and for gender-reassignment procedures.

Furthermore, a rotational "skin swap" scrotal skin flap is an **indispensable substitute for penile skin** when this has been used as a urethral substitute (Turner-Warwick, 1968, 1989a, b). The underlap/overlap principle of preventing penile shaft fistulas by using a flap of subcutaneous tissue that is much wider than the skin strip is shown in Figure 14-7.

Foreskin. A pedicled island foreskin (PIFS) procedure is the natural source of vascularized "wet" skin.

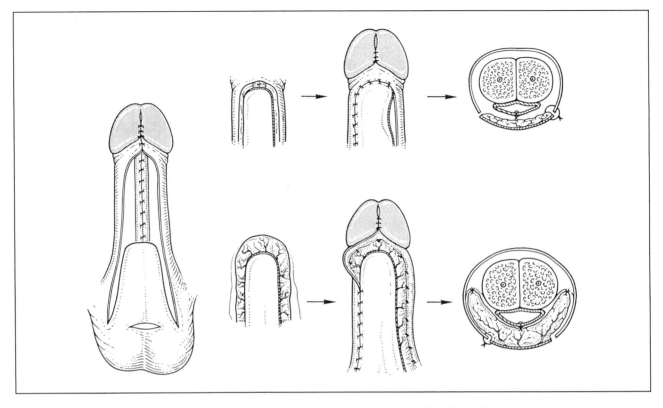

Figure 14-7. *The prevention of fistulas by underlap/overlap overclosure. A. If the width of the subcutaneous tissue of the scrotal rotation flap is not much wider than the skin strip, the potential leak track is short. B. The width of the subcutaneous tissue should be at least twice as wide as the skin strip to provide good underlap/overlap leak-proof security. (Copyright 1986 by the Institute of Urology.)*

In an uncircumcised patient, a unilaterally pedicled PIFS graft can be mobilized for bulbourethral substitution (Turner-Warwick, 1972); however, the extensive mobilization of a unilateral pedicle required to enable it to reach the posterior bulbar urethra can render it rather precarious (Fig. 14-8).

The Penile Skin. Pedicled inlays of penile skin (PIPS) have proved a relatively reliable substitute for the penile urethra in circumcised patients over many years. In the two-stage Duplay procedure, it is "rolled-in" on a long lateral (LATPIPS) pedicle that provides good vascularization; the LATPIPS pedicle, also can be used as a one-stage procedure (Orandi, 1972).

BIPIPS Urethroplasty. The bilaterally based pedicled island penile skin (BIPIPS) procedure (Turner-Warwick, 1989a 1993a) was the natural development of our UNIPIPS onlay augmentation bulbopenile urethroplasty (Turner-Warwick, 1972). It was designed to facilitate the use of penile skin in circumcised patients by reducing the length of the pedicle required to enable a PIPS graft to reach the bulbomembranous urethra and

also to improve the reliability of its blood supply by basing it bilaterally (Fig. 14-9).

Even in circumcised patients, the length of the ventral penile skin between the glans and the scrotum is sufficient to replace the whole length of the bulbomembranous urethra—this is due to the combination of the extraordinary mobility of the subcutaneous tissue and vascularization of the penile skin as well as to the easily demonstrable fact that minimal traction on the glans penis is sufficient to enable it to reach back as far as the anus.

Thus the BIPIPS procedure for the reployment of relatively moisture-resistant and virtually hairless ventral penile skin has particular advantages:

1. Its broad, bilaterally vascularized subcutaneous pedicle provides a more reliable blood supply than a long unilateral pedicle.
2. In uncircumcised patients, the ventral penile skin is long enough to replace most of the penile urethra, in addition to the bulbar urethra. Even in circumcised patients, the ventral skin of the penis is long enough to reconstruct the whole length of the bulbar urethra.

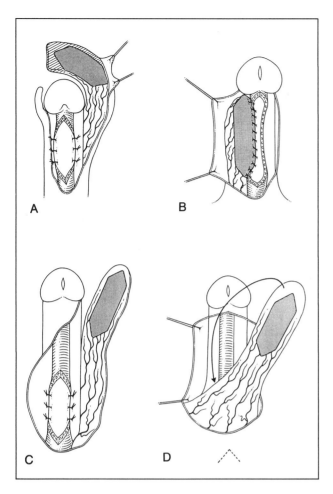

Figure 14-8. *One-stage pedicled island penile skin (PIPS) plasty. A. Pedicled island foreskin (PIFS) plasty for terminal hypospadiac urethroplasty (Duckett, 1970). B. Laterally pedicled island penile skin (LATPIPS) plasty for one-stage penile Duplay urethroplasty (Orandi, 1972). C. Unilaterally pedicled island penile skin (UNIPIPS) plasty for bulbopenile urethroplasty (Turner-Warwick, 1972). D. Bilaterally pedicled island penile skin (BIPIPS-TWARS) plasty for bulbomembranous urethroplasty (Turner-Warwick, 1989). (Copyright 1987 by the Institute of Urology.)*

3. Retrogradely invaginated, the hairless distal apex of the pedicled ventral penile skin island easily reaches the membranous and even the bladder neck. The retrograde paraurethral course of the BIPIPS pedicle facilitates overclosure of a redeployment spongioplasty (when this is possible) and of the bulbospongiosus muscle; this helps to prevent sacculation of the substitution reconstruction, and it may restore postvoiding evacuation and ejaculation.

4. In uncircumcised patients, it is often possible to close the consequent ventral penile skin defect by a spiral redeployment of the residual dorsal penile skin—alternatively, a scrotal rotation flap can be used for

this because the vascular pedicle of a BIPIPS graft is quite separate from that of the scrotal skin, and consequently, their vascularization is unimpaired by the combination of a double redeployment "skin swap" procedure.

5. Most important, in the relatively unusual event of a proximal or distal junctional neourethral restenosis, it is often possible to resolve this by a simple redeployment and reanastomosis because—unlike other substitution procedures—an extensive PIPS graft failure is rare, and it is easily remobilizable.

"Combination" Urethroplasty—The Principle of the Augmented Roof-Strip Procedure

When the whole circumference of several centimeters of the bulbar urethra has been lost as a result of trauma or previous surgery (see Fig. 14-6), a circumferential substitution is usually necessary. However, the incidence of complications resulting from the inherent shortcomings of skin substitution can be reduced by limiting the proportion of its contribution to the neourethral circumference, i.e., using it in "combination" to avoid a circumferential substitution whenever possible (Turner-Warwick, 1968, 1972, 1989a, b).

The basic principle is the creation of a "fixed, flat" roof strip about 1.5 cm wide—preferably by anastomotic redeployment of the urethra; the remaining half of the neourethral circumference is completed by a substitution graft.

1. A spongiofibrotic urethral roofstrip is less likely to develop a secondary narrowing contraction if it is laterally spread and fixed flat by suture anchoring of its lateral margins.

2. Even if part of the augmenting neourethral overclosure graft should fail, restenosis is unlikely to result because—on the basis of the Hamilton Russell (1914) buried-strip principle—tissue overclosing an established epithelial roofstrip does not cross-adhere and so tends to reepithelialize by induced regeneration.

The Creation of a Bulbar Urethral Roof Strip and Redeployment Spongioplasty.
A neourethral roof strip in the bulbar area can be created by several procedures (Fig. 14-10). When the length of the strictured lumen is not too long, it is best achieved by anastomotic redeployment; for longer strictures, its width can sometimes be augmented by multiple longitudinal fenestrating incisions which are "held open" by the lateral anchoring sutures so that the epithelial defects have

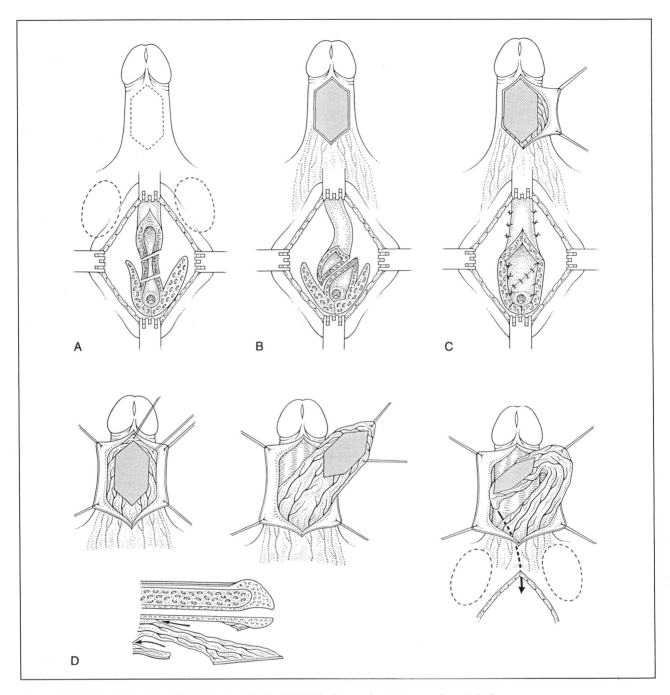

Figure 14-9. *The bilaterally pedicled island penile skin (BIPIPS) bulbar urethroplasty procedure. A, B, C. Reconstruction of a dorsal urethral roof-strip (when possible). D. Mobilization of an island of ventral penile skin based proximally on a broad, bilaterally vascularized subcutaneous pedicle. E, F. Redeployment of the BIPIPS graft by retrograde inversion. G. Perineal overclosure and scrotal skin advancement to cover penile skin defect. (Copyright 1986 by the Institute of Urology.)*

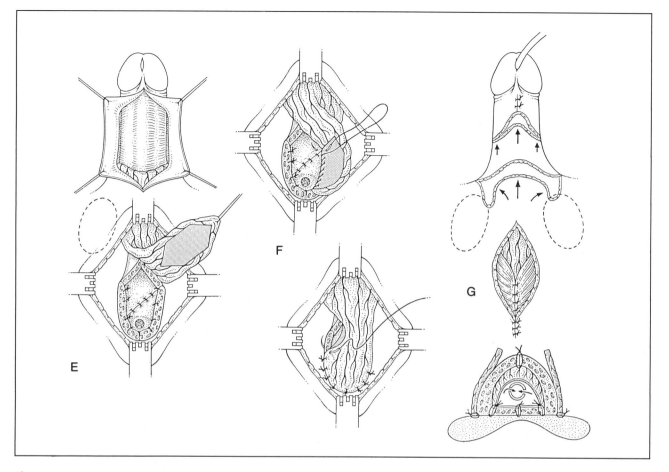

Figure 14-9. (*Continued*)

to heal by regeneration. Occasionally, when a scroto-urethral inlay for a particularly complex bulbomembranous stricture proves unstable due to eczematous "stenosing scrotitis" during the interval stage, a roof strip of generous proportions can be created with a free skin graft, and the final-stage closure can be deferred until the healing of this is observed to be stable.

An anastomotic redeployment roof strip is achieved by mobilizing the bulbar urethra from the bulbomembranous junction to the base of the penis and transecting it at the point of maximum narrowing of the lumen, thus increasing the width of the roof strip by a side-to-side overlap anastomosis (Fig. 14-11). Because the urethral lumen is dorsally eccentric within the bulbar spongy tissue, this involves a **definitive lateral spongioplasty** (Turner-Warwick, 1973, 1989)—the reflection of posteriorly based flaps of the excess bulk of spongy tissue by sharp dissection with excision of any areas of spongiofibrosis within them. Any normally supple spongy tissue that remains is redeployed lateral to

the fixed flat roof strip for subsequent overclosure support on the basis of its main posterior blood supply.

There is an important additional maneuver that reduces the risk of posterior junctional stenosis when a bulbar stricture extends posteriorly, close to the sphincter mechanism. The posterior extent of the incision separating the spongioplasty flaps is extended lateral to the bulbomembranous urethral junction so that this can be "funnelled open" by two anterolateral fixation sutures and by three additional ones posteriorly in the the midline and laterally through the bulbar spongioplasty flap.

The Substitution Augmentation of a Bulbar Roof-Strip "Combination" Urethroplasty. Completion of the neourethral circumference overclosing a roof strip is preferably achieved on a one-stage basis by a BIPIPS graft whenever the quality of both the roof strip and the penile skin is appropriate—otherwise, a two-stage drop-back scrotourethral inlay is advisable.

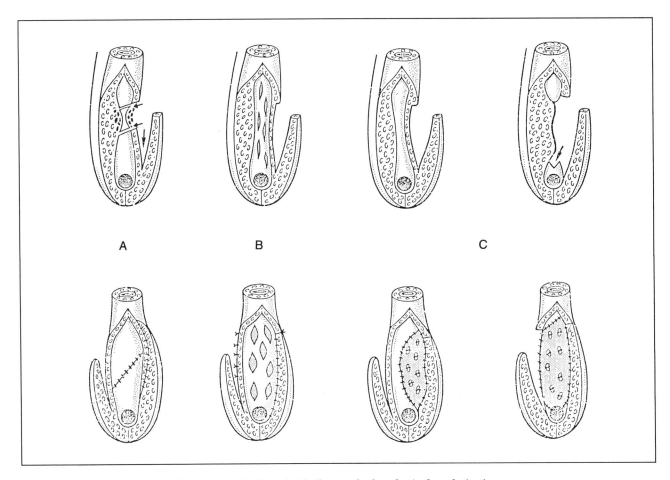

Figure 14-10. *The options for the creation of a fixed flat bulbar urethral roof strip for substitution augmentation. A. Mobilization of the bulbar urethra, excision of the stricture, and restoration of urethral roof-strip continuity by an oblique reanastomosis with a lateral redeployment spongioplasty. B. "Tesselation" of the urethral roof strip with lateral fixation to induce regeneration of the uroepithelium. C. Full-thickness free graft of penile skin. (Copyright 1986 by the Institute of Urology.)*

Two-Stage Scrotourethral Inlay Urethroplasty

The two-stage scrotal drop-back procedure (Fig. 14-12) is described in detail elsewhere (Turner-Warwick, 1968, 1989a); however, there are a few important principles that require emphasis. The scrotal drop-back is achieved by dividing the perineal skin vertically, by a midline incision, and closing this horizontally. Before making the secondary inlay-urethrostomy incision in the scrotal skin, it is important to ensure that the bulk of the intertesticular subcutaneous tissue drops back, behind the inlay, to provide well-vascularized support for the posterior skin bridge.

The Management and Duration of the "Interval" Stage.

The term *two-stage* applied to a scrotourethral inlay urethrostomy is to some extent a misnomer because it fails to emphasize that the key to the success in this type of reconstruction for the more complex bulbomembranous strictures is the meticulous management of the interval, which involves an additional interval stage procedure. The prime purpose of the open first-stage inlay is to provide access for (1) direct observation of the healing of the fixed, flat roof strip of a "combination" procedure, (2) the local rearrangement of the scrotal inlay or adjustment of the urethral roof strip, and (3) hair follicle destruction in the area of the inlay that will be used to complete the neourethral circumference of the "combination" reconstruction.

The duration of the interval between the first stage and the final closure depends on the time it takes to establish a stable time-proven stricture-free inlay: the reliability of the procedure depends on this.

When a two-stage scrotourethral inlay is used as part of a combination procedure, its success is primarily dependent on the roof strip, and therefore, its closure may be undertaken as soon as the healing of this strip is

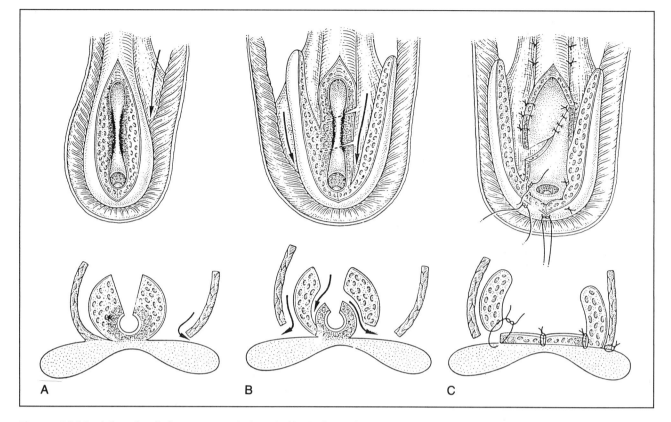

Figure 14-11. *A lateral redeployment spongioplasty is required to achieve a fixed flat roof strip by anastomotic redeployment in the bulbar area because of the dorsal eccentricity of its lumen within the spongy tissue. A. The lumen of the mobilized bulbar urethra is opened, and the midline origin of the bulbospongiosus muscle is detached. B. The excess bulk of the lateral spongy tissue is dissected free, preserving its posterior blood supply and leaving a layer about 3 to 4 mm thick around the urethral lumen for its vascular support. C. After the excision of the tightly strictured segment, the continuity of a spongiofibrotic urethral roof strip is restored by an oblique anastomosis, and it is fixed flat by lateral anchor sutures. Note that the posterior extent of the angle of the spongioplasty dissection enables the lumen of the subsphincteric proximal bulbar urethra to be spread open by anchor sutures to avoid the development of a restenosis at the posterior end of the augmenting skin graft—two sutures anterolaterally and also three posteriorly—inserted through the whole thickness of the posterior spongioplasty flap. (Copyright 1982 by the Institute of Urology.)*

observed to be satisfactory. This is so because only a small margin of the scrotal skin inlay is required to augment the urethral circumference, so the time-proven quality of this is less important to the result than it is when scrotal skin is used without a definitive roof strip—nevertheless, its neourethral margin should be carefully epilated.

Free-Graft Urethroplasty

When well-vascularized penile skin is available for a urethral reconstruction, introduction of the additional risk of restenosis due to a partial "failure of take" of a free graft may be difficult to justify. However, if the survival of a pedicled penile skin inlay is likely to be precarious as a result of compromised vascularization (commonly resulting from the failure of multiple previous surgical endeavors in the area of the penile urethra), it is sometimes safer to use it on a free-graft basis for a retrievoplasty (Turner-Warwick, 1993b).

The immediate survival of a full-thickness skin graft depends primarily on diffusion (not on a vascular "hookup," which is a later development) and consequently on the proximity of the basal epithelial cells to the graft bed and the quality of the nutrient vascularization of this bed. Meticulous subdermal cleaning of a free skin graft (a process that is sometimes erroneously referred to as "defatting" because there is virtually no fat under the penile skin) is facilitated by spread fixing it on

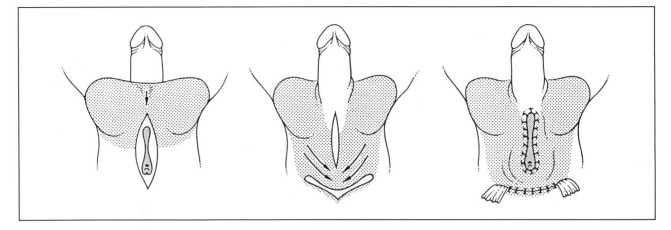

Figure 14-12. *A scrotal drop-back is achieved by a midline perineal incision and closing this horizontally. Before making the secondary inlay urethrostomy incision in the dropped-back scrotal skin, it is important to ensure that the bulk of the intertesticular subcutaneous tissue drops back, behind the inlay, to provide well-vascularized support for the posterior skin bridge. (Copyright 1968 by the Institute of Urology.)*

an adhesive surface such as that of a sterile sharps-disposal Discardopad (used by operating room staff for the collection and counting of used suture needles). The prevention of subgraft serosanguineous accumulations is equally important.

When a full-thickness skin graft is used to reconstruct the whole circumference of the urethra, it is important to maintain the neourethral caliber by a stenting* catheter during the immediate postoperative healing period. A fenestrated catheter may be preferable to one with a solid shaft because this facilitates—rather than obstructs—the free drainage of the healing tissue exudates (Turner-Warwick, 1973) (Fig. 14-13).

Although commonly used as a stenting catheter, a balloon-retained Foley catheter is inadvisable after a urethral reconstruction because not only does it have a solid shaft, but the accidental traction-removal of a fully inflated balloon risks disruption of a neourethral graft and even its elective removal may be sufficient to dislocate a free graft as a result of stretch corrugations of the surface of a fully deflated balloon. It is generally safer to retain a urethral catheter with a sling suture to a button on the abdominal wall after any urethral reconstruction (see Fig. 14-13), and a simple technique for the synchronous insertion of this and a suprapubic catheter is illustrated in Figure 14-14.

The foreskin or penile skin is the generally preferred donor site. When there is a paucity of penile skin and a long graft is required, a full-thickness graft from the

*The term *stent* is used to describe a device intended to maintain the lumen caliber of a surgically recreated space during the postoperative healing period. Dr. Stent was a pioneer faciomaxillary surgeon who devised a wax-mold "stenting basis" to locate a split skin graft lining of a neomaxillary sinus.

groin or the inner aspect of the arm can be used. However, although the dermis of these areas is thinner than that of most integumental skin areas, it is very much thicker than that of the penis. Furthermore, the underlying subcutaneous tissue is fat-laden so that subdermal cleaning is particularly important. Closely fenestrated "tessellation" of the graft is also helpful to achieve drainage of subgraft exudates, the accumulation of which compromises a successful graft "take." It also somewhat reduces the compromising thickness of the dermis and induces reepithelialization of the "windows."

Buccal skin is an excellent substitute for relatively small areas of urethral substitution such as hypospadiac glans-meatoplasty corrections. Bladder urothelium also can be used on a free-graft basis for anterior urethral substitution, but it tends to become protuberant and "sticky" if it is exposed at a neomeatus.

Spongiosupported Skin-Patch Plasty. When it is used for retrieval surgery, a full-thickness skin graft often has to be based on the residual periurethral muscle or adventitial tissue; however, spongy tissue provides a particularly good bed for a free graft, and a spongiosupported reconstruction is, in fact, the closest approximation to the recreation of a normal urethra in which the uroepithelium is applied virtually directly to the vascular spaces of the spongy tissue (Fig. 14-15). Thus patch spongioplasty is particularly appropriate for the creation or recreation of a near-perfect glans meatoplasty (Turner-Warwick, 1993a, b), and it is sometimes an appropriate alternative to a BIPIPS augmentation of a redeployment bulbar urethral roof strip when there is sufficient residual normal spongioplasty tissue after excision of the spongiofibrosis.

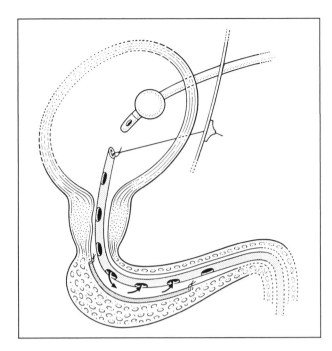

Figure 14-13. *Urine drainage after urethral reconstruction is most safely achieved by the combination of a suprapubic and a sling-stitch-retained fenestrated urethral catheter. The fenestrations in the urethral catheter shaft ensure positive drainage of the exudates and also facilitate postoperative contrast studies to exclude suture line extravasation before its removal—the "cathetergram." The use of a balloon-retained urethral catheter is a source of occasional complications caused by the accidental withdrawal of an undeflated balloon or by the obstructed drainage of exudates by the standard shaft and consequent pericatheter infection. A plastic catheter is preferable for fenestrating because its lumen is relatively large compared with that of a silicone/rubber catheter. The length of the fenestrated area of the shaft is tailored to the circumstances; it rarely needs to extend distal to the penoscrotal junction. For the simple drainage of a bulbar urethroplasty, size 14 to 16 French is generally appropriate for an adult, but a larger one is required to stent a free graft. The fenestrations are simply made by sharp bending a catheter and cutting off the projecting kink angle of the flattened fold with scissors. (Copyright 1987 by the Institute of Urology.)*

Reoperative Bulbar Urethral Surgery

Stricture operations that fail almost always complicate a subsequent definitive "retrievoplasty"—some affect it only slightly, some critically, and some disastrously. This should be recognized in determining the initial treatment. For instance, extension of the minimal spongiofibrosis associated with a short straddle-injury bulbar stricture by a relatively unreliable optical urethrotomy may preclude an anastomotic repair and necessitate a substitution retrievoplasty, which has a much higher inherent incidence of restenosis. The failure of a definitive reconstruction not only involves significant secondary scarring and an extension of the spongiofibrotic abnormality but also commonly compromises the residual tissue available for a substitution reconstruction.

The Surgical Anatomy of the Posterior Sphincter-Active Urethra

The Sphincter Mechanisms of the Posterior Urethra

An accurate knowledge of the functional anatomy of the sphincter mechanisms is essential to the success of posterior urethral surgery because its whole length is sphincter-active—from the internal meatus down to the membranobulbar urethral junction.

The feasibility of almost every posterior urethral surgical procedure—such as the resolution of prostatic obstruction, the repair of sphincter-strictures, and the anastomotic reconstruction of subprostatic pelvic fracture urethral distraction-defects—depends on the **independent function of the proximal bladder neck and of the distal urethral sphincter mechanisms, each of which is competent and independently capable of maintaining continence in the absence of the other** (Turner-Warwick, 1973, 1981, 1983a, 1989a).

The **bladder-neck sphincter** is functional from the internal meatus down to the level of the verumontanum, and in the male, it is reliably competent—provided it is not surgically damaged or rendered incompetent by unstable detrusor contractions.

The **distal sphincter mechanism** is about 2.5 cm long, but it is only 3 to 4 mm thick; it forms the whole thickness of the membranous urethra and extends upward, through the apical prostatic capsule, to the verumontanum. The competence of this distal urethral mechanism is, in fact, entirely dependent on the sphincter muscles within this 3- to 4-mm thickness of the membranous and supramembranous urethra because there is no periurethral "external sphincter" mechanism external to it—either anteriorly or laterally (Chilton and Turner-Warwick, 1985). Behind it, in the midline, the medial margins of the pelvic floor levators insert into the perineal body—but these muscles are only capable of momentary occlusion of the urethra and are quite incapable of maintaining continence (Turner-Warwick, 1979, 1981, 1983a).

The Pubo-Urethral Space—The Urogenital Hiatus in the Pelvic Levator Diaphragm and the Myth of the "Urogenital Diaphragm"

The anatomic entity of the pubo-urethral space within the urogenital hiatus in the pelvic floor is, in fact, located exactly in the supposed position of the mythical "urogenital diaphragm" (Turner-Warwick, 1981, 1983a, 1991). Only minimal mobilization of the bulbar urethra, from a perineal approach, is required to enable a

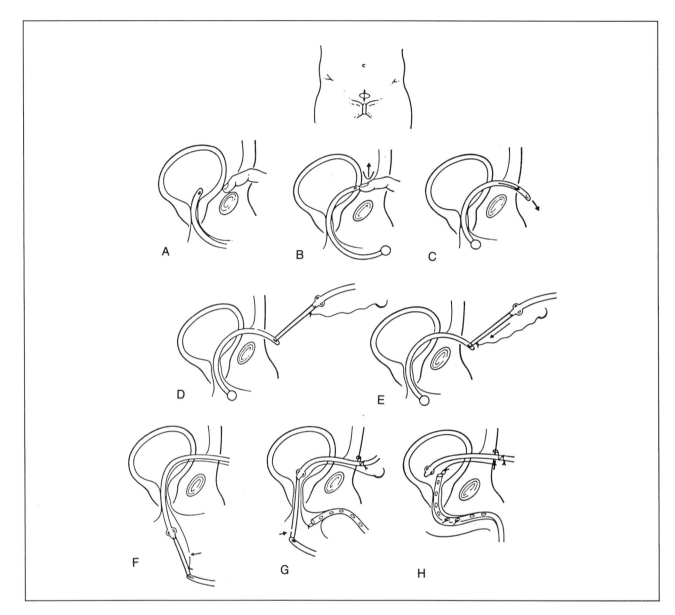

Figure 14-14. *The Turner-Warwick "pull-in" procedure for the synchronous introduction of a supra-pubic catheter and a sling stitch to retain a fenestrated urethral catheter—using an eyelet-tip Hey-Groves half-circle urethral sound. A. Finger introduced into the retropubic space through a minimal suprapubic incision (3 cm horizontal skin, 3 cm vertical midline in rectus sheath, Mayo scissors pushed through rectus muscle into retropubic space and opened.) B. Fingertip in the retropubic space feels the back of the pubis, deflects the peritoneum upward, and feels the tip of the sound in the bladder—which is simply pushed through the bladder wall (C). D. A monofilm nylon suture is passed through the tip of the suprapubic catheter and the eyelet of the sound to create a 20-cm pull-in loop. E. The knot is pushed to the tip of the sound. F. The suprapubic catheter is pulled out through the posterior urethra into the urethrostomy to ensure that it is not merely invaginating the fundus of the bladder. G. The sling stitch is cut, and its end is tied through the terminal hole of the fenestrated catheter to retain it with a button on the abdominal surface. H. The suprapubic catheter is pulled back so that its end lies in the bladder base, where—after checking that it drains freely—it is retained with a skin stitch. The pull-in nylon loop is then cut and withdrawn. (Copyright 1987 by the Institute of Urology.)*

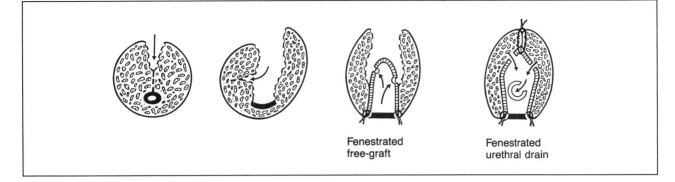

Fenestrated
free-graft

Fenestrated
urethral drain

Figure 14-15. *Full-thickness skin-patch spongioplasty. Normal spongy tissue provides a particularly good basis for a free graft. A spongiosupported reconstruction is, in fact, the closest approximation to the recreation of a normal structure of the urethra in which the uroepithelium is applied virtually directly to the vascular spaces of the spongy tissue. (Copyright 1983 by the Institute of Urology.)*

fingertip to be inserted into it—between the membranous urethra and the subpubic arch—and up to the level of the puboprostatic ligamentous bundle that forms its roof (Fig. 14-16).

Detailed anatomic studies (Chilton and Turner-Warwick, 1985) confirmed that the only muscles of the pelvic floor that relate directly to the membranous urethra are the posteriorly located pubourethral elements of the pelvic levators and the transverse perineii that insert into the perineal body adherent to its posterior surface.

The *nervi erigentes*, which innervate the erection mechanism of the penile corpora, lie in close posterolateral relationship to the membranous urethra, and injury to them may result in impotence; they are particularly at risk during sphincter-relaxing urethrotomy incisions in the 4 and 8 o'clock positions and also in the course of a posterior prerectal surgical exposure of the prostatomembranous urethra facilitated by the "exaggerated lithotomy" position.

Despite relatively recent recognition, the pubourethral space is highly relevant to urethral reconstruction in this area and to the variations in the site of subprostatic urethral rupture and the extent of the hematoma associated with pelvic fracture urethral injuries (Turner-Warwick, 1989a, 1991). The pubourethral space is of particular importance to reoperative reconstructions involving the bulbomembranous urethra because it is easy to develop surgically and the external approach to the membranous urethra and the apex of the prostate that it provides enables the distal extent of the distal sphincter mechanism to be identified and preserved most accurately.

Thus the traditional description of a urogenital diaphragm—enclosing a bulk of striated external sphincter

muscle and encircling the membranous urethra—is totally imaginary and inaccurate; there is no supporting sphincter musculature anterior or lateral to the membranous urethra.

Regrettably, even a cursory review of current literature and illustrations shows that an extraordinary number of urologists still suppose that there is an "external sphincter" external to the membranous urethra—within the confines of an erroneously conceived "urogenital diaphragm." The false confidence engendered by this erroneous belief has resulted in the distal sphincter being treated in a most cavalier manner by generations of surgeons—not only during prostatectomy procedures (the transvesical, the Millin retropubic, the so-called radical total prostatectomy, and even the TUR) but also by the treatment of sphincter-strictures by internal urethrotomy, which carries a high risk of incontinence (see Fig. 14-5) (Turner-Warwick, 1981, 1983a, 1991).

Posterior Urethral Strictures

Unfortunately, the term *posterior urethral stricture* is still widely used to include **both** simple **sphincter-strictures** and subprostatic **pelvic fracture urethral distraction-defects** (PFUDDs). This is confusing because they—and the principles of their surgical resolution—are entirely different. Logically, the term *urethral stricture* should be used to indicate a narrowing of urethral continuity—not a gap.

Simple continuity strictures of the membranous urethra are commonly the result of an internal urethral injury (prostatic surgery, instrumentation, indwelling catheters, or tumor invasion); they are best referred to as

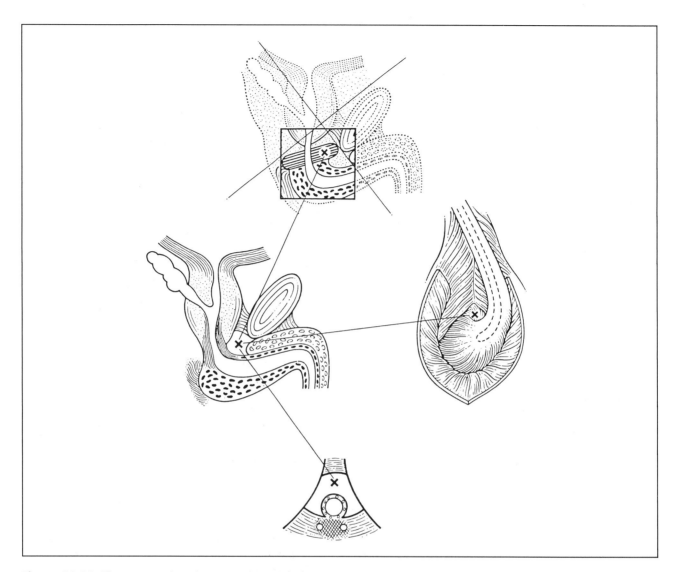

Figure 14-16. *The concept of a sphincter muscle containing "urogenital diaphragm" is completely erroneous. The distal urethral sphincter mechanism is entirely contained within the 3- to 4-mm thickness of the wall of the membranous and supramembraneous urethra, and this relates anteriorly to the "pubourethral space" in the "urogenital hiatus" of the pelvic floor diaphragm between the pubic origins of the levator muscles. (Copyright 1982 by the Institute of Urology.)*

sphincter-strictures (Turner-Warwick, 1983b, 1989, 1991) because this emphasizes that although the function is generally impaired to a variable extent, the distal urethral sphincter mechanism has not been destroyed.

The **primary aim** of the treatment of a sphincter-stricture must be the **preservation of the residual distal sphincteric function**, just as the primary aim of the management of a pelvic fracture urethral distraction-defect (PFUDD) is the preservation or functional reconstruction of **the only residual sphincter mechanism at the bladder neck** because in all but the most minimal lesions the function of the intramural distal urethral

sphincter is destroyed by the subprostatic urethral rupture through its mechanism (Turner-Warwick, 1968, 1973, 1983b).

Postprostatectomy Sphincter-Strictures

Postprostatectomy distal sphincter-strictures are common, and they present particular problems because

1. They are located in the only sphincter mechanism that remains after prostatectomy ablation of the bladder neck (whether transurethral or enucleation).

2. The injury that created the distal sphincter-stricture, and often its subsequent treatment, also damages its functional competence to a greater or lesser extent.
3. They tend to restenose particularly rapidly—presumably accelerated by the natural sphincter occlusion of their lumen.

Hence they are much the most difficult of all strictures to manage, and the prime consideration must be preservation of the all-important residual intrinsic sphincteric function rather than the definitive resolution of the stricture itself.

The Significance of the Distinction between "Supple" and "Rigid" Sphincter-Strictures

There is a wide variation in the extent of sphincter damage associated with sphincter-strictures. At one extreme, when a sphincter-stricture is the result of simple erosion and denudation of its epithelial lining, the sphincter mechanism may be almost undamaged and "supple" so that, like a normal distal sphincter, it can be overdilated to a caliber of 32 to 36 Ch without significant diminution of the urinary control. On the other hand, densely fibrotic, "rigid" sphincter-strictures are generally associated with sphincter damage that is so severe that even the simple atraumatic passage of a 16-Ch dilator may render it temporarily incompetent and the patient incontinent.

There are, of course, all gradations between these extremes, and these are identified by observing the result of judiciously progressive recalibrations—using simple **expansion** of the Otis instrument **without** its knife blade.

Once identified by appropriate recalibrations, the safest treatment procedure for the more rigid sphincter-deficient stricture is simple, frequent, small-caliber dilation—often this is best achieved by teaching the patient to pass a soft olive-tipped plastic dilator as frequently as necessary to ensure an effortless passage—sometimes as often as once a week or more (Turner-Warwick, 1981, 1983a).

The potential disasters of treating a postprostatectomy sphincter-stricture by internal urethrotomy should be self-evident (see Fig. 14-5). If a patient is not immediately rendered incontinent as a result of transecting the 3- to 4-mm thickness of the intramural distal sphincter mechanism, secondary fibrosis may convert a supple mechanism into one that is rigid and relatively complex. Unfortunately, largely perhaps as a result of the common misconceptions about the thickness of the external sphincter among traditionally trained urologists, sphincter-stricture urethrotomy is still an all too common disaster.

Occasionally, after most careful thought and discussion, a patient with a supple sphincter-stricture that is proving difficult to manage by dilation may elect to accept the small but inherent risk of incontinence involved in a definitive repair procedure; when the bulbar urethra is normal, the best option for this is the push-in bulbar sleeve procedure with spongiospongioplasty revascularization in case the implantation of a peribulbar artificial sphincter is subsequently necessary (Turner-Warwick, 1983b) (Fig. 14-17).

Pelvic Fracture Urethral Injuries

Hemorrhage, Hematoma, and Hematoma Fibrosis

All pelvic fracture injuries result in the development of a pelvic floor hematoma, the size of which varies from minimal to massive and lethal. The urethra is injured in about 10 percent of pelvic fracture injuries, and in the adult, the usual location of this is within the 2 cm of the relatively unsupported subprostatic membranous urethra, which relates to the pubourethral space anteriorly (Turner-Warwick, 1981, 1989)—not to a fictious "urogenital diaphragm." When the membranous urethra is also torn across, a hematoma develops between the distracted ends of the prostatic and bulbar urethra—naturally, the size of this depends on the extent of the prostatic dislocation, and accordingly, it may or may not be in continuity with the pelvic floor hematoma; various combinations of this are illustrated in Figure 14-18.

Circumferential injuries to the subprostatic urethra almost always result in occlusion unless a false passage is created and maintained—between the prostatic urethra proximally and the bulbar urethra distally—through the intervening hematoma which eventually consolidates to form dense hematoma fibrosis of varying extent. In reality, therefore, the consequent stenosis is a pelvic fracture urethral distraction-defect, or PHUDD—not a urethral continuity stricture. The end results of these may be short or long, and they may be simple or complex (Fig. 14-19).

Surprisingly, the surgical significance of hematoma fibrosis is rarely discussed and often underestimated, but in reality, this is the factor that should properly determine the extent of the operative procedure required for the anastomotic restoration of urethral continuity—indeed, the remarkable reliability of this procedure is largely dependent on the resolution of the

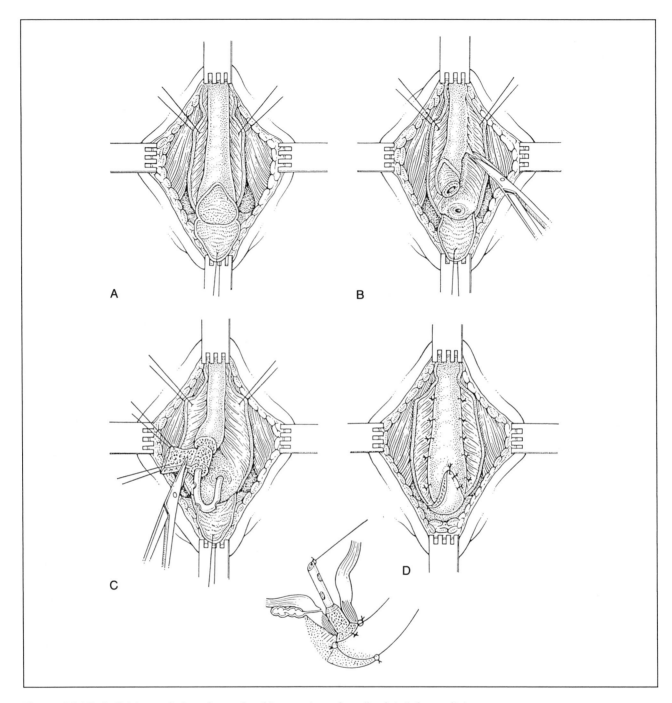

Figure 14-17. *Definitive resolution of a supple sphincter stricture by a "push-in" sleeve relining procedure. A. Posterior flap spongioplasty. B. Transection and mobilization of the bulbar urethra. Dilation of the supple sphincter stricture to 32 to 34 French. C. Trimming of the spongiosus to form a supple "push-in" sleeve inlay about 5 mm thick. D. Sleeve inlay retained by sutures around the "collar" of untrimmed spongy tissue. Spongiospongioplasty revascularization by posterior spongioplasty flap. (Copyright 1978 by the Institute of Urology.)*

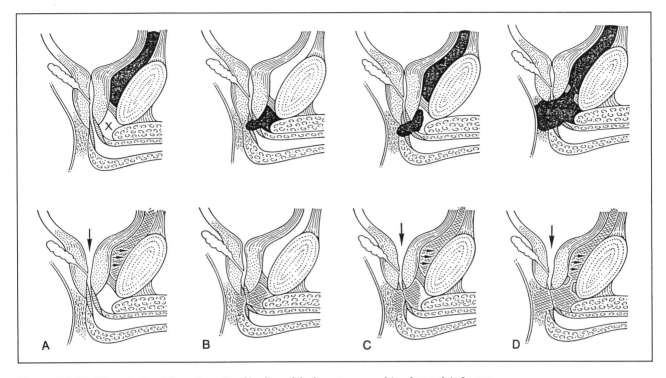

Figure 14-18. *The extent and the end results of healing of the hematoma resulting from pelvic fracture urethral injuries. A. Hematoma fibrosis resulting from resolution of a pelvic floor hematoma commonly tethers a normal mechanism to the inner aspect of the pelvis. As the hematoma retracts, it pulls the bladder neck open, rendering it incompetent. B. Minor degrees of subprostatic urethral rupture can result in the development of a hematoma confined to the "pubourethral space." This commonly results in a short urethral distraction defect and localized hematoma fibrosis. C. The combination of a pelvic floor hematoma and a "pubourethral space" hematoma naturally tends to result in the combination of an incompetent bladder neck mechanism and a short subprostatic urethral defect associated with minimal fibrosis. D. A confluent retropubic/subprostatic hematoma associated with rupture of the puboprostatic ligaments results in a complex urethral distraction defect associated with extensive hematoma fibrosis. (Copyright 1986 by the Institute of Urology.)*

complicating features that are often associated with this dense fibrosis (Turner-Warwick, 1973, 1977, 1989b).

Simple Distraction Stenosis

The most common end result of a subprostatic urethral injury is the development of a relatively short prostatobulbar urethral gap. Usually, such a simple short-gap defect can be resolved by a relatively simple perineal approach anastomotic repair—provided it is not associated with an extensive hematoma fibrosis and provided the bladder neck mechanism is occlusive and competent.

Complex Distraction-Defects

A complex PFUDD generally requires a perineoabdominal approach to resolve one or more of its features

shown in Figure 14-19; the urologic management of the initial injury should endeavor to avoid the development of these complications. Most of the features of a complex urethral distraction-defect stem from an unreduced major dislocation and the consequently extensive eventual hematoma fibrosis—if the eventual outcome of a severe prostatic dislocation injury is only a simple distraction stenosis that can be resolved by a perineal approach repair, it is a generally acceptable result of the initial treatment, provided its achievement has not increased the risk of impotence.

The two centimeters of the sphincter-active membranous urethra below the prostate relate, anteriorly, to the pubourethral space (Fig. 14-20); a subprostatic rupture can occur at any point within this relatively unsupported 2 cm, but most commonly it is close to the apex, and it is rather unusual to find more than 1 cm of intact

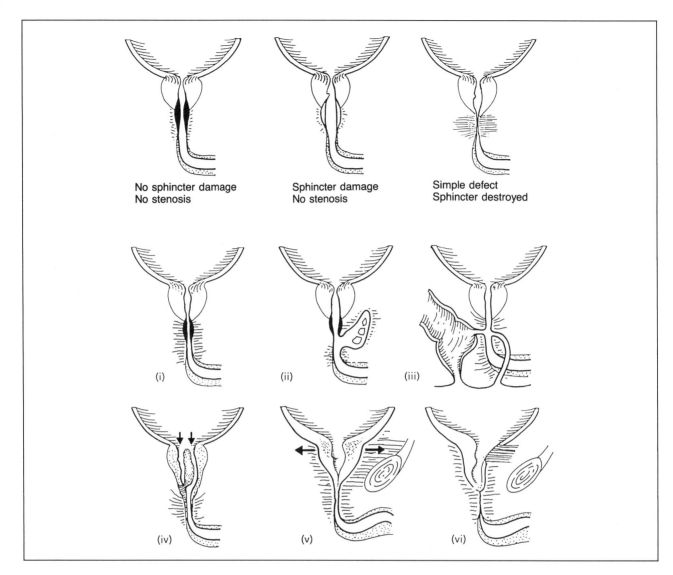

No sphincter damage
No stenosis

Sphincter damage
No stenosis

Simple defect
Sphincter destroyed

(i)   (ii)   (iii)

(iv)   (v)   (vi)

Figure 14-19. *The end results of pelvic fracture urethral injuries. Subprostatic urethral injuries commonly destroy the distal urethral sphincter function and result in the development of a simple distraction gap that usually can be resolved by a perineal-approach repair. Complex distraction injuries require an abdominoperineal-approach repair to resolve (i) a long distraction defect, (ii) a distraction sacculation, (iii) fistulas extending into the perineum, thigh, lower abdomen, or rectum, (iv) false passage into bladder base, incompetence of the only remaining sphincter mechanism at bladder neck level due to hematoma fibrosis retraction (v) or to sphincter damage (vi). (Copyright 1987 by the Institute of Urology.)*

membranous urethra distal to it—usually no more than a few millimeters (Turner-Warwick, 1989a). Thus the competence of the distal urethral mechanism is almost invariably destroyed by a subprostatic pelvic fracture urethral rupture so that, after restoration of urethral continuity, continence is entirely dependent on the bladder neck mechanism (Turner-Warwick, 1968, 1977, 1979). Reported claims of persistent distal sphincter function after bulboprostatic anastomosis are generally based on videocystourethrographic or electromyographic evidence of pubourethral levator activity.

The Bladder Neck Mechanism

A normal male bladder neck mechanism is generally reliably competent unless it is rendered incompetent by unstable detrusor contractions; patients whose continence is dependent on it usually have satisfactory uri-

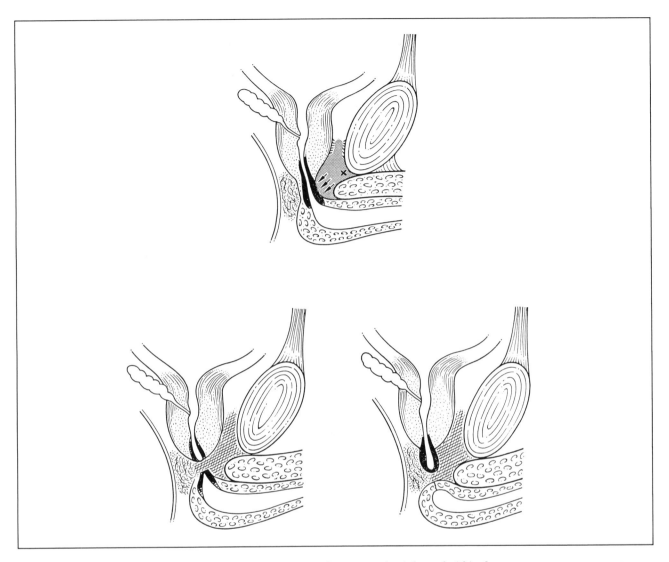

Figure 14-20. *A subprostatic rupture of the sphincter-active membranous urethra is located within the "weak-link area" of its relation to the puboprostatic space. This is usually close to the apex of the prostate, but sometimes it is a centimeter or more distal to it. A circumferential rupture almost always destroys the functional occlusion of the distal urethral sphincter mechanism. (Copyright 1987 by the Institute of Urology.)*

nary control, although, of course, in the absence of the distal urethral sphincter they are unable to instantly interrupt their voiding stream if their pubourethral levator sling is also damaged.

Bladder Neck Incompetence

The bladder neck may be damaged by a pelvic fracture injury, but the most common cause of its incompetence is the circumferential tethering of an **uninjured** mechanism by the natural shrinkage/replacement of an extensive pelvic floor hematoma by hematoma fibrosis (Fig. 14-21). In such cases, it is usually possible to restore its functional competence by mobilizing it meticulously

by removal of the dense hematoma fibrosis anchoring it to the pubis anteriorly and laterally; naturally, the reliability of this procedure depends on prevention of secondary fibrotic reimmobilization by occluding the consequent paraprostatic dead-space cavity with a supple omental pedicle graft which preserves the functional mobility of the liberated sphincter mechanism.

Internal Urethrotomy

A trial of urethrotomy may be appropriate in some minimal subprostatic pelvic fracture urethral injuries; however, a urethrotomy is only likely to succeed when the

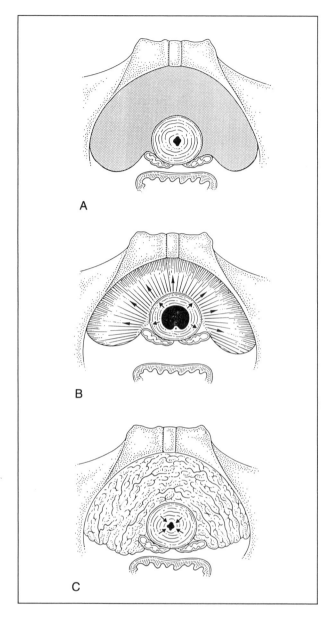

Figure 14-21. *The most common cause of bladder-neck sphincter incompetence after a pelvic fracture is retraction of a normal mechanism by hematoma fibrosis (B) resulting from the retraction of a surrounding pelvic floor hematoma (A). Competence is often restorable by excision of the hematoma fibrosis and its replacement by supple omentus (C). (Copyright 1984 by the Institute of Urology.)*

incision can be extended into a supple expandable tissue plane. Unfortunately, the pubourethral space is usually obliterated by dense hematoma fibrosis after pelvic fracture urethral injuries, so a simple incision into this tends to close immediately—hence it is most unlikely that any but the most minimal PFUDD will respond to satisfactory internal urethrotomy (Fig. 14-22). Furthermore, a distal extension of a urethrotomy into the normal proxi-

mal bulbar spongy tissue results in spongiofibrotic scarring and a reduction in the effective length of the mobilized bulbar urethra which may compromise an anastomotic retrievoplasty. A **dorsal** urethrotomy scar dictates the need for a **dorsal** spatulation and, consequently, a 180-degree rotation of the mobilized bulbar urethra in order to achieve its anastomosis with the **anterior** aspect of the apical prostatic urethra (Turner-Warwick, 1989b). Overenthusiasm for an extensive urethrotomy conducted on a "dead reckoning" basis and sometimes described as "cutting for the light" (of a suprapubic urethroscope)—and sometimes without light—can be disastrous (Turner-Warwick, 1989b).

The Shortcomings of Substitution Procedures

However, in a personal series of more than 600 PFUDD repairs, **provided the whole length of the bulbar urethra was normal**, it has almost invariably been possible to restore stricture-free urethral continuity by a deferred one-stage spatulated-overlap bulboprostatic anastomosis; the long-term reliability of this procedure is so good that the cause of any complications—and certainly any anastomotic restenosis—must be sought and reviewed. The inevitable incidence of complications inherent in all substitution procedures should never be introduced unless there is a specific indication in an individual case. However, the failure of a previous surgical repair of a PFUDD usually damages the previously normal bulbar urethra so that the reoperative procedure is likely to require a substitution procedure.

The Perineoabdominal Progression-Approach (PAPA) Procedure

The four-option progression-approach bulboprostatic anastomotic procedure that I advocate (Turner-Warwick, 1973, 1977, 1989) differs in significant detail from that described by Waterhouse et al. (1974)—total pubectomy has rarely been necessary, and I particularly emphasize the importance of complete clearance of the hematoma fibrosis and all fistulous tracts anterolaterally—as well as the obliteration of the consequent para-anastomotic dead space by redeployed omental support. Because it is a multiprocedural operation, it cannot be described as a single entity but only by outlining the principles of the various individual component procedures that may or may not be required—according to the findings at the time of operation. Careful attention to detail in every respect is essential to the avoidance of predictable complications (Turner-Warwick, 1989).

There are four distinct progression-approach options for the restoration of urethral continuity by the

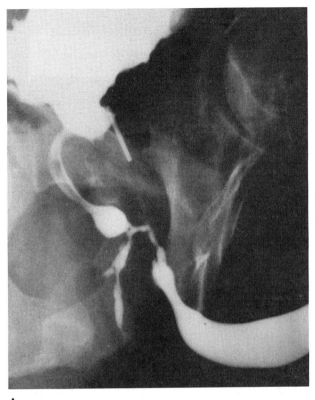
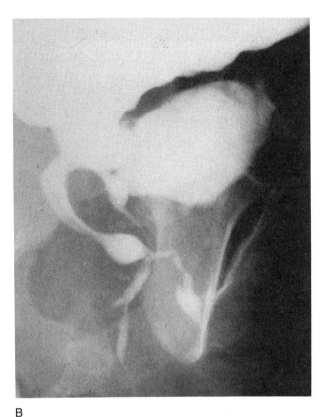

A   B

Figure 14-22. *A subprostatic urethral distraction defect with a perineal fistula disastrously complicated by iatrogenic incontinence. The only remaining sphincter mechanism at the bladder neck was transected by a grossly overenthusiastic "cutting-for-the-light" optical urethrotomy that was clearly more in the nature of "dead reckoning"—leaving* in situ *the broken knife blade, embedded in the dense hematofibrosis, as evidence of the misdemeanor. The retrievoplasty involved excision of the mass of the hematofibrosis and the broken knife blade with an omentum-supported sphincteroplasty of the bladder neck and a relatively simple anastomotic restoration of prostatobulbar urethral continuity. The patient is continent and stricture-free 8 years later. (Copyright 1987 by the Institute of Urology.)*

PAPA procedure: the perineal and three perineoabdominal procedures—retropubic, partial pubectomy, and the total pubectomy. These are summarized in Figure 14-23, and the technical details are recorded elsewhere (Turner-Warwick, 1986, 1989a).

The principles of the TITBAPIT procedure are just important to progression-approach reoperative PFUDD reconstruction as they are to elective first-time reconstructions, but of course, the likelihood of finding an undamaged bulbar urethra suitable for an anastomotic restoration of urethral continuity is naturally somewhat less.

Fixed-Flat Spatulated Bulbo-Prostatic Anastomosis

The remarkable reliability of anastomotic bulbo-prostatic restoration of urethral continuity is fundamentally dependent on meticulous technique. The inherent tendency of a spongy urethral anastomosis to contract and restenose can be prevented by the combination of an overlap spatulation and lateral spread-flat fixation. Because the subverumontanal urethra is usually more or less concentric within the apical tissue of the prostate, a wedge-shaped resection of the anterolateral sector of this is usually required to achieve the necessary fixed-flat spatulation (Fig. 14-24). Occasionally, however, the anterior commissure of the subverumontanal prostate is relatively deficient. Because the normal caliber of both the apical prostatic urethra and the posterior bulbar urethra is in the region of 25 French, the eventual caliber of an efficient overlap anastomosis should be 25 + 25 = 50 French—this short segment of augmented caliber persists as a small localized bulbar dilatation on follow-up urography, overtly excluding restenosis at the anastomosis.

Mobilization of the Bulbar Urethra to Achieve Its Tension-Free Approximation to the Prostate

After division of the bulbar urethra immediately below the subprostatic hematoma fibrosis, mobilization of a

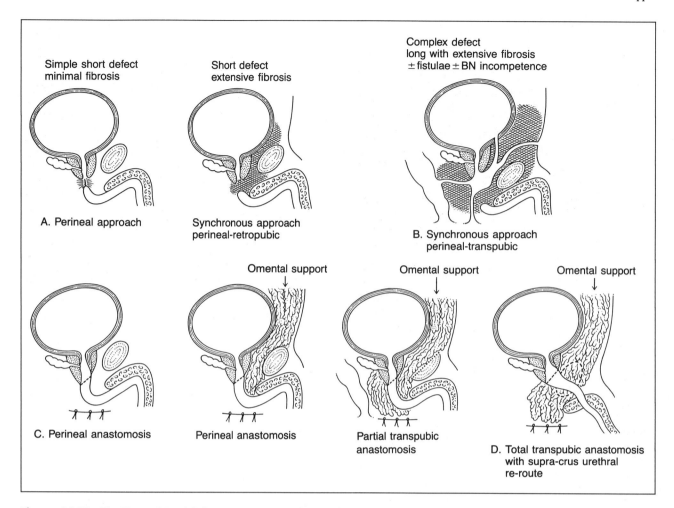

Figure 14-23. *The Turner-Warwick four-option perineoabdominal progression-approach (PAPA) procedures for the resolution of pelvic fracture urethral distraction defects, according to the findings at operation. A. The perineal approach. B. The perineoretropubic (P-R) procedure (perineal anastomosis with retropubic excision of hematoma fibrosis and omental support). C. The perineal partial-pubectomy (PPP) procedure (for abdominal-access anastomosis with omental support). D. The total pubectomy (TP) procedure (for supracrural rerouting of the mobilized urethra to reach a high prostatic dislocation, with omental support). (Copyright 1987 by the Institute of Urology.)*

normal bulbar urethra to the base of the penis generally achieves 4 to 5 cm of elastic lengthening—this is usually sufficient to achieve a tension-free 2-cm spatulated overlap anastomosis with the apical prostatic urethra after bridging a gap of 2.0 to 2.5 cm without rerouting (Fig. 14-25).

When the prostatobulbar gap is longer than 2 to 3 cm—as a result of a high dislocation of the prostate—or when the available elongation of the mobilized bulbar urethra has been foreshortened by damage due to previous surgical procedure, it may be necessary to reroute the mobilized bulbar urethra transpubically, over the penile crus on one side, to enable it to be anastomosed to a high-lying prostate. It is rarely necessary to

remove the whole of the pubis simply to gain adequate access for a bulboprostatic anastomosis from above—a partial resection of its posterior margin with a Capener's gouge is usually sufficient (Turner-Warwick, 1973, 1977, 1989a and b). With the exception of the rare coincidence of pubic osteomyelitis, the occasional need for supracrural urethral rerouting is virtually the only indication for a total pubectomy approach in the Turner-Warwick four-option PAPA approach procedure.

The posterior spongioplasty flap that is created by the preliminary separation of the eccentric bulk of the spongy tissue can be used to revascularize the mobilized bulbar urethra posteriorly by simple spongiospongioplasty overclosure after "windowing" its capsule (see

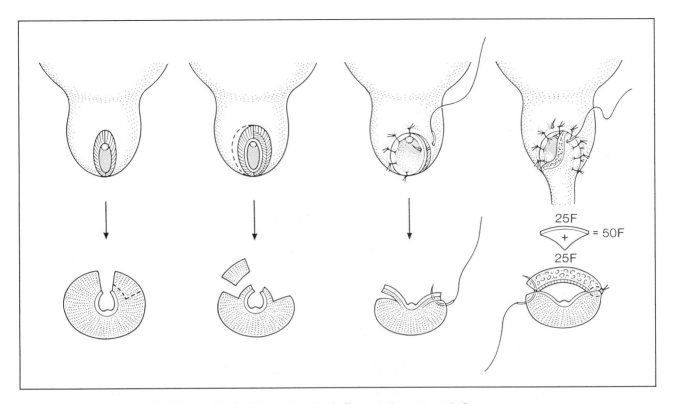

Figure 14-24. *The principles of a spatulated stricture-preventing bulboprostatic anastomosis. Because the urethra below the verumontanum is generally surrounded by apical prostatic tissue, an anterolateral wedge resection of this is required to enable it to be spread flat and anchored laterally to achieve a broad anastomosis to the spatulated proximal end of the mobilized bulbar urethra. This results in a permanent bulb-shaped augmentation of the caliber of the urethral lumen in the area of the spatulated overlap. (Copyright 1984 by the Institute of Urology.)*

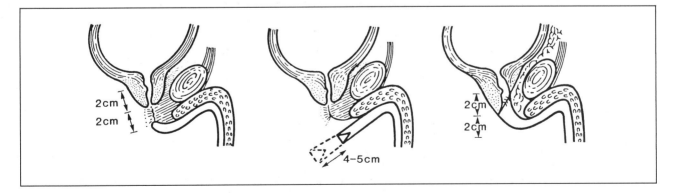

Figure 14-25. *The natural elasticity of the normal bulbar urethra generally provides 4 to 5 cm of lengthening after mobilizing it from the membranous urethra to the base of the penis—thus enabling a 3-cm or more subprostatic gap to be bridged with a 2-cm overlap anastomosis. An extended mobilization onto the penile shaft should never be undertaken to gain additional length because it not only compromises its retrograde vascularization but also creates penile curvature chordee. (Copyright 1982 by the Institute of Urology.)*

Fig. 14-17). This is particularly important when the bladder neck mechanism is damaged and an artificial sphincter is required because, otherwise, the fitting of its cuff around the bulbar urethra compromises the retrograde blood flow, and this increases the risk of erosion.

Complications Resulting from an Overextended Mobilization of the Bulbopenile Urethra

Any endeavor to obtain additional urethral length for tension-free approximation of the bulbar urethra to the prostate by **an extended mobilization of the penile urethra** is fundamentally contraindicated.

1. The available longitudinal elasticity of the penile urethra is naturally extended during an erection, and any attempt to gain extra urethral length by mobilizing the penile urethra tends to result in a curvature chordee of the penile shaft (Turner-Warwick, 1986, 1989a and b) (Fig. 14-26).
2. The spongy tissue of the bulbar urethra receives its main blood supply from the posterior bulbar vessels. When these are divided by a proximal urethral transection, the retrograde blood flow along the normal bulbopenile spongy tissue derived from its distal collateral vascular communications is usually sufficient to maintain its viability (Fig. 14-27). However, the vascularization may be critically impaired by an overextensive mobilization of the urethra onto the penile shaft and also by extensive spongiofibrosis resulting from previous urethritis or urethral surgery—resulting in spongionecrotic loss of the posterior bulbar urethra that necessitates a substitution retrievoplasty (Fig. 14-28).

Hematoma Fibrosis, False Passages, and Their Excision. The hematoma fibrosis created by the organization of a sizable pelvic floor hematoma forms a cast around dislocated but largely undamaged structures like a "concrete boot." Thus, once the incarcerated prostatic tissue is liberated, it is quite normal and supple. The meticulous and complete excision of all the anterolateral paraanastomotic hematoma fibrosis is a time-consuming procedure that I sometimes refer to as a "Michael Angelo procedure" because "the beauty is hidden in the marble"—however, it is a particularly important component of a reliable complication-free restoration of prostatobulbar urethral continuity.

Occlusion of the Paraanastomotic Dead-Space by Pedicled Omental Support. When the paraurethral fibrosis associated with a short-gap defect is minimal, it can be removed and the anastomosis completed through a

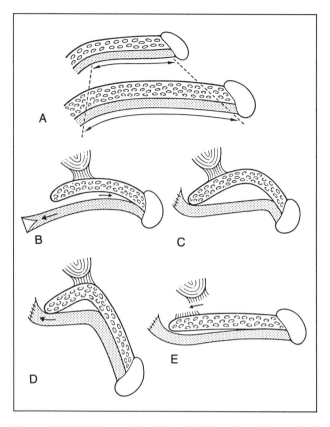

Figure 14-26. *The mechanical principles of anterior urethral mobilization. The available elastic lengthening of the penile urethra is naturally somewhat stretched during an erection (A). Endeavors to obtain additional urethral length for an anastomotic repair by mobilizing the penile urethra (B) result in penile curvature chordee (C). Angulation chordee after bulbar urethral mobilization (D) can be reduced by division of the angulating fulcrum created by the adventitial element of the suspensory ligament (E); this does not result in any significant disability of the erection. (Copyright 1984 by the Institute of Urology.)*

perineal approach. However, the removal of any but a minimally extensive hematoma fibrosis associated with a urethral distraction-defect creates a sizable dead-space cavity because the fibro-osseous walls of this cavity are rigid and cannot collapse. Serosanguineous exudates accumulating within this dead space around a bulboprostatic anastomotic suture line predispose to the complications of suture-line leakage, fistulation, and eventual restenosis due to its organization and fibrosis.

The reliability of an anastomotic repair of a complex pelvic fracture urethral defect is greatly increased by the routine obliteration of any significant perianastomotic dead space with a pedicled omental graft (Turner-Warwick, 1973, 1976, 1977). Omental wrapping not only reduces the incidence of anastomotic compli-

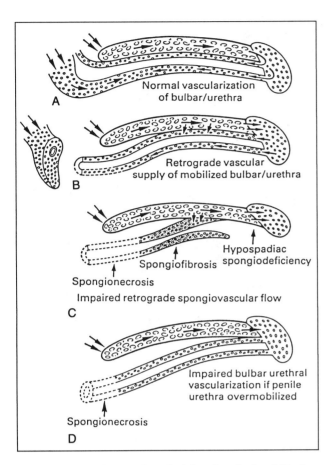

Figure 14-27. *The vascular principles of urethral mobilization. After division of the main posteriorly entering bulbar arteries, vascularization of the proximal end of the mobilized bulbar urethra is dependent on the retrograde blood supply along its spongy tissue (A, B). Ischemic necrosis of the proximal end of the mobilized urethra may result when the retrograde blood supply is compromised by hypospadiac maldevelopment (C), incidental spongiofibrosis, or division of distal collateral vessels by mobilization of the penile urethra (D). (Copyright 1984 by the Institute of Urology.)*

cations to practically zero but also is fundamental to the functional success of bladder-neck sphincteroplasty (Turner-Warwick, 1973, 1986, 1989, 1993b)—the Turner-Warwick PAPA procedure was specifically developed to achieve this. One of three definitive omental pedicle mobilization procedures is required to enable the omental apron to reach the perineum (Fig. 14-29)—these are detailed elsewhere (Turner-Warwick, 1976, 1989).

Impotence. The erection mechanism may be damaged by pelvic fracture injuries that do not result in urethral injury—the incidence is higher when the urethra is ruptured and much higher when the prostate is grossly dislocated (Turner-Warwick, 1977, 1983, 1989). The Brindley procedure for the investigation of impotence by intracorporal papaverine injections has shown that pelvic fracture erection failure is more often the result of damage to its neural than to its vascular mechanism. Owing to the posterolateral proximity of the nervi erigentes to the subprostatic urethra, which are somewhat tethered within the fibrotic perineal body, it is probable that most subprostatic dislocations are associated with some degree of injury to the neural mechanisms of potency, irrespective of whether they result in an overt impairment of erection or not. Any local operation, immediate or deferred, in the area of a secondary hematoma fibrosis behind the apex of the prostate must carry some risk of critically extending any primary local neuropathy associated with the original injury—particularly if it involves dissection or separation of the tissue planes behind the apex of the prostate. A strictly anterior approach to surgical repairs in this area is therefore advocated, using the perineoabdominal progression-approach (PAPA) operating position/procedure and avoiding any disturbance or mobilization of the posterolateral retroprostatic tissue plane and the posterolateral angle of the pubourethral space whenever possible. Unfortunately, the traditional exaggerated lithotomy position tends to encourage such a posterior approach.

The Perineo-Abdominal Progression-Approach (PAPA) Operating Position and Procedure

The perineo-abdominal operating position (Fig. 14-30) is essential for the "four-option" PAPA procedure (see Fig. 14-23). When an abdominal approach is required, a midline abdominal incision should always be used because it may be necessary to extend this up to the xiphisternum to obtain access for mobilization of the right gastroepiploic vascular pedicle of the omentum from the stomach to enable a short-apron omentum to be repositioned in the pelvis.

Shortcomings of the Limited-Option Perineal/Pubectomy Approach Procedures

A synchronous cystogram and retrograde urethrogram—the "up-and-down-agram"—reveals most of the features that identify a PFUDD as "complex"—and consequently requiring a synchronous perineoabdominal approach repair. However, it is fundamentally important to appreciate that the radiographic demonstration of a short-gap prostatobulbar urethral defect is not a valid basis for a surgical assumption that it is "simple"

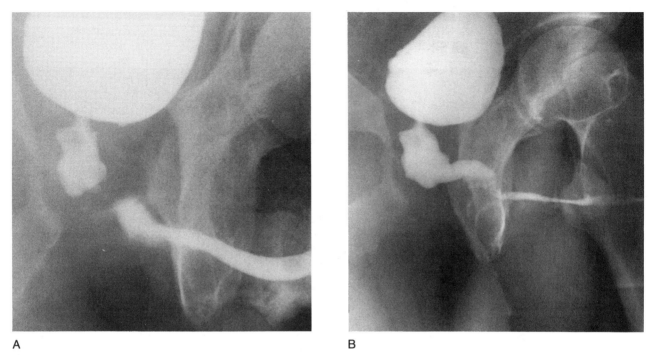

A
B

Figure 14-28. *A. Spongionecrosis of the proximal bulbar urethra resulting from ischemia due to over-mobilization of the penile urethra commonly results in a prostatobulbar urethral defect. B. A circumferential PIPS substitution retrievoplasty was required to restore urethral continuity. (Copyright 1992 by the Institute of Urology.)*

and consequently appropriate for a perineal-approach repair; this can only be determined accurately by the operative findings at the time of reconstruction. Hence preoperative "gapometry" has limited value, and it is irrelevant to the planning of a PAPA procedure (Turner-Warwick, 1973, 1976, 1983, 1989).

However, in many urologic units, the choice of access for the repair of pelvic fracture urethral defects is commonly limited to two antipodal-approach procedures—the simple perineal and the formal total pubectomy (transpubic)—without intermediate options that extend an inadequate exposure on the one hand and avoid an unnecessarily extensive bone resection and its occasionally attendant complications on the other. This shortcoming is often augmented by the use of quite different operating positions—the exaggerated lithotomy position that is often favored for a perineal approach procedure is singularly ill-adapted to perioperative extension of the procedure to a pubectomy procedure when the need for this becomes apparent in the course of the operation. Consequently, a surgeon using these either/or approach procedures has to elect, preoperatively, which to use—although the factors on

which the decision should be properly based may not become apparent until they are revealed in the course of the operation.

While a perineal-approach procedure may be appropriate for the majority of pelvic fracture urethral distraction-defects—because they are most commonly "simple"—some reports record an incidence of complications such as anastomotic fistulas, restenosis, and incontinence that I would regard as unacceptable—many of these are avoidable by use of the appropriate progression-approach and omental-wrap procedures. Thus, however "simple" a short-gap pelvic fracture urethral defect may appear to be, I strongly advocate the reservation of appropriate operating time, surgical experience, and cross-matched blood to enable a perineal-approach procedure to be immediately extended into a synchronous abdominal-approach procedure if the operative findings so indicate. Only thus can one avoid the occasional disaster of failure to achieve a satisfactory anastomotic repair that is stricture-free in the long term because of an unexpected encounter with an extensive block of solid hematoma fibrosis "concrete" around a beguilingly short-gap defect.

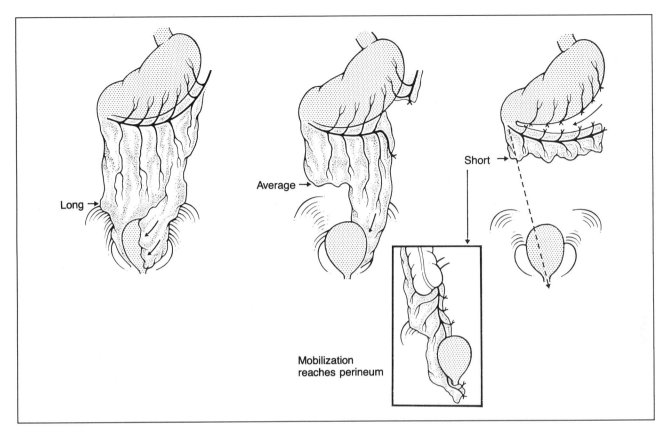

Figure 14-29. *In about 30 percent of cases, the omental apron is long enough to reach the perineum after its simple separation from the transverse colon and mesocolon—in another 30 percent, an additional division of its minor left gastric epiploic pedicle is required. In 40 percent, a formal mobilization of the whole length of its major right gastroepiploic vascular pedicle from the stomach is required—in such cases the pedicle should be protected by positioning it behind the mobilized right colon. (Copyright 1963 by the Institute of Urology.)*

Urinary Continence and Restoration of Bladder-Neck Sphincter Function

Because the function of the distal sphincter mechanism is generally destroyed by a urethral distraction injury, urinary continence thereafter is fundamentally dependent on the bladder-neck function. It is important to evaluate the potential of its competence preoperatively and to include an appropriate functional restoration procedure as part of the repair when necessary (Turner-Warwick, 1986, 1989a and b, 1991, 1993a). Thus failure to demonstrate the prostatic urethra by preoperative cystography is often regarded as a nuisance because it precludes measurement of the "prostatobulbar urethral gap," but it is, in reality, reassuring evidence of the competence of the bladder neck—while a mechanism that remains open during bladder filling indicates that it is incompetent.

The most common cause of incompetence of the bladder-neck sphincter after a pelvic fracture is external circumferential tethering of a normal uninjured mechanism by the contraction of retropubic hematoma fibrosis (see Fig. 14-22). The endoscopic appearances of this are those of a fixedly open but otherwise normal circular and unscarred bladder-neck mechanism; its simple mobilization, by resection of the fibrosis anteriorly and laterally, together with its replacement by a supple omental pedicle wrap, is often all that is necessary to restore its competence. However, a bladder neck that has sector scarring usually requires a definitive reduction sphincteroplasty (Turner-Warwick, 1986, 1989, 1989). Thus, whenever a bladder neck appears to be incompetent on preoperative cystourethrography, I advocate one of the synchronous perineo-abdominal procedures and a bladder-neck sphincteroplasty in an endeavor to avoid the need for an artificial sphincter

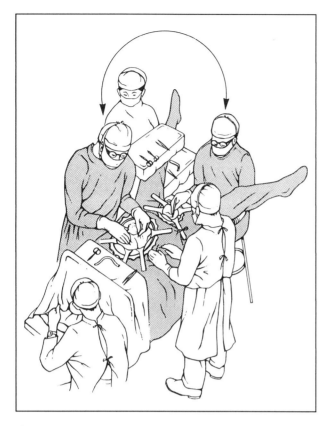

Figure 14-30. *The perineo-abdominal progression-approach (PAPA)-operating position is preferred for all perineal and pelvic surgical procedures. It is essential for the Turner-Warwick "four-option" progression procedure for the resolution of pelvic fracture urethral distraction defects. Irrespective of the apparent simplicity or complexity of the urethral injury preoperatively and the anticipated extent of the procedure, the patient is positioned on the operating table for a synchronous perineo-abdominal procedure, tilted slightly head downward, legs widely abducted, and with only moderate flexion. The patient is prepared and draped with a single sterile operating field; this facilitates the progression from a perineal to a perineo-abdominal approach—with or without partial or total resection of the pubic bone—according to the findings as the operation proceeds. For the perineal approach, the surgeon is seated with the scrub nurse and the instrument table immediately to the right (or left, if left-handed). If a perineal-approach repair proves difficult or inappropriate, the surgeon moves round to the abdominal-approach position, and the scrub nurse and the instrument table move between the legs. The universal Turner-Warwick perineo-abdominal ring retractors provide excellent exposure without the need for a retracting assistant. The surgeon repositions—from the abdomen to the perineum and back—as often as required in the course of the operation. It is unnecessary to have two surgeons for a synchronous approach. (Copyright 1984 by the Institute of Urology.)*

(Turner-Warwick, 1986, 1989a and b; Turner-Warwick and Kirby, 1993).

The preoperative identification of bladder-neck incompetence is particularly important in short-gap defects because this is, in itself, a definitive indication of the need for a synchronous lower-abdominal exploration, even if the urethral distraction-defect is otherwise apparently suitable for perineal-approach repair. Retropubic fibrosis resulting from an independent pelvic floor hematoma which is not in continuity with the minimal fibrosis associated with a short-gap urethral lesion (see Fig. 14-18) may not be identifiable during a simple perineal repair, and failure to check this and to attend to it appropriately results in avoidable incontinence. The "retropubic option" of the progression-approach procedures was specifically developed for the resolution of this type of short-gap stenosis; in this procedure, the actual anastomotic restoration of urethral continuity is usually achieved from the perineum (Turner-Warwick, 1983, 1986, 1989).

Retrieval Bulbo-Prostatic Reanastomotic Repair

Remobilization of the bulbar urethra is usually possible after a previous anastomotic repair so that most **short** bulboprostatic anastomotic restenoses can be resolved by a reanastomotic repair. However, a longer defect due to loss of the proximal bulbar urethra (see Fig. 14-27)—a situation that not uncommonly results from ischemia due to overextensive mobilization of the penile urethra in an endeavor to gain extra length for a bulbo-prostatic anastomotic repair—unfortunately requires a circumferential substitution reconstruction.

Rectal Fistula

A coincident rectal fistula is not an uncommon feature of complex pelvic fracture urethral injuries—there have been more than 30 in our series. If a fistula is not already protected by a defunctioning colostomy, a preoperative bowel preparation and a perioperative temporary loop ileostomy are required. In the majority of cases, the fistulous track into the rectum is quite small so that, after appropriate resection of the hematoma fibrosis associated with the urethral distraction-defect down to the rectal wall and the restoration of urethral continuity, the simple occlusion of the dead space by the omental pedicle graft is often sufficient to occlude the fistula orifice without a formal suture closure (Fig. 14-31).

The Results of Urethroplasty

Most publications have recorded the results of one individual operation, and this tends to underemphasize the

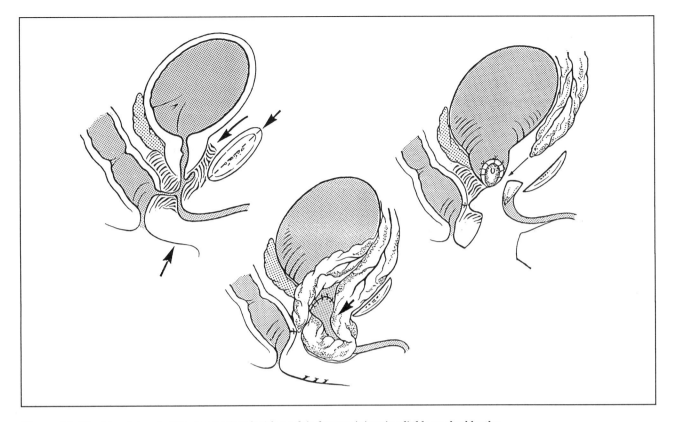

Figure 14-31. *A prostatorectal fistula associated with a pelvic fracture injury is reliably resolved by the Turner-Warwick omentum-supported bulbo-prostatic anastomotic repair. If the fistulous track is small, as it often is, a formal suture closure is usually unnecessary. (Copyright 1972 by the Institute of Urology.)*

fundamental importance of selecting the most appropriate procedure for the particular stricture. However, Webster et al. (1985) reviewed the management of 100 cases of urethral stricture. The results of 29 anastomotic repairs of traumatic strictures were recorded with only 1 failure; 34 full-thickness skin-graft repairs with 5 failures; 13 pedicled island grafts with 1 failure; 24 two-stage repairs of complex full-length strictures with 2 failures; the overall failure rate of 9 percent might have been reduced by a third if free-graft repairs of extragenital skin had not been used. These are the realistic expectations of the results of appropriately selected definitive repairs of urethral strictures and distraction-defects in a specializing unit.

Our own experience indicates that a failure rate greater than 5 percent within 5 years after a urethral substitution procedure—and almost any restenosis after a one-stage anastomotic repair—should cause reconstructive surgeons to reflect on ways to improve their results. But these two procedures are quite different. A satisfactory spatulated anastomosis of normal urethra to normal urethra that is stable after 2 years is likely to

remain so—almost indefinitely. However, because there is no perfect substitute for the urethra in the long term, even if a substitution urethroplasty is satisfactory after 5 years, there is a continuing incidence of restenosis in the region of about 1 percent per year.

The Results of the Progression-Approach Pelvic Fracture Urethral Distraction-Defect Repair Procedure

Although a progression-approach repair of a complex urethral distraction injury may take several hours when an abdominal extension is necessary, it must be one of the most cost-effective multi-major procedural operations because it provides an extraordinarily high expectation that a young suprapubic-catheter-dependent urologic cripple will, within about 3 weeks, be voiding freely with satisfactory urinary control and without the need for any further routine urethral instrumentation or long-term follow-up supervision.

The observations in this chapter are based on a personal series of more than 650 PFUDD reconstructions between 1960 and 1992. However, it is important to recognize that the case mix of the patients treated in different specialist centers is variously skewed by the selection factors involved in their particular tertiary referral patterns. Naturally, patients who can be managed conservatively tend not to be referred to a specializing center. Those who have to travel long distances, especially those from overseas, tend to be the more complicated ones—often, unfortunately, as a result of many previous surgical failures. Thus the incidence of abdominal progression procedures in our series reflects this— and also our endeavor to restore the function of an overtly incompetent only remaining sphincter mechanism at the bladder neck. A successful sphincteroplasty is obviously preferable to an artificial sphincter (Turner-Warwick and Kirby, 1993)—especially for overseas patients who cannot afford one. Most PFUDD accident patients have low-income, high-injury-risk jobs—and the great majority of road accident injuries are pedestrians—not car drivers.

Thus the relatively high incidence of abdominal progression procedures in our series—compared to that of Webster et al.—does not indicate a marked difference in our surgical philosophies because we are in broad agreement—however, we do differ significantly from the Waterhouse transpubic approach as the routine alternative to a perineal approach.

An analysis of 308 consecutive cases at the Middlesex and St. Peter's Hospitals between 1974 and 1991 emphasizes the relevant perspectives of some points. The selection of the aliquot of 308 patients for analysis from our series of more than 600 was simply and fairly based on their country of origin (particularly the United Kingdom, Australasia, and certain European countries) because this made an acceptable follow-up possible. Of these 308 patients, 183 had had one or more (sometimes many) previous surgical failures—and so required a retrievoplasty—162 by anastomosis and 21 by substitution. Of the 287 (162 + 125) patients who had an anastomotic repair, the known incidence of recurrent stenosis over periods of 1 to 16 years has been 7—only 2 of these were located at the anastomosis; the remaining 5 were late-developing bulbopenile strictures—all in the group of 162 patients who had had previous operations. This probably reflected an underlying subclinical spongiofibrosis resulting from the earlier treatment. The low incidence of restenosis at the anastomosis, and the absence of any fistulas, must surely be further testimony to the extraordinary efficiency of the vascularized omental support. The success of our endeavor to improve the functional incompetence of the bladder-neck sphincter by bladder-neck lysis omental wrap (LOW) procedure

has been in the region of 75 percent or more and by a reduction sphincteroplasty for a sector defect about 60 percent or more—but our analysis of these data is not yet complete.

Reference to personal publications in this chapter is made to provide the background of personal viewpoints and statements—no one is more conscious than we are of the contributions of many friends and colleagues across the world who are interested in and have contributed greatly to this most intriguing field of surgery. We are also particularly grateful to the many—worldwide— who have most graciously referred the patients that created the series of several thousand reconstructions upon which this communication is based—and indeed, no less, to the patients themselves.

Conclusions

Times have changed—and urology is not what it was. It is no longer possible for a general urologist to have an indepth competence in more than one or two of the many expanding subspecialist fields—pediatric urology, oncology, reconstruction and functional restoration, renal stone surgery, gynecourology, spinal injuries, transplantation, fertility and andrology, and so on. The advances in definitive reconstructive procedures have naturally stemmed from subspecialization.

While some techniques for the resolution of urethral strictures—such as internal urethrotomy—are rightly regarded as "general urologic" procedures, the problems involved in definitive urethral and sphincter reconstruction should not be underestimated. Any operative procedure that fails—however well intentioned and however well performed—inevitably complicates a subsequent retrievoplasty. Surgeons who do not have a special additional experience of reconstructive procedures, and a particular aptitude for them, must be advised that "having a go" at complex problems cannot be in the best interest of their patients. The importance of this should not overlooked—there should be no brave surgeons—just brave patients.

Although interdisciplinary cooperation is often admirable for the occasional case—"committee surgery"—involving a urologic, a gynecologic, colorectal, and plastic surgeons—it is surely an outdated concept of reconstructive pelvic surgery for routine procedures. Effective reconstructive urinary tract surgery often involves pelvic surgery as a whole, and this should be regarded as a "horizontal" surgical specialty with appropriate training—in much the same way that other regional specialties have developed—such as hand surgery and head and neck surgery. However, while there can be no question of a particular "right" way of doing any surgical procedure, there are certainly many "wrong" ways. The avoidance of complications and the need for retrieval procedures are the essence of good surgery, and this is essentially a personal matter because many contrarily conceived procedures work quite satisfactorily in the hands of others.

Thus, in addition to a training in "general urology," surgeons undertaking urinary tract reconstruction should have an additional period of training in plastic surgical techniques and tissue handling and a particular personal aptitude for meticulous surgical minutiae. Furthermore, they should have an instinctive inclination to adopt and to adapt procedures, according to the findings at the time of operation—specializing reconstructive surgeons are rarely able to precisely predict the procedure most appropriate for the repair of a particular stricture preoperatively. Furthermore, reconstructive surgery is time consuming but rarely urgent, in the medical sense—consequently, it has a relatively low priority in a busy urologic service unit. To specialize exclusively, reconstructive surgeons require a "protected" working environment in association with colleagues who are themselves enthusiastically oriented to the care of the various urgencies of cancer, stones, and emergencies. Unfortunately, there are as yet remarkably few such coordinated referral units in the world.

Bibliography

Chilton, C, and Turner-Warwick, R. The relationship of the distal sphincter mechanism to the pelvic floor musculature. Ann R Coll Surg 67:54, 1985.

Hamilton Russell, R. The treatment of urethral strictures by excision Br J Surg 2:375, 1914.

Milroy, EJG, et al. A new treatment for urethral strictures—A permanently implanted stent. J Urol 141:1120, 1989.

Orandi, A. One-stage urethroplasty—A four-year follow-up. J Urol 107:977, 1972.

Turner-Warwick, R. The repair of urethral strictures in the region of the membranous urethra. J Urol 100:303, 1968.

Turner-Warwick, R. The use of pedicle grafts in the repair of urinary tract fistulae. Br J Urol 44:644, 1972.

Turner-Warwick, R. Observations on the treatment of traumatic urethral injuries and the value of the fenestrated urethral catheter. Br J Surg 60:775, 1973.

Turner-Warwick, R. The use of the omental pedicle graft in urinary tract reconstructions. J Urol 116:341, 1976.

Turner-Warwick, R. Complex traumatic strictures. J Urol 118:546, 1977.

Turner-Warwick, R. Clinical urodynamics. Urol Clin North Am 6:13, 1979.

Turner-Warwick, R. The sphincter mechanisms—The avoidance of postprostatectomy incontinence. In W Webber and D Jonas (eds), Die Post-Operative Harninkontinenz des Mannes Internationales Symposium. Stuttgart: Thieme, 1981, pp 17–33.

Turner-Warwick, R. The sphincter mechanisms: Their relation to prostatic enlargment and its treatment. In F Hinman and GD Chisholm (eds), Benign Prostatic Hypertrophy. New York: Springer-Verlag, 1983a, pp 809–828.

Turner-Warwick, R. Postprostatectomy sphincter-strictures. In F Hinman and GD Chisholm (eds), Benign Prostatic Hypertrophy. New York: Springer-Verlag, 1983b, pp 979–984.

Turner-Warwick, R. Urethral stricture surgery. In AR Mundy (ed), Current Operative Urology. New York: Churchill Livingstone, 1989a, pp 215–218.

Turner-Warwick, R. The prevention of complications of urethral injuries. Urol Clin North Am 16:335, 1989b.

Turner-Warwick, R. The anatomical basis of functional reconstruction of the urethra. In M Droller (ed), Anatomical Approach to the Surgical Management of Urological Disease. St Louis: Mosby–Year Book, 1991, chap 60.

Turner-Warwick, R. The principles of urethroplasty. In GF Webster, R Kirby, and L King (eds), Reconstructive Urological Surgery. Oxford: Blackwell, 1993a, chap 46.

Turner-Warwick, R. The principles of hypospadiac and epispadiac retrievoplasty. In GF Webster, R Kirby, and L King (eds), Reconstructive Urological Surgery. Oxford: Blackwell, 1993b, chap 55.

Turner-Warwick, R, and Kirby, R. The principles of sphincteroplasty. In GF Webster, R Kirby, and L King (eds), Reconstructive Urological Surgery. Oxford: Blackwell, 1993, chap 48.

Turner-Warwick, R, Wynne, EJC, and Handley Ashken, M. The use of the omentum in the repair and reconstruction of the urinary tract. Br J Surg 54:849, 1967.

Waterhouse, K, et al. Transpubic repair of membranous urethral strictures. J Urol 111:188, 1974.

Webster, GD, Koefoot, RB, and Sihelnik, SA. The urethroplasty management of 100 cases of urethral stricture—A rationale for procedure selection. J Urol 134:892, 1985.

Stress Incontinence

ERNEST M. SUSSMAN
DEBORAH R. ERICKSON
SHLOMO RAZ

Recurrent stress urinary incontinence (RSUI) is not an uncommon problem in female urology. After the original anti-incontinence procedure, anywhere from 5 to 40 percent of women will be bothered by either a persistence or recurrence of their stress urinary incontinence (SUI) which will, in some situations, actually become worse than their preoperative status. The goal of this chapter will be to discuss the pathophysiology and classification of recurrent stress urinary incontinence and specifically the reoperative surgery that we recommend. Conservative and medical interventions are outside the realm of this chapter and will not be emphasized. The various modalities for treating both recurrent anatomic (hypermobility) and intrinsic (poor urethral coaptation) stress urinary incontinence will be highlighted.

Etiology of Recurrent Incontinence

An important point to remember is that the condition of genuine stress urinary incontinence is the loss of urine per urethra coincident with an increase in intraabdominal pressure in the absence of any involuntary detrusor activity. Stress urinary incontinence may be due to malposition of the normal sphincteric unit (anatomic incontinence, AI) or due to dysfunction of the sphincteric unit (intrinsic sphincteric dysfunction, ISD) as a result of paralysis, radiation, trauma, or multiple surgeries.

Aside from stress urinary incontinence other sources for urethral loss of urine include urgency incontinence and urethral diverticula (Table 15-1). Watery discharge per vagina after an anti-incontinence procedure is not always from the urethral meatus, and other causes for the extraurethral drainage (leakage) must be ruled out

during the process of performing a detailed workup for recurrent stress urinary incontinence. This will become obvious if diligently searched for and includes (1) genitourinary fistulas (vesicovaginal, ureterovaginal, and urethrovaginal), (2) fallopian tube discharge, and (3) congenital abnormalities such as ureteral ectopia.

Nonstress Incontinence

Urgency Incontinence

Urgency incontinence is an abnormal loss of urine per urethra caused by involuntary detrusor contractions and exists in between 15 and 30 percent of patients undergoing stress urinary incontinence surgery. Reportedly, between 60 and 85 percent of these patients should have resolution or a vast improvement of their urinary incontinence after an anti-incontinence procedure. On the other hand, de novo urinary incontinence after surgery for stress urinary incontinence has been reported in between 5 and 15 percent of most reported series. Careful history taking along with a properly performed urodynamic assessment should identify these patients both preoperatively and postoperatively. The most important diagnostic maneuver in patients with urinary incontinence is to accurately identify stress urinary incontinence preoperatively before any anti-incontinence surgery is undertaken (see diagnosis section). Anticholinergic medication (oxybutynin, hyoscyamine sulfate, or propantheline bromide) with or without the addition of imipramine hydrochloride or estrogen has been helpful in this subgroup of patients in controlling their urinary incontinence. Urinary tract infections, occult carcinoma in situ, iatrogenic intra-

Table 15-1. *Etiology of Incontinence*

Per urethra
  Stress
    Anatomic incontinence (AI)
    Intrinsic sphincter dysfunction (ISD)
  Urge incontinence
  Urethral diverticula
  Overflow incontinence
  Congenital (epispadias, ureteral ectopia)
Extraurethral
  Fistulas (vesicovaginal, urethrovaginal, ureterovaginal)
  Hydrops tubae profluens
  Congenital (ureteral ectopia, vaginal cysts)

---

vesical suture placement, and neurologic lesions must be ruled out before assigning a patient into this subgroup of idiopathic bladder instability.

Diverticula

Urethral diverticula as a cause of urinary incontinence are extremely rare. Patients will frequently complain of lower tract irritative voiding symptoms along with postvoid dribbling. An anterior vaginal wall mass may be palpated which after milking of the urethra can cause urine from the diverticular sac to be expressed at the external meatus. A diverticulum can occasionally be found coexistent with anatomic stress urinary incontinence. Our preference for repair in this situation would be to combine a formal diverticular repair along with the Raz bladder neck suspension (BNS); however, other techniques may be employed depending on surgeon preference. This is done, of course, only in those patients whose stress urinary incontinence is due to anatomic incontinence. The key in this combined approach is to perform the bladder neck suspension first, transferring the nonabsorbable sutures suprapubically before completing the diverticular repair to diminish the chances for retropubic space infection. We have not had any increase in the number of complications using this maneuver. If intrinsic sphincter dysfunction is the cause for the recurrent stress urinary incontinence, then a staged procedure performing the diverticulectomy first with some form of urethral compressive manuever to follow would be more appropriate (see treatment for intrinsic sphincter dysfunction).

Fistulas

A vesicovaginal fistula (VVF) should be highly suspected as a cause of extraurethral urinary leakage especially after a hysterectomy. Patients with recurrent stress urinary incontinence also may have a vesicovaginal fistula which may actually mask their stress urinary incontinence component. The diagnosis is made either with a cystogram or with the intravesical administration of any of the available vital dyes and a vaginally placed tampon.

Urethrovaginal fistulas may be more difficult to diagnose; however, a high index of suspicion should suggest this entity. Patients usually will complain of alterations in their urinary stream and have leakage per vagina after urination. Physical examination, voiding cystography, cystoscopy, and/or vaginoscopy can help confirm the diagnosis.

Ureterovaginal fistulas can occur alone or in combination with a vesicovaginal fistula. Ureteral genitourinary fistulas also can be diagnosed utilizing the pad-tampon test after either an oral urine colorizing agent (phenazopyridine) or intravenous agent (indigo carmine) is administered. A positive test here, in the face of a negative pad-tampon test after intravesical dye administration, thus ruling out a vesicovaginal fistula, is almost confirmatory. Intravenous urography may demonstrate complete or partial obstruction and establish the diagnosis; however, retrograde studies are frequently necessary to fully delineate this abnormal communication.

Hydrops Tubae Profluens

Another rare form of vaginal drainage is hydrosalpinx, which is an abnormal fallopian tubovaginal leakage into the vaginal cuff after an abdominal hysterectomy. Leach et al. described two of these cases, one of which was found in coexistence with stress urinary incontinence. Diagnosis may be demonstrated with the aid of a negative oral phenazopyridine test proving the urine not to be the source of leakage. Vaginoscopy and a vaginogram are then used to locate this abnormal communication. Treatment consists of a transperitoneal repair and Burch colposuspension if coexisting stress urinary incontinence is present.

Congenital

Congenital abnormalities, including ureteral ectopia, should rarely persist into the elderly population without escaping detection. Young adolescents or even teenage girls with presumed stress urinary incontinence should be evaluated carefully for these rare forms of incontinence. Antegrade contrast studies along with voiding cystography can aid in the detection of these abnormalities.

Pathophysiology of Recurrent Stress Urinary Incontinence

As with stress urinary incontinence, the pathophysiology of recurrent stress urinary incontinence must be considered in the context of either of two types: (1) anatomic incontinence due to displacement or hypermobility of the sphincteric unit or (2) intrinsic sphincter dysfunction due to malfunction of the normal sphincteric unit as a result of radiation, multiple surgery, trauma, or neurologic disease.

When the patient with recurrent stress urinary incontinence presents after having had a bladder neck suspension for anatomic incontinence and the patient was well selected, the key factor in determining the pathophysiology of these operative failures is whether or not the bladder neck is adequately supported and whether the operation helped at all. This can best be determined by combining the history and physical examination, with voiding cystourethrography (see diagnosis section). Within this context, *recurrent* stress urinary incontinence signifies that the bladder neck suspension was initially curative, while *persistent* stress urinary incontinence indicates that the stress urinary incontinence was never helped. Three clinical scenarios are possible: (1) recurrent stress urinary incontinence with good support, (2) recurrent stress urinary incontinence with recurrent hypermobility, and (3) persistent stress urinary incontinence with or without hypermobility (the operation never helped).

If a patient has good support of the bladder neck after a bladder neck suspension and has persistent or recurrent incontinence, then the following diagnoses must be entertained in the pathophysiologic differential diagnoses of this abnormal urethral incontinence: (1) urinary incontinence, (2) intrinsic pathology, including foreign bodies or suture material, and most important, (3) underlying intrinsic sphincter dysfunction.

If the patient develops recurrent stress urinary incontinence after a prolonged period of clinical cure and has a bladder neck that is hypermobile, then certainly failure from either suture breakage or erosion from the paraurethral tissues is the most common cause. Factors that may predispose to recurrent stress urinary incontinence in these scenarios include (1) type of suture material (absorbable material has a higher tendency to fail), (2) quality of the tissues that are incorporated in the suspension, and (3) unusual physical stresses (chronic coughing or obesity).

If the patient with poor support has persistent stress urinary incontinence, that is, never having gained benefit from the bladder neck suspension, then most probably the sutures were never properly placed in the paraurethral tissues surrounding the bladder neck. Rarely, inadequate suture tension also may contribute to this scenario. We have referred to these paraurethral tissues as the so-called good stuff that supports the bladder neck

and proximal urethra. These tissues represent the urethropelvic ligaments that reside lateral to the bladder neck. Anatomically, the urethropelvic ligament is a condensation of the periurethral and endopelvic fasciae that provides support of the above-mentioned structures to the tendinous arc on the lateral pelvic sidewall.

In patients with failure after a urethral sling or artificial urinary sphincter for intrinsic sphincter dysfunction, the above-mentioned factors for recurrent stress urinary incontinence in a patient with good bladder neck support following a bladder neck suspension for anatomic incontinence can be included. Failure to adequately compress the urethra during the initial operative procedure, however, is usually the source of the recurrent stress urinary incontinence in these patients with intrinsic sphincter dysfunction.

Diagnosis

Patients with recurrent stress urinary incontinence must be evaluated in a very thorough manner, which should include a history, physical examination, urinalysis, cystoscopy, and radiographic and urodynamic evaluation. The clinician again should keep in mind any of the above-mentioned differential diagnoses for extraurethral vaginal leakage.

History

Patients will subjectively report their incontinence, and most of the time it will become evident what type they have. Frequently, the clinician may need to prompt the patient as to the nature of the incontinence. Stress urinary incontinence due to anatomic incontinence typically occurs only at the time of stress, and characteristically, patients are dry in the supine position. On the other hand, intrinsic sphincter dysfunction may produce stress urinary incontinence caused by minor exertional forces such as with positional changes or even with stressful maneuvers in the supine position. One careful distinction in the evaluation is to discern genuine stress urinary incontinence from stress-induced instability producing the incontinence. With stress urinary incontinence, the patient will lose urine simultaneously with increases in intraabdominal pressure. With the later entity, the incontinence will follow the stressful maneuver in approximately 10 to 20 seconds.

Overflow incontinence will typically present with continual incontinence that may be severe, requiring numerous pads per day. Nocturnal enuresis is typically present. Vaginal fullness or introital bulging is a characteristic complaint if vaginal prolapse is present (cystocele, enterocele, uterine prolapse, and/or rectocele).

Physical Examination

The best way to diagnose stress urinary incontinence is to observe the loss of urine at the external urethral meatus when the patient is asked to strain or cough with a full bladder (Marshall test). If the recurrent stress urinary incontinence is due to anatomic incontinence, manual elevation of the bladder neck should provide continence again with the same stressful maneuvers. When performing this test, one should make sure that only the tissues lateral to the bladder neck are being elevated. If the urethra and bladder neck themselves are elevated, this might inadvertently produce periurethral compression instead of paraurethral elevation. By this we mean that the urethral lumen can become compressed and mask intrinsic sphincter dysfunction as the underlying cause for the recurrent stress urinary incontinence. In fact, patients who have a poor urethra (ISD) usually will have relatively good support of their bladder neck. Incontinence can be elicited most of the time in the lithotomy position; however, a standing examination may be required when the history is suggestive of stress urinary incontinence and a negative examination in the lithotomy position is encountered.

Careful examination of the anterior vaginal wall also should be performed to detect other conditions producing or contributing to the incontinence, such as a diverticulum or fistula. Other forms of vaginal prolapse, as mentioned above, also should be assessed because these conditions may require concomitant correction. We have found that examining the patient with the lower half of a vaginal speculum held posteriorly helps one to assess the degree of bladder neck hypermobility and cystocele. With the speculum held anteriorly, enteroceles or rectoceles can be detected.

Cystoscopy

While not diagnostic, cystoscopy is certainly complementary in assessing the degree of bladder neck hypermobility and intrinsic urethral integrity. In patients with anatomic incontinence, bladder neck hypermobility can be appreciated while viewing with the 0- or 30-degree lens during straining maneuvers. In contrast, endoscopy demonstrates that patients with intrinsic sphincter dysfunction quite frequently have a poorly coapting lumen even without straining. Of course, endoscopy is invaluable in detecting occult urologic lesions that may be associated with or the cause of recurrent incontinence.

Urodynamics

Urodynamic evaluations have proved helpful in the workup of these complex cases of recurrent stress urinary incontinence. Cystometrograms (CMGs) can be separated categorically into three functions of the bladder that provide an assessment of filling, storing, and voiding phases. Filling cystometrograms are helpful in assessing compliance, detrusor stability, and/or intact sensation. The storage phase of the cystometrogram is necessary because this is where we test for competence of the urethral continence mechanisms. Voiding-phase pressure-flow studies may suggest iatrogenic obstruction from previous surgery or other difficulties with emptying. Experimentally, static and dynamic urethral pressure profile determinations have shown considerable overlap between the different types of stress urinary incontinence and have not proved useful in guiding therapy.

Voiding Cystourethrography

Lateral voiding cystourethrograms (VCUGs) with a urethral catheter in place can be very helpful in defining the anatomy of the bladder and urethra. Funneling and hypermobility of the bladder neck on straining maneuvers are more consistent with anatomic incontinence as the cause for recurrent stress urinary incontinence. An open bladder neck or urinary leakage at rest (or with low Valsalva pressures) is more suggestive of intrinsic sphincter dysfunction. Unfortunately, without simultaneous urodynamic monitoring, bladder and rectal pressures are not recorded. Because of this, the clinician cannot be sure whether increases in intravesical pressure, produced during provocative maneuvers, are due to abdominal or detrusor contributions. The voiding cystourethrogram is helpful, however, in the detection of other pathology such as fistulas, diverticula, and degree of cystocele, if present.

Videourodynamics

While we realize that this study is not readily available in most clinical centers, it is very helpful in certain situations of complex recurrent stress urinary incontinence. Simultaneous urodynamic and fluoroscopic monitoring of intravesical pressures along with bladder neck morphology will frequently distinguish whether recurrent stress urinary incontinence is due to anatomic incontinence or intrinsic sphincter dysfunction. As mentioned above, patients with stress urinary incontinence due to anatomic incontinence will usually have funneling of the bladder neck with increases in intraabdominal pressures (Fig. 15-1). Conversely, patients with intrinsic sphincter dysfunction demonstrate either an open bladder neck at rest or funneling with low Valsalva pressures (Fig. 15-2).

If the patient with recurrent stress urinary incontinence also has a component of obstruction, the voiding phase of the cystogram will occasionally demonstrate high voiding pressures and a fixed and/or kinked urethra with relatively poor support of the bladder neck region. These patients are found to have had a suspension of urethra (usually midurethra) rather than the bladder neck, which is still hypermobile. These clinical scenarios have been found to occur most commonly after the Marshall-Marchetti-Krantz retropubic and Stamey transvaginal bladder neck suspensions in which inadvertent placement of the suspending sutures are either too medially near the urethra or too distal away from the bladder neck. The management of these patients will be discussed under urinary retention.

Physiology of Anti-Incontinence Surgery

While the goal of surgery for anatomic incontinence is reposition of the sphincteric unit to a well-supported retropubic position, the goal of surgery for intrinsic sphincter dysfunction is to provide coaptation, support, and compression to the damaged sphincteric unit (Table 15-2). The basis for continence after a bladder neck suspension for anatomic incontinence is not completely understood, but several factors may participate:

1. The urethra is moved from a low, dependent position to a higher, supported location, making the bladder

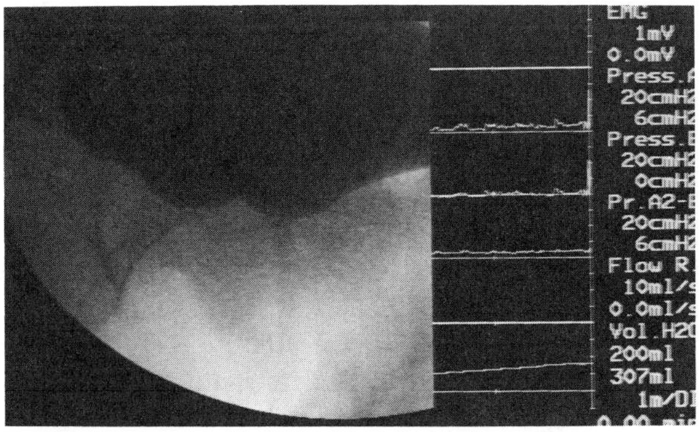

Figure 15-2. *Cystogram phase of video study revealing "beaking" of the bladder neck at rest. (Note: Stress urinary incontinence is clearly demonstrated in the standing position.)*

base the most dependent portion of the bladder. Changes in intraabdominal pressure in the standing position are transmitted to the bladder base and not to the bladder neck, thus protecting the sphincteric unit.

2. A true valvular effect is created. Increases in intraabdominal forces in the presence of a well-supported urethra allow the bladder base to rotate posteriorly, increasing urethral resistance. Evidence for this the-

Table 15-2. *Physiology of Anti-Incontinence Surgery*

Anatomic incontinence (AI)
    Alteration in pressure distribution
    Valvular effect
    Equal pressure transmissions
    Backboard effect
Intrinsic sphincter dysfunction (ISD)
    Provide compression

Figure 15-1. *A. Videourodynamic study demonstrating a normal bladder configuration at rest* (A = *vesical pressure;* B = *abdominal pressure; and* C = *detrusor pressure). B. Same patient during straining maneuvers showing funneling of bladder neck (note Valsalva pressure of 62 cmH₂O).*

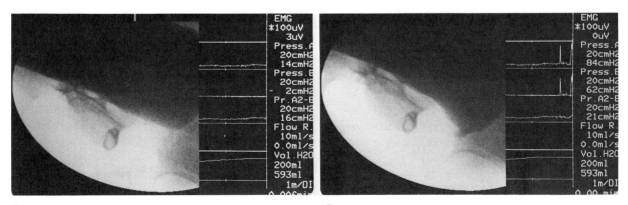

A   B

ory is based on the clinical observation that elevation of the bladder base in patients supposedly cured by a bladder neck suspension may recreate stress urinary incontinence.

3. Reposition of the bladder neck into the higher position improves transmission of increases in intraabdominal pressure to the sphincteric unit, thus keeping the pressure in this zone higher than that of the bladder.

4. Suspending sutures to the urethropelvic ligaments provide a backboard effect for more effective compression of the sphincteric unit at the time of stress.

In the intrinsic sphincter dysfunction group, the patient has a poorly coapting urethra and thus has such a poor resistance that even the slightest movements or increases in intraabdominal pressures will produce incontinence. The intrinsic sphincteric unit is thought of characteristically as being made up of a specific urethral architecture and composition.

The vital structures contributing to continence in this region include (1) mucosal infoldings and spongy tissue (from submucosal vasculature), (2) smooth muscle, (3) intrinsic and extrinsic skeletal musculature, and (4) the periurethral envelope. Surgery for intrinsic sphincter dysfunction attempts to compensate for deficiencies in these contributors to the passive continence mechanisms by providing better coaptation.

Treatment

The best chance of surgical cure for the stress incontinent patient is that derived from the first operation. The choice as to which approach to use initially should be based on the particular expertise of the surgeon along with consideration as to the need for concomitant procedures. Many cases of recurrent stress urinary incontinence are complicated by periurethral fibrosis and fixation of various parts of the bladder and urethra to the retropubic area. In deciding which repair to perform, several factors should be taken into consideration before the most appropriate procedure is chosen. These factors include (1) severity of incontinence, (2) factors leading to intrinsic sphincter dysfunction (numerous failed repairs, radiation, pelvic trauma, and congenital factors), (3) presence of associated vaginal pathology (cystocele, enterocele, uterine prolapse, and/or rectocele), and (4) presence of obstruction.

Of the above-mentioned factors, the most important is deciding whether the recurrent stress urinary incontinence is the result of recurrent bladder neck hy-

permobility producing anatomic incontinence or a poorly coapting urethra producing intrinsic sphincter dysfunction (Table 15-3). Procedures for correcting the former aim to restore the bladder neck to its original retropubic position. The presence and degree of cystocele also will affect the type of reoperative approach that should be planned. The remainder of this chapter will focus first on those retropubic procedures which have been described for reoperative surgery on the stress urinary incontinence patient, followed by transvaginal approaches for recurrent stress urinary incontinence. Lastly, interventions for intrinsic sphincter dysfunction that essentially compress the poorly compliant urethra will be discussed.

Reoperation for Anatomic Incontinence

Retropubic Procedures

Retropubic operations for recurrent stress urinary incontinence are quite common and, again, are used depending on the experience of the individual surgeon and the need for additional procedures. All these procedures aim to effectively increase urethral resistance by tightening the musculofascial planes supporting the proximal urethra into a higher retropubic position. The Marshall-Marchetti-Krantz (MMK) retropubic suspension, the paravaginal repair, and the Burch suspension procedures are the most common.

Lee et al. in 1975 reported on their reoperative experience employing the Marshall-Marchetti-Krantz suspension in 36 patients, all of whom had undergone at least one prior Marshall-Marchetti-Krantz procedure. Anatomically, 24 (66 percent) of the patients demonstrated a significant recurrence of their cystourethrocele

Table 15-3. *Treatment for Recurrent Stress Urinary Incontinence*

Anatomic incontinence
  Retropubic
    Marshall-Marchetti-Krantz
    Paravaginal repairs
    Burch
  Needle
    Stamey
    Raz
    Gittes
Intrinsic sphincter dysfunction
  Periurethral injections
  Artificial urinary sphincters
  Sling procedures
    Autologous or synthetic
    Vaginal wall (Raz)
  Bladder neck reconstruction

preoperatively. Intraoperative observations of the degree of scarring and fixation indicated that only the anterior bladder or bladder neck was initially suspended instead of the better-supporting tissues just lateral to the urethra. In this series by Lee et al., 32 (88 percent) of 36 patients are continent with a mean follow-up of 4.5 years. Two patients initially continent recurred and required a secondary vaginal plication.

It is extremely important when performing either an initial or a redo Marshall-Marchetti-Krantz procedure not to place the suspending sutures too close to the urethra. In reoperative cases, careful dissection down over the bladder neck and anterior urethral regions is necessary to free any obstructive adhesions or urethral kinks that might have been produced iatrogenically. Usually, these sutures were placed periurethrally instead of in the good tissues lateral to the bladder neck, as mentioned earlier, and cause fixation with difficult emptying. Inadvertent bladder or urethral injury can be minimized by either placing fingers in the vagina or by performing a cystotomy for more control.

According to these authors, another advantage to performing a cystotomy is to check for underlying intrinsic urethral incompetence otherwise missed by routine preoperative endoscopic and radiographic assessments. Normally, the urethra should be snug around a 16 or 18 French Foley catheter. If this is not found intraoperatively, they then advocate urethral plication after extending their previously created anterior cystotomy through the bladder neck over the urethra almost to the level of the external meatus. This maneuver, which is actually Lee's modification of the Marshall-Marchetti-Krantz procedure, also should work for recurrent stress urinary incontinence caused by bladder neck hypermobility complicated by intrinsic sphincter dysfunction.

Paravaginal suspensions as pioneered by Turner-Warwick are based on the premise that a weakness in the paravaginal endopelvic fascia, that is, the connection of the pubocervical or endopelvic fascia to the lateral pelvic sidewall at the tendinous arc, is defective. Pathophysiologically, the levator musculature in these patients with bladder neck hypermobility is a lax, weak unit causing secondary deficiencies in the normally supportive endopelvic fascia.

The Richardson paravaginal repair is based on the same theory of defective lateral support as proposed by Turner-Warwick; however, the insertion of the endopelvic fascia to the tendinous arc over the iliopectineal line is not taken down in this modification. Richardson et al. in 1980 reported on their 6-year experience with this repair in 233 patients, 53 (23 percent) of whom were

reoperative patients who had undergone either a retropubic or vaginal repair. Their overall cure rate with no stress urinary incontinence was 88 percent, with follow-up ranging from between 2 and 8 years; however, they did not separate their results into the initial and reoperative cases.

Cowan et al. in 1979 reported on their experience with the Burch colposuspension in 77 patients, 23 of whom were having reoperations for recurrent stress urinary incontinence. They reported an overall success rate of 93 percent with 1.5 to 3.5 years of follow-up. Unfortunately, they also did not separate their results with respect to the initial and reoperative patients. For review, the Burch suspension relies on resuspending the paravaginal tissues to the pectineal or Cooper's ligament. Of the reported complications, enterocele formation seems to be the highest with all these retropubic suspensions at between 10 and 17 percent.

Needle Procedures

The initial work of Peyrera began the advent of transvaginal needle bladder neck suspensions for stress urinary incontinence. Since that time, modifications in this basic principle have led to a host of needle suspensions for the correction of stress urinary incontinence due to anatomic incontinence, including the Cobb-Ragde, Stamey, Raz, and Gittes procedures. At the University of California at Los Angeles, we perform the Raz procedure (modified Pereyra) for all our reoperative cases unless they require concomitant abdominal procedures such as augmentation cystoplasty or ureteral reimplantation, necessitating an abdominal or retropubic approach.

Schaeffer, in his 1980 review article concerning the treatment of recurrent stress urinary incontinence, stated that the Stamey bladder neck suspension was his preference for the initial treatment of stress urinary incontinence along with his reoperative cases. He reported in conjunction with Stamey a 91 percent cure rate in 203 patients with a minimum follow-up of 6 months. In accordance with the results of needle suspensions from most reported series, most failures occurred within 1 year. Of the patient population, 188 prior procedures had been performed.

At the University of California at Los Angeles, we perform the Raz bladder neck suspension for all patients with either new-onset, persistent, or recurrent stress urinary incontinence. This operation is indicated for those patients whose stress urinary incontinence is due to anatomic incontinence with or without low-grade cystoceles and, most important, no evidence for intrinsic sphincter dysfunction. Leach and Raz in 1984 reviewed

54 patients who were referred to our institution for persistent or recurrent incontinence after one or more failed operative procedures. Of these patients, 14 had a poorly complaint or "pipe stem" urethra and underwent an additional urethral reconstructive procedure to improve coaptation. With a minimum follow-up of 24 months, 94 percent of these patients were totally continent.

We are soon to report our updated experience with over 300 patients undergoing the Raz bladder neck suspension since 1984 with an average follow-up of 16 months. Sixty percent of these were operations for recurrent stress urinary incontinence. Our overall results for this subgroup indicate that 84 percent of these patients were totally cured (no stress urinary incontinence), while 8.5 percent were almost perfect (rare stress urinary incontinence, no protection), providing satisfactory results in over 92 percent of this reoperative patient population. Interestingly, there was no statistical difference in the cure of stress urinary incontinence between patients undergoing the Raz bladder neck suspension as their initial or reoperative procedure.

Raz Bladder Neck Suspension for Anatomic Incontinence

Step 1: With the patient in the modified lithotomy position, silk sutures are used for libial retraction after the usual prepping procedures. A Lowsley retractor is used to facilitate placement of a suprapubic Foley catheter. Another 16 French Foley catheter is placed per urethra, and the anterior vaginal wall is grasped with an Allis clamp at the midurethral level (halfway between the bladder neck and external meatus).

Step 2 (Fig. 15-3): Normal saline is injected in the proposed inverted-U incision site with the apex of the U just inferior to the Allis clamp. The arms of the U should stay just 1 cm medial to the lateral vaginal walls and extend just inferior to the bladder neck level.

Step 3: After the inverted-U incision, Metzenbaum scissors are used to dissect the vaginal wall off the underlying glistening periurethral fascia to the point where this fascia meets the undersurface of the pubic bone at the tendinous arc (the periurethral fascia at this level is now termed the *urethropelvic ligament*).

Step 4 (Fig. 15-4): Heavy curved Mayo scissors are used to pierce the urethropelvic ligament just underneath the bone with the tips pointing toward the ipsilateral shoulder, thus entering the retropubic space. Blunt dissection and, if need be, sharp dissection are required to mobilize the urethropelvic ligament off the pubic bone from the level of the bladder neck to the ischial spine.

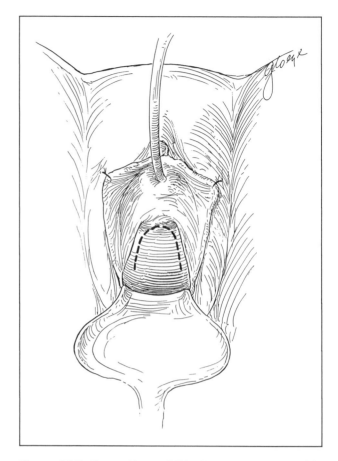

Figure 15-3. *Proposed inverted-U incision site. (Note: Apex of the incision is at the midurethral level.)*

Step 5 (Fig. 15-5): A no. 1 polypropylene suture on a no. 5 or no. 6 Mayo needle (Ethicon, special order) is then used to take several helical bites at the level of the bladder neck of both the urethropelvic ligaments and the vaginal wall without taking the epithelium. The key to our procedure lies in (1) taking the medial edge of the urethropelvic ligaments and (2) taking the vaginal wall underneath the incision to include the pubocervical fasciae. At this point, the strength of the anchor is tested by applying traction to the suture and being able to rock the patient on the table.

Step 6 (Fig. 15-6): The next step involves transference of the sutures to the suprapubic space. A small transverse suprapubic incision is made just over the superior edge of the symphysis pubis down to the level of the rectus fascia. With a finger inserted into the retropubic space, the double-pronged needle (Cook urological, Spencer, Ind.) is passed into this space, staying just underneath the posterior surface of the symphysis. While maintaining finger control of the tips, the needle

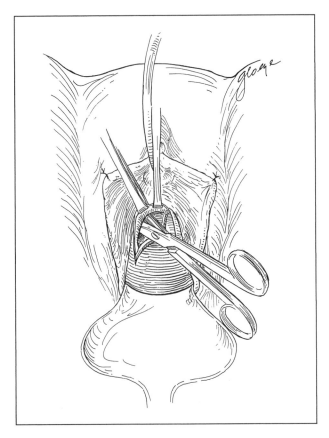

Figure 15-4. *Curved Mayo scissors piercing the urethropelvic ligament just underneath the inferior ramus of the pubis.*

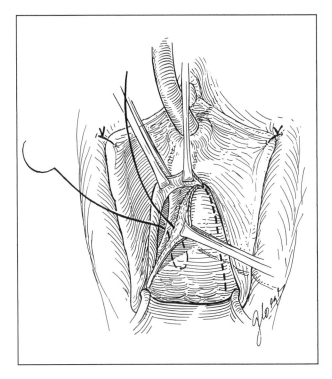

Figure 15-5. *Prolene suture incorporates the urethropelvic ligament and vaginal wall without its epithelium.*

is guided out through the vaginal vault, and the sutures are transferred to the suprapubic space.

Step 7: After an intravenous injection of indigo carmine, cystoscopy is carried out to check for (1) inadvertent suture placement, (2) ureteral efflux, and (3) bladder neck elevation and coaptation upon traction of the suprapubic sutures.

Step 8 (Fig. 15-7): The vaginal incision is closed with a running 2-0 absorbable suture. A vaginal pack with antibiotic ointment is placed. The polypropylene sutures are tied first individually and then to the contralateral mate. The suprapubic incision is closed subcuticularly, and the suprapubic tube is secured.

Postoperative Care

Intravenous antibiotics are continued for 24 hours, and then an oral cephalosporin is begun. The vaginal pack and the urethral Foley catheter are removed on the first postoperative morning. Following this, the suprapubic tube is plugged, and the patient is asked to check residuals every 4 hours. The suprapubic tube is removed after

the postvoid residuals are less than 60 cc, which usually takes 1 to 2 weeks.

Reoperation for Intrinsic Sphincter Dysfunction

If a patient has been determined to have recurrent stress urinary incontinence based on intrinsic sphincteric dysfunction, therapy should be chosen accordingly to provide the necessary coaptation for this defect. The available modalities for management of this type of recurrent stress urinary incontinence include (1) periurethral injection of an inert substance (collagen or Teflon), (2) an artificial urinary sphincter, (3) sling procedures, and (4) bladder neck reconstruction.

Periurethral injections of collagen or Teflon may be an alternative to reoperation for patients with recurrent stress urinary incontinence due to intrinsic sphincter dysfunction. Cure rates for Teflon are reported to be between 21 and 70 percent. Collagen is a biodegradable substance that is presumed to be replaced by the patient's own collagen. Unfortunately, we do not know the long-lasting effects of this substance, and reports indicate that the collagen is disappearing in the tissues.

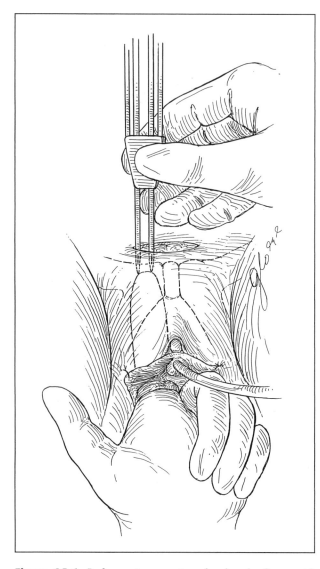

Figure 15-6. *Prolene sutures are transferred under finger guidance. (Note: The index finger is in the retropubic space just behind the symphysis pubis.)*

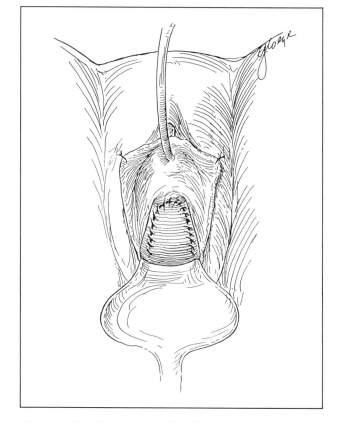

Figure 15-7. *The vaginal wall is closed in a running fashion.*

Although potentially useful, it has not been approved yet by the Food and Drug Administration (FDA).

Artificial urinary sphincters for recurrent stress urinary incontinence have met with mixed results. Obviously, surgical expertise in the handling of prosthetic devices is mandatory, especially in these reoperative settings. Problems thus far with this device include (1) ischemic atrophy from excessive coaptation, (2) revisions for recurrent stress urinary incontinence due to inadequate closing pressures, and (3) mechanical malfunction. Mention will only be made of several articles that deal specifically with the management of recurrent

stress urinary incontinence using the Scott AS-800 artificial urinary sphincter.

Diokno et al. in 1987 reported on 32 women who had placement of this device by means of the suprapubic route for recurrent stress urinary incontinence after a failed bladder neck suspension. Of the 32 devices implanted, 31 were functioning with an average follow-up of 2.5 years, although this required a 21 percent reoperation rate for mechanical complications. Ninety-one percent of these patients were dry without pads. Appell in 1988 reported on his experience with the transvaginal insertion of an artificial sphincter in patients for recurrent stress urinary incontinence, all of whom had undergone at least two prior surgical procedures. As of this report, all patients were dry; however, three patients did require revisionary surgery for mechanical complications. Interestingly, there were no instances of infection, cuff erosion, or detrusor instability.

Sling Procedures

The remainder of this chapter will cover sling procedures for recurrent stress urinary incontinence caused by intrinsic sphincter dysfunction. Autologous materials include vaginal wall, rectus fascia, fasciae latae, and round ligaments. Synthetic materials used as slings include Marlex, Mersilene, and Gore-Tex. Our preference for repair is the vaginal wall sling to be described. This procedure is contraindicated in patients who have either an extremely short vagina or a marginal vaginal length but who desire to remain sexually active. In either case, we would then perform a rectus fascia sling as described by McGuire.

Raz in 1989 described a new sling technique called the *vaginal wall sling*. The vaginal wall is autologous tissue, which is desirable in that there is no need for an extravaginal harvesting incision, thus minimizing morbidity. In addition, the vaginal island graft allows for this type of sling to be tailored precisely to the width and length of the urethra. The 32 patients in this initial report were followed from 10 to 28 months. Of these patients, 26 had sphincter dysfunction based purely on intrinsic urethral factors, while the remainder had a neurogenic basis for their incompetent proximal urethra. Within this subgroup of 26, 22 patients underwent a total of 97 prior anti-incontinence procedures. Of these 22 reoperative cases, 20 resulted in an excellent outcome, that is, no incontinence. Two patients failed the procedure. An updated report to be published shortly from our institution reviews an additional 65 patients with intrinsic sphincter dysfunction who had this sling procedure, 48 having had at least one prior anti-incontinence procedure. Within this group of 48, 90.7 percent are totally dry with a mean follow-up of 24 months. An additional 3.7 percent have only rare incontinence, giving a satisfactory result in over 94 percent of this reoperative group. Of note is that 83 percent of these patients had temporary obstructive voiding symptoms postoperatively, with 5.5 percent requiring continual clean intermittent catheterization for urinary retention.

Vaginal Wall Sling: Operative Technique

Step 1: Preoperative preparation is carried out as above for the Raz bladder neck suspension, and the suprapubic and urethral Foley catheters are placed in the same fashion.

Step 2 (Fig. 15-8): Normal saline is injected in an inverted-U fashion, this time with the apex of the U inferior to the external meatus. The incision is carried out, and again, the glistening periurethral fascia is dissected toward the pubic bone as above. Also, the urethropelvic ligament is pierced and freed up from the

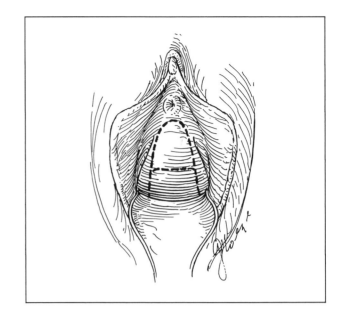

Figure 15-8. *The vaginal wall island is outlined anteriorly (A) with the future flap for coverage located posteriorly (B).*

undersurface of the pubic bone from the bladder neck toward the ischial spine.

Step 3: A transverse incision is made at the level of the bladder neck joining the lateral borders of the original incision. This creates a rectangular island of anterior vaginal wall that underlies the bladder neck and urethra. The size of this island is tailored easily to the length and caliber of the urethra.

Step 4 (Fig. 15-9): The proximal vaginal wall is then undermined to create a flap that will be advanced to cover the vaginal island sling at a later step.

Step 5 (Fig. 15-10): The four corners of the vaginal wall island are then anchored with individual no. 1 polypropylene sutures. The set close to the bladder neck will incorporate (1) the urethropelvic ligament, (2) the periurethral fascia, and (3) the full thickness of the vaginal wall epithelium in that order. The distal set of sutures will incorporate only the full-thickness corner of the vaginal wall along with the periurethral fascia at that level.

Step 6: Transference of the sutures with the aid of the double-pronged needle and cystoscopy are carried out as described above for the Raz bladder neck suspension.

Step 7 (Fig. 15-11): The proximal vaginal wall flap is then advanced over the sling to provide an epithelial cover and restore the integrity of the anterior vaginal wall using a 2-0 polyglactin suture.

Step 8: The polypropylene sutures are then tied, and the suprapubic wound is closed as above. All Foley cath-

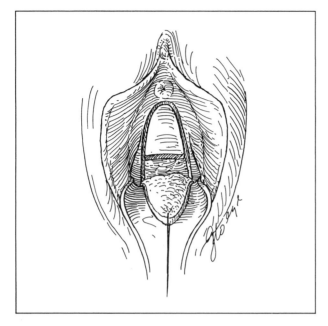

Figure 15-9. *The posterior vaginal flap is created by sharp dissection.*

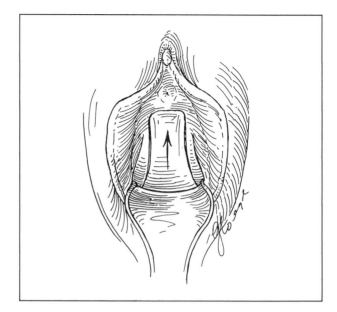

Figure 15-11. *The posterior flap is now advanced to cover the sling.*

eters and the vaginal packing are maintained in exactly the same way. Postoperative care is identical.

Urinary Retention

All approaches for the correction of stress urinary incontinence, whether done retropubically or transvaginally, have the potential to produce obstructive voiding symptoms. Complete urinary retention or obstructive voiding with overflow incontinence is rare in the routine bladder neck suspension procedure. Whether a suprapubic tube is left indwelling or intermittent catheterization is instituted immediately postoperatively, most patients will void with insignificant postvoid residuals (less than 60 cc) within 1 to 2 weeks. Patients may require longer intervals before voiding to completion, especially after sling procedures. The patient's medications should be reviewed thoroughly along with a carefully performed neurologic evaluation.

This condition has not been a problem in our patient population, and the majority of patients with this condition could have been predicted preoperatively on a neurologic basis. If retention is indeed due to the bladder neck suspension, then three causes for this iatrogenic obstruction need to be considered: (1) sutures are too close to the urethra, (2) sutures are tied too tightly and (3) the sutures have been placed midurethrally.

Figure 15-10. *The four quadrant sutures have been placed as described. (Note: All sutures also should incorporate the periurethral fasciae.)*

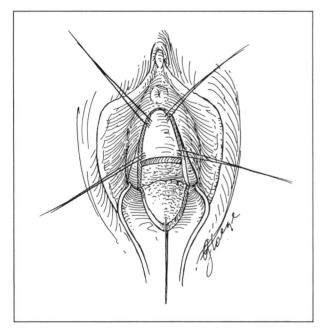

Reoperation for Retention after Bladder Neck Suspension

Regardless of which needle bladder neck suspension is performed, too much tension on the suspending sutures may be the etiologic agent. This can be corrected suprapubically by initially taking down one set of sutures, and if this is still not curative, the other set must be taken down. If the patient is still obstructed or is found to have recurrent stress urinary incontinence associated with the obstructed state, then urethrolysis with a takedown of the previous suspension sutures and repeat bladder neck suspension will be required. Only the retropubic and Raz bladder neck suspensions will afford the necessary exposure to accomplish this task.

Utilizing the Raz bladder neck suspension in these reoperative cases, the dissection of the anterior vaginal wall should proceed in the normal fashion with entry into the retropubic space after adequate dissection of the glistening periurethral fascia from the overlying vaginal wall epithelium. After the retropubic space is entered, blunt and sharp dissections of the anterior aspect of the urethra are carried out with care to stay right on the posterior surface of the symphysis pubis. The old suspending sutures should be cut at this time and removed, although removal is not mandatory if technically unfeasible. After these maneuvers, the surgeon's finger should be able to pass anteriorly around the urethra and bladder neck region, ensuring their total freedom from adhesions. The operation then proceeds in the normal fashion.

If the transvaginal approach fails or indications exist for an open operation, then we will perform urethrolysis transabdominally. Several technical points deserve emphasis here. Careful dissection between the anterior urethra and undersurface of the pubic bone is mandatory to obtain total freedom of the urethra in the retropubic space. If the lateral support of the bladder neck region is intact in a continent patient, then only urethrolysis with interposition of a pedicle-based omental flap is carried out. If recurrent stress urinary incontinence is also present or poor support of the bladder neck is demonstrated, then resuspension is indicated.

Recurrent Stress Urinary Incontinence with Cystocele

The presence of a significant cystocele complicating recurrent stress urinary incontinence changes our method of repair; however, we still prefer to approach these complicated cases transvaginally. Cystoceles are graded depending on the degree of descent toward the vaginal introitus in the standing position. A *grade I* cystocele involves a bladder neck with minimal hypermobility and is what is found most commonly clinically. *Grade II* cystoceles descend further toward the vaginal introitus. A *grade III* cystocele comes outside the introitus with straining, while a *grade IV* cystocele (severe anterior wall prolapse) is outside the introitus at rest. If the patient has recurrent stress urinary incontinence and either a grade II or III cystocele, we use the four-corner bladder neck suspension. This procedure, in addition to suspending the urethropelvic ligaments for bladder neck support, also suspends the pubocervical fasciae and cardinal ligaments for cystocele reduction. If the patient has recurrent stress urinary incontinence and a severe cystourethrocele (grade IV), we perform a formal cystocele repair and bladder neck suspension consisting of (1) reapproximation of the pubocervical fasciae across the midline to repair the bladder herniation through the central defect, (2) suspension of the bladder neck, pubocervical fasciae, and cardinal ligaments to correct the urethral and bladder hypermobility caused by the lateral or paravaginal deficit, and (3) reapproximation of the cardinal and sacrouterine ligaments across the midline to support the bladder base.

Summary

Recurrent stress urinary incontinence can be quite distressing to both patient and physician, and reoperations in this subgroup of patients prove to be technically demanding at times. Behavior modification and medical therapy involving such measures as Kegel exercises and alpha-adrenergic agonists may be helpful at times in patients who present initially with mild stress urinary incontinence; however; these conservative interventions are even less effective in cases of recurrent stress urinary incontinence.

After the clinician determines that the patient's leakage is indeed due to recurrent stress urinary incontinence, the most important diagnostic maneuver is to differentiate between anatomic incontinence (hypermobility) and intrinsic sphincter dysfunction (poor urethra) as the etiology for the recurrent stress urinary incontinence. With the former cause, a bladder neck suspending procedure should correct the problem. If the patient has a bad urethra, we prefer to provide the patient with better coaptation and feel that a sling procedure gives the best and most long-lasting results. The experience of the surgeon and the need for additional procedures (enterocele repair, hysterectomy, urethrolysis, and/or augmentation cystoplasty) will dictate the necessary approach. We hope that with the ever-expanding field of female urology and continual modifications in current surgical techniques, better and longer-lasting results will be encountered, thus obviating the need for reoperative surgery.

Bibliography

Bent, AE. Management of recurrent genuine stress urinary incontinence. Clin Obstet Gynecol 33(2):358, 1990.

Bent, AE, and Ostergard, DR. Recurrent stress incontinence. Postgrad Med 83(7):113, 1988.

Leach, GE, and Raz, S. Modified Pereyra bladder neck suspension after previously failed anti-incontinence surgery: Surgical technique and results with long-term follow up. Urology 23(4):359, 1984.

Leach, GE, et al. Surgery for pelvic prolapse. Semin Urol 4(1):43, 1986.

Lee, RA, and Symmonds, RE. Repeat Marshall-Marchetti procedure for recurrent stress urinary incontinence. Am J Obstet Gynecol 122(2):219, 1975.

Raz, S. Modified bladder neck suspension for female stress incontinence. Urology 17:82, 1981.

Raz, S, Klutke, CG, and Golomb, J. Four-corner bladder and urethral suspension for moderate cystocele. J Urol 142:712, 1989.

Raz, S, Maggio, AJ, Jr, and Kaufman, JJ. Why Marshall-Marchetti operation works . . . or does not. Urology 14(2):154, 1979.

Raz, S, et al. Vaginal wall sling. J Urol 141:43, 1989.

Schaeffer, AJ. Treatment of recurrent urinary incontinence. Clin Obstet Gynecol 27(2):459, 1984.

Siegel, AL, and Raz, S. Surgical treatment of anatomical stress incontinence. Neurourol Urodyn 7:569, 1988.

Stamey, TA. Endoscopic suspension of the vesical neck for urinary incontinence in females. Ann Surg 192(4):465, 1980.

Staskin, DR. Complications of female anti-incontinence surgery. In Complications of Urologic Surgery: Prevention and Management, 2d ed. Philadelphia: Saunders, 1990, pp 514–515.

16

Failed Hypospadias Repair

MICHAEL A. KEATING
JOHN W. DUCKETT, JR.

The correction of hypospadias remains one of the most challenging problems encountered by today's urologists. Unfortunately, despite the apparent advantages of modern medicine and contemporary urethroplasties, complications still occur in even the best of hands. And, although their incidence appears to be decreasing, each failed primary repair bears frustrating testimony to the anatomic and technical nuances of the anomaly being addressed. Complications also serve to remind hypospadiologists that their ultimate goal, devising a procedure that affords maximal correction while risking minimal morbidity, remains a grail not yet achieved, although some progress has been made.

Twenty years ago, surgeons were unable to assess the presence of chordee at one sitting, and sequenced two-stage repairs provided the standard. Although fairly effective, these urethroplasties suffered from their inability to project the neourethra beyond the level of the coronal sulcus. As a consequence, surgeries were commonly deferred in boys with distal or "grade 1" hypospadias because the results were often no better or sometimes worse than the presenting hypospadias. Today's surgical objectives have been redefined by our better understanding of chordee and the surgical plasticity of the glans penis as well as the arrival of novel one-stage urethroplasties. Regardless of the severity of the anomaly, these objectives include (1) straightening of the penis by orthoplasty (resection of chordee), (2) restoration of the neomeatus to the tip of the glans, (3) construction of a hairless urethra having a uniform caliber, (4) creation of a symmetrical glans and penile shaft, and most important, (5) normalization of voiding and erections. In short, our goal is to reconstruct a penis that is functionally and cosmetically normal.

The implications of these revised surgical objectives are obvious. Recommending surgery for the child with severe chordee and proximal hypospadias who would sit to void if left uncorrected could always be done without hesitation. However, the majority of hypospadias (70 percent or more) are glanular or coronal variants that sometimes affect boys who would remain functionally normal if surgery were deferred. Nevertheless, the psychological aftermath of uncorrected hypospadias has been well documented, while others ultimately develop functional problems from underappreciated chordee or meatal stenosis. It is understandably impossible to predict which child will have problems later in development. However, the cosmetic, functional, and potential psychological benefits of today's urethroplasties outweigh their risks, and correction is recommended for all but the most distal hypospadias variants. When the inevitable complication appears, the family or patient should be reassured that the *objectives cited above remain the aim of any reoperations* that might become necessary.

Successful Urethroplasty

Successful reoperations for the failed hypospadias repair will have their basis in a thorough understanding of the principles of primary urethroplasty as well as the etiologies of their attendant complications. As a consequence, an overview of the guidelines in selection, technique, and postoperative management used to optimize our results with primary repairs is germane to the discussion.

Technique Selection

Many of the complications of hypospadias surgery seen in consultation stem as much from *errors in design and application* as from faulty technique. Selecting a urethroplasty properly tailored to the individual's anatomy is at least as important to maximizing one's results as technical ability or even experience. Adaptability is crucial. Hypospadias must be considered a spectrum of anomalies whose correction requires any one of a variety of techniques. As a consequence, the application of a "favorite repair" that provides excellent results for one variant might concede inevitable complications to another. Today's hypospadiologist must be able to perform a variety of urethroplasties as well as be familiar with their limitations and potential complications. An algorithm for primary urethroplasty is shown in Figure 16-1.

Briefly, the meatal advancement and glanuloplasty (MAGPI) repair is ideal for most *distal (glandular and coronal) hypospadias without chordee* (Duckett, 1981a). Dissatisfaction with the repair undoubtedly stems from its application in unsuitable candidates. The MAGPI's apparent simplicity belies a complex sequence of tissue transfers required of the technique. Success depends on the respective mobilities of both the dorsal urethral plate (the ventral penile shaft skin distal to the meatus) and the ventral urethra, as well as the pliability of the glans. When the plate or urethra is immobile or the glans is fish-mouthed or noncompliant, urethral retrusion and glans breakdown become an inevitable consequence of tension. Alternative repairs such as the pyramid procedure (Duckett, 1989) or the onlay island flap (OIF) (Elder, 1987a) should be used if anatomy is unfavorable. When properly deployed, however, the cosmetic and functional results of the MAGPI are excellent. We have used the repair in over 1000 boys with a complication rate of less than 1 percent (Duckett, 1992a).

Figure 16-1. *Algorithm for hypospadias repair. Technique selection is crucial to avoiding reoperations.*

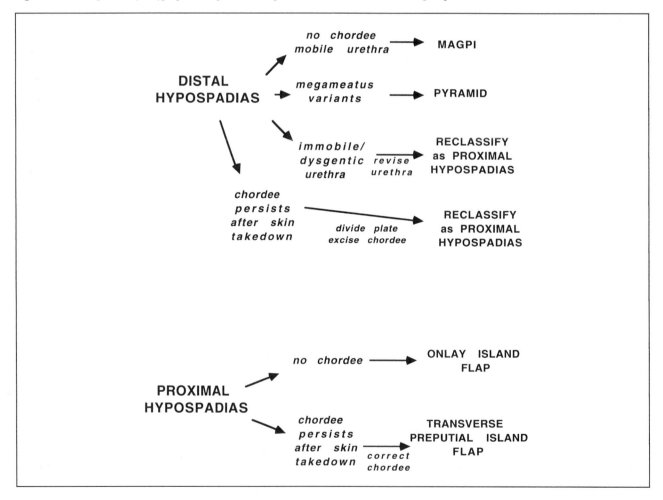

Midshaft and proximal hypospadias without chordee and most *distal variants not amenable to MAGPI* are ideal candidates for the onlay island flap urethroplasty. Our preference for the onlay island flap stems from its technical ease, vascularity to the neourethra which is predictable and dependable, and preservation of ventral shaft skin that enables a midline, raphelike closure in most cases. In addition, the onlay island flap can be adapted to more proximal variants if need be. Perimeatal-based flaps (the Mathieu or flip-flap procedure) also can be used to correct many distal and midshaft variants but have drawbacks. Flip-flaps rely on vascularity from perimeatal tissues that are sometimes deficient, are limited in length (since hair-bearing skin below the penoscrotal junction should not be included in their construction), and often leave significant skin defects of the ventral penis that require complex flap coverage. In one recent review, a slightly lower complication rate occurred with the onlay island flap than with perimeatal-based flaps when applied to similar hypospadias (Hollowell, 1990).

The tubularized transverse preputial island flap (TPIF), or Duckett, procedure remains the best option for *proximal hypospadias with chordee* (Duckett, 1981b). However, the decision to apply the transverse preputial island flap is not made until other surgical options are considered. Until recently, when preoperative chordee was present, the urethra was rotely circumscribed with the initial skin incisions, and pericorporal dissections were performed behind the urethral plate. We have since noted that in many instances, severe curvature often results from superficial chordee rather than from tethering by the urethral plate or deeper dysgenetic tissues positioned along the corporal bodies. As a consequence, we now begin virtually every hypospadias repair by *preserving* the plate, taking down the shaft skin, and *then* performing a saline erection to assess chordee. The degree of curvature that can be corrected simply by mobilizing the shaft skin with its underlying fibrous dartos fascia and releasing the aberrant insertions of the hooded prepuce that cause glans tilt is revealing.

Using this sequence, when the penis is straightened and the tissues of the urethral plate are healthy and well developed, the onlay island flap can be applied to even very proximal hypospadias. Otherwise, the plate must be divided, the urethra mobilized to clear the corpora of any offending tissues, and a transverse preputial island flap used to complete the repair. Complication rates for the tubularized flap are higher than with the onlay flap, and the technical benefits of the latter are real. Preservation of the urethral plate by using dorsal plication sutures with *mild or moderate* residual chordee remains

controversial, but the early experience with this approach has been favorable (Hollowell, 1990).

The intricacies of these urethroplasties are thoroughly reviewed elsewhere and will not be discussed here (Duckett, 1981a and b; Elder, 1987). However, portions of individual repairs will be used to illustrate principles in technique that apply to reoperative urethroplasties, especially in the context of complications to which they are particularly prone.

Preoperative Evaluation

A thorough history and examination are performed on every patient. Technical details of all prior genital surgeries, including circumcision, can play an important role in limiting the possible options in repair. Operative records are sometimes helpful and should be obtained. The examination includes assessments of penile size, glanular configuration, position of the meatus, and quality and quantity of excess shaft skin. Other problems that must be addressed, including meatal stenosis, chordee, and penile torsion, are also noted. Finally, cryptorchidism is occasionally overlooked by an earlier surgeon, should raise the question of intersex, and requires further evaluation.

A voiding study or retrograde urethrogram provides useful documentation of complex complications, but meatal stenosis or urethral strictures can make catheterization difficult or impossible. When these are present, radiographs are deferred until a less traumatic evaluation can be completed at surgery. Urinary ultrasounds are reserved for boys who have developmental abnormalities of other organ systems in concert with hypospadias. These suggest a "common hit" in embryogenesis that also might affect the kidneys and/or ureters. Otherwise, the incidence of surgically significant upper tract abnormalities found with hypospadias is probably no greater than that of the general population.

Timing of Surgery

Advancements in anesthesia and microsurgical technique have enabled surgery in progressively younger children. The optimal time for correcting hypospadias occurs between 6 and 18 months of age. This window in development precedes the onset of genital awareness (about 18 months of age) and leaves the child amnestic for the repair. Fortunately, most infant penises are large enough to allow functional and cosmetic results similar to those achieved in older children and adults without increased morbidity (Duckett, 1992b). In addition, the infant is more easily managed and parental anxiety is lessened using this approach.

One of the most common errors we see in referred cases stems from the timing of reoperative surgery. Other than local care, the initial management of most complications of urethroplasty is predicated on patience. Complications are understandably upsetting for everyone involved, including the surgeon, but nothing is more deleterious than premature attempts at "making things right." Corrective surgery should not be planned until optimal healing has occurred, which is usually *no earlier than 6 months*. In patients who have had multiple prior surgeries, it is not uncommon to defer reoperations for up to a year. Another advantage of doing primary urethroplasties in infancy is that complications can still be repaired within the optimal psychological window.

Principles in Technique

The chances for success with reoperative hypospadias repairs are optimized by applying the principles and instruments used by plastic surgeons. Castroviejo needle holders, fine iris scissors, and surgical magnification with loupes are invaluable. Skin hooks, traction sutures (5-0 silks), and fine (0.5 jeweler's) forceps are also used to minimize trauma to the delicate tissues.

Bleeding poses a problem, whether it occurs during surgery or presents as a hematoma afterwards. Dry fields are desirable, but not at the cost of excessive cauterization, causing tissue damage and vascular thrombosis, both risk factors for infection. Individual vessels are grasped and cauterized with low current. Tissues intended for the construction or coverage of a neourethra are left undisturbed. Subcutaneous lidocaine (1%, maximum dosage 5 mg/kg) with epinephrine (1:100,000) placed along the proposed incisions and into the glans itself provides excellent hemostasis. A tourniquet is also effective, but we rarely find this necessary when epinephrine is used. Bleeding in the latter stages of a case is often caused by a full bladder compromising venous return rather than the loss of epinephrine's vasoconstrictive effects.

Persistent chordee should be an avoidable complication. Artificial erections confirm orthoplasty before constructing a primary neourethra or completing reoperations. Tethering fibers must be excised completely from the corporal bodies, extending the dissection into the glans if necessary. When mild or moderate curvature persists, dorsal plications are simple and effective. The neurovascular bundles are identified, elevated, and preserved by lateral to medial dissections of Buck's fascia. Two transverse incisions, spaced 8 to 10 mm apart, on the dorsolateral aspect of each corpora are made in the tunica opposite the point of greatest curvature. A nonab-

sorbable suture is then used to approximate the outer edges of the incisions. Braided suture (4-0 Tevdek or Ticron) is preferred because its knots are inocuous (Fig. 16-2). Dorsal plications sacrifice little in the way of penile length and have provided excellent results with extended follow-up. Dermal grafts are reserved for phalluses with severe curvature (Horton, 1973).

Neourethras are constructed or repaired with fine absorbable sutures (6-0 or 7-0 polydiaxanone) that cause little inflammation. Anastomoses are spatulated to minimize stenosis, and tubularized neourethras are placed with their closures against the shaft of the penis to maximize coverage. Suture lines are inverted lumenally with hopes of lessening the chances of fistula. Completed repairs are tested for leaks by instilling saline through a feeding tube while proximally occluding the urethra, and interrupted stitches are used to shore up any weaknesses. Additional layers of tissue coverage aid vascularization, eliminate crossing suture lines, and reduce the chances of fistula formation. These layers can be harvested from deepithelialized prepuce or the subcutaneous layers of adjacent shaft skin or scrotum with more proximal repairs (Retik, 1988) (Fig. 16-3). A flap of tunica vaginalis from an adjacent gonad also can be used to provide an effective buttress of a repair. The importance of multiple-layered closures to urethroplasties has been dramatically emphasized by a recent report where one fistula occurred in over 200 primary repairs by applying double-layered closures of the neourethra (Kass, 1990).

Figure 16-2. *Dorsal plications effectively correct persistent chordee and sacrifice little penile length. Neurovascular bundles are mobilized with Buck's fascia, and sutures (inset) buried as incisions in the tunica are reapproximated. (Reproduced with permission of the University of Indiana.)*

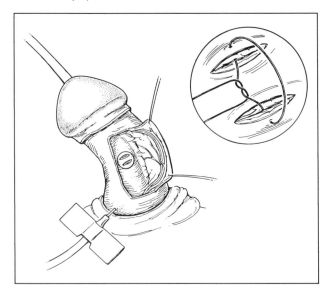

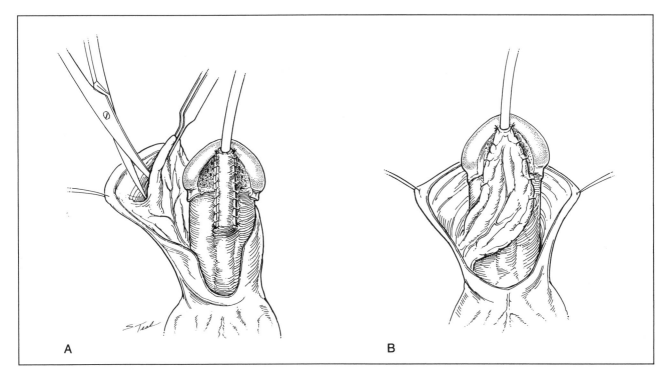

Figure 16-3. *Preputial subcutaneous wrap. Subcutaneous tissues (A) are easily mobilized from beneath the prepuce to (B) provide additional vascularized coverage of urethroplasties (in this case a perimeatal-based flap). (Reproduced with permission of the University of Indiana.)*

Sizing the neourethra is critical to the success of any repair. An acceptably reconstructed urethra walks a fine line between stricture and diverticulum. A lumenal size of no. 10 French is planned for the smallest boys, while no. 18 or 20 French is adequate for the older male. Intermittent calibration using a bougie à boule ensures adequate patency of the meatus, urethra, and proximal anastomosis. The glansplasty also can threaten the underlying *neourethra*. When a glans tunnel is used, a generous buttonhole of epithelium and deeper spongiosal tissue should be removed to create an uncompromising hiatus. If a glans split is planned, it is also helpful to excise some deeper tissues before reconstructing the glans in two layers.

Meticulous skin coverage completes the repair. Tension-free reapproximation is done using fine (6-0 or 7-0) chromic sutures for the skin and meatus. Subcutaneous sutures have been used recently to help avoid the unsightly epithelialized suture tracts that occurred with other forms of closure. Covering reoperative surgeries can be particularly challenging. In these cases, the lines of previous skin closure often can be appreciated, and every attempt should be made to continue to work along

them. This preserves vascularity and avoids the creation of isolated "islands" of skin devoid of blood supply. Many urethroplasties can be completed using single ventral midline closures. The medial approximation of ventrolateral shaft skin is made possible by splitting the prepuce dorsally. The cosmetic results are excellent, and concerns about recurrent chordee have been unfounded. Byars method provides effective coverage of significant ventral skin defects, but more complex Z-plasties tend to disrupt vascular patterns, increase the risks of skin loss, and should be avoided if possible.

Perioperative and Postoperative Management

We now perform virtually every repair on an outpatient basis, except when free grafts are used, and have not experienced increased morbidity. Preoperative parental teaching and simplified dressings and drainage have been instrumental in this regard. A urinalysis should be checked and a broad-spectrum antibiotic (cephalosporin) given at the beginning of each reoperative case. Infections should be treated before proceeding to surgery. Peripubertal and postpubertal boys are at an increased risk for infection, and Betadine showers are given to lower colonization of the perineum. Trimethoprim/sulfamethoxazol is given to suppress the bacteriuria that accompanies urinary drainage and is continued for a few days after the tube is removed to cover any residual infection/colonization.

Dressings accomplish three functions: (1) immobilization of the penis and drainage tube, (2) protection of delicate suture lines, and (3) containment of edema and bleeding until swelling begins to subside 48 hours after surgery. Transparent, permeable dressings such as Op-Site are ideal and apply adequate compression without undue tension. The repair is kept dry for 4 to 5 days until warm soaks are begun. This loosens the dressing and enables its removal at home. As an alternative, Xeroform gauze can be used to wrap the penis, which is then snugly sandwiched between two pads of Telfa and secured to the abdominal wall with a sheet of Op-Site.

We continue to divert every primary urethroplasty, with the exception of the MAGPI, and all but the most minor secondary repairs. A no. 6 French Silastic tube (reinforced ventriculoperitoneal shunt tubing) that lies proximal to the external sphincter and allows continual egress of urine has been very effective for younger boys. This soft tube is well tolerated, and bladder spasms are not as common as with other catheters. Diapers and open drainage are not well tolerated by older boys and men. As an alternative, a soft Silastic no. 13 French urethral splent that lies across the repair but distal to the external urethra or a suprapubic tube allows for spontaneous voiding. Diversion is continued for approximately 7 to 10 days, depending on the extensiveness of the repair and interval assessments of its healing. Our trials with leaving urethroplasties undiverted have generally resulted in children who experience considerable discomfort with voiding. In addition, some have returned a few years later with fistulas that were only appreciated once toilet training was begun and voiding could be observed.

Managing Early Complications

Early postoperative problems, including hematoma, skin loss, and infection, are fairly common. Fortunately, most require no more than supportive measures and do not require surgical revision with continued healing.

Hematomas threaten the integrity of repairs. Bleeding tendencies usually become evident at the completion of the case. Most stop with application of the dressing, but if a hematoma is appreciated beforehand, it should be evacuated. When concerns about bleeding persist, a tiny Penrose or Mini-Vac suction drain can be left subcutaneously. Hematomas that appear after the dressing is removed usually organize and resolve, but serial checks are required lest they become infected.

Skin loss is caused by progressive ischemia and usually does not become apparent until the dressing is removed. Vascularized flap procedures (TPIF and OIF) may be particularly prone in this regard, and careful mobilization of their pedicles should be done to avoid compromising the overlying shaft skin. Perioperative fluorescein can be used to assess the viability of tissues. When ischemia is suspected, affected tissue should be excised until its revised edges bleed. Hematomas, excessive tension, and constrictive dressings also can cause skin loss. In cases where skin loss and wound separation occur, defects usually fill with granulation tissue. The penis is forgiving and generally reepithelializes with little scarring. Skin grafting is rarely necessary unless a number of prior complications and surgeries have occurred. Multiple layers of urethral coverage assume additional importance when skin viability is equivocal, especially if free grafts are used.

Wound infections typically affect ischemic skin, are usually superficial, and should respond to local measures, including sitz baths and topical antibiotics. When a more serious infection is suspected, the wound should be opened to establish drainage and a culture sent. Systemic antibiotics are given to stem the progression of the process, while debridement also occasionally becomes necessary.

Urethrocutaneous fistulas are the most nettlesome problem that occur early after surgery. One or more of the risk factors cited above usually can be implicated in their formation. Acutely, fistulas present after urinary diversion has been discontinued and leakage of a ventral suture line or multiple streams are noted. Secondary blowouts of proximal suture lines sometimes cause fistulas, and the meatus should be checked for stenosis or plugging with secretions. Reestablishing drainage with a suprapubic tube or Foley catheter rarely results in a fistula's spontaneous closure. As the tract matures, the affected penis may exhibit an impressive amount of induration and swelling. The family should be made aware that further problems with healing may perpetrate additional breakdown of the repair. They also should be reassured that the cosmetic appearance of the penis will improve dramatically as the reaction subsides. Again, attempts at correcting fistulas, glans breakdowns, or wound separations should be deferred until the penis has fully healed, usually in 6 months.

Reoperations for Persistent Complications

Urethrocutaneous Fistulas

Fistulas represent the most common complication of hypospadias surgery. The majority can be managed with simple excision and closure, although the position, size, and number of fistulas influence the preference in repair. Identification of any occult fistulas can be made by injecting saline into the urethra under pressure. Before addressing the fistula(s), stenosis or strictures of the distal urethra and meatus must be ruled out. Cystoscopy is not done routinely. Instead, the urethra can be assessed adequately and less traumatically for valvelike flaps or diverticula by calibration with a bougie à boule. When distal obstruction is present, it also should be corrected. However, the swelling that inevitably results distally potentially jeopardizes the proximal fistula repair with higher voiding pressures. To avoid potential blowouts, urinary diversion becomes necessary, whereas diversion is usually not required of simple fistula closure alone.

A no. 3 French feeding tube is placed in the fistula and is sutured to its rim. The ostium of the fistula can then be circumscribed and its tract carefully dissected to the urethra using the tube for traction. Fistulas often have very aberrant courses and commonly tunnel obliquely in the subcutaneous tissues for several millimeters. After mobilization, the tract is excised flush with the urethra. Turbulence from urethral redundancy poses a risk factor to fistula recurrence. In cases where an adjoining diverticulum or megalourethra is present, the urethra also should be revised. After excising the fistula, the edges of healthy urethra are inverted using fine (6-0 or 7-0) polydiaxanone sutures. Additional layers of adjacent subcutaneous tissues are mobilized to help buttress the urethrostomy. Minor rotational flaps or V-Y advancements of the shaft skin provide useful coverage of most fistulas and help eliminate overlapping suture lines (Fig. 16-4). Such flaps should be mobilized adequately to *avoid tension*, perhaps the most common cause of failure with repairs of simple fistulas, where success rates of 95 to 98 percent are expected in most cases.

Particularly challenging exceptions are *fistulas positioned near the meatus or along the adjacent coronal sulcus.* Here, the surrounding skin is often less vascularized and affords minimal mobilization. Recurrent fistulas or sloughs of the skin bridge that exists between the tract and fistula are commonplace. As an alternative, we commonly prefer bringing this type of fistula in continuity with the meatus by incising the skin between the two.

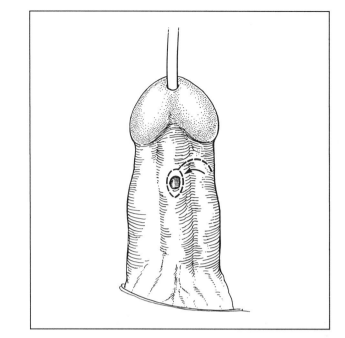

Figure 16-4. *Smaller fistulas usually can be corrected with simple excision and closure. V-Y flap advancements or rotational flaps (shown) provide effective coverage of repair. (Reproduced with permission of the University of Indiana.)*

The resulting defect can then be repaired by tubularization of the urethral plate with techniques such as the pyramid procedure, a urethral advancement, or even an onlay flap of redundant shaft skin.

Larger fistulas sometimes demand more complex urethroplasties. Simple Johanson-type turn-ins can be effective, but care must be taken to avoid urethral narrowing and stricture at the site of the closure (Fig. 16-5). When the potential for lumenal compromise exists, a patch flap of redundant penile skin is preferred (see onlay island principle below). This maneuver is especially helpful when fistulas are associated with distal urethral strictures that also must be corrected.

Finally, when *multiple fistulas* are present, it is often difficult or even impossible to repair them individually. The closure of one fistula can jeopardize the repair of another. Close proximity can lead to tension or compromised blood supply. As an alternative, it is often better to incise the tissue between the tracts, creating one large fistula. This can then be repaired using a turn-in or onlay flap technique.

Urethral Strictures

Urethral strictures usually become apparent during the first few months after surgery. Typical presentations

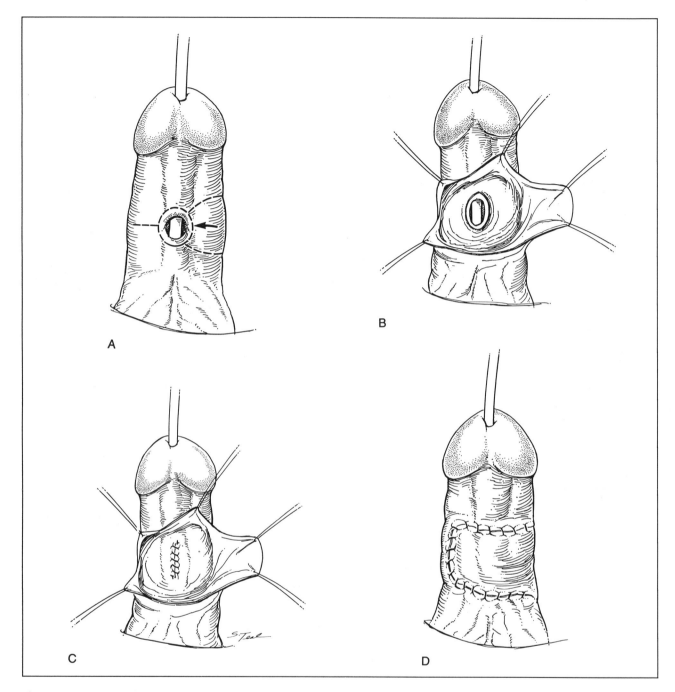

Figure 16-5. *Johanson-type repair. A. Large fistula and lines of incision for its flap coverage (arrow) outlined. B. Fistula has been circumscribed and adjacent flap mobilized. C. Closure completed, being careful not to compromise urethral lumen. D. Completed repair. (Reproduced with permission of the University of Indiana.)*

include dysuria, infection, hematuria, and decreased force of stream with straining to void. Strictures occur at any position along urethroplasties but most commonly affect their anastomosis with the dystopic meatus. Inadequate spatulation, incorporation of dysgenetic tissue, and angulation of tubularized pedicle flaps have all been implicated in their prevalence at this level. The latter can be avoided by tacking the spongiosum of the proximal urethra to the corporal bodies before anastomosing the flap. In other instances, infection, fistulization, or ischemia can lead to scarring of the neourethra. Finally, adequate neourethral sizing is mandatory to avoid iatrogenic narrowing.

A number of "less invasive" methods have been used for management of strictures, although their success is somewhat unpredictable. Dilation is sometimes successful for minor strictures. When the stricture is more extensive or has recurred, direct visual urethrotomy provides another alternative in treatment. Success rates with urethrotomy for all types of childhood strictures have been as high as 80 percent (Noe, 1983). However, this modality is not as effective for posturethroplasty strictures, where technical miscalculations or vascular mishaps are seemingly not as amenable to simple incisions. Repeated urethrotomies should be avoided to minimize the corporal fibrosis that undoubtedly results from the technique.

While dilation or urethrotomy can provide tempor-

ary panaceas of obstruction, recurrent or extensive strictures usually require formal urethroplasty. This should be avoided in the setting of a recent urethrotomy or traumatic dilation. If severe symptoms of obstruction persist despite recent manipulations, a suprapubic tube or even perineal urethrostomy is recommended to allow affected tissues to heal. Primary excision with reanastomosis is rarely, if ever, used for this type of stricture. The mobilization of previous urethroplasties is technically difficult, can further compromise vascularity, and also risks penile foreshortening. As an alternative, we prefer onlay-flap urethroplasties that preserve the viability of the urethral plate for smaller strictures. Tubularized flaps are used to bridge the more extensive defects that remain when longer strictures must be excised. One-stage repairs are preferred whenever vascularized flaps can be harvested from redundant penile skin (Fig. 16-6). Otherwise, Johanson's staged procedure remains a useful alternative for extensive or recurrent strictures (Johanson, 1953). Bladder and buccal mucosal grafts also have been used for strictures with some success, although experience with posturethroplasty strictures is limited (Hendren, 1986).

Meatal Stenosis

The distal manifestation of stricture, meatal stenosis, can be caused by transient edema, ischemia with scar-

Figure 16-6. *Onlay island flap repair of urethral stricture. A. Stricture of penile urethra, typically occurring at the site of the original meatus. B. Stricture opened with its ends spatulated. Redundant shaft skin yields vascularized flap. C. Flap is "patched" onto the stricture, restoring normal caliber to urethra. (Reproduced with permission of the University of Indiana.)*

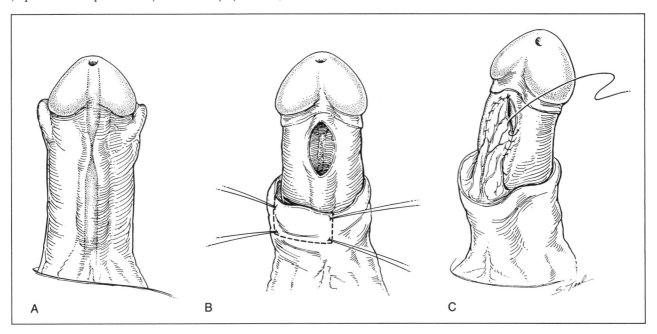

A   B   C

ring, or a poorly constructed glans tunnel or wrap. Meatal dilations have not been part of our routine post-operative management. However, if stenosis is suspected, daily meatal dilations with the tip of an ophthalmic ointment tube or fine feeding tube have been successful in resolving the problem for some patients. For others, a formal meatoplasty becomes necessary to resolve persistent obstruction. The scarred meatus is incised dorsally or ventrally, depending on its position relative to the tip of the glans. The defect that is created in the now widely opened meatus is closed by reapproximating the urethral mucosa to the skin in a Heinecke-Mikulicz fashion, in effect advancing the urethra. More extensive degrees of stenosis occasionally can involve the entire distal glanular neourethra. In these cases, the glans must be filleted open and an onlay island or meatal-based flap used to augment the strictured segment, covering it with generously mobilized glans wings (Jordan, 1987).

Balanitis xerotica obliterans (BXO) describes an idiopathic condition that occasionally involves the reconstructed meatus after hypospadias surgery. Balanitis xerotica obliterans is heralded by chronic inflammation of the dermis causing hyperkeratosis and a pale halo of toughened skin around the meatus. Pruritus or urethral discharge sometimes occurs, and unremitting meatal stenosis is commonplace. Steroid injections or topical testosterone are occasionally helpful, but excision with reconstruction is ultimately required of most affected urethras.

Meatal Regression

The retrusive meatus is an avoidable sequelae of the MAGPI urethroplasty applied to inappropriate variants having inadequate urethral and glanular mobility (see above). Regression also can occur with any other urethroplasty where breakdown of the distal neourethra and its overlying glans occurs. Symptoms are not usually a problem, although deflection of the stream is common. Nevertheless, the cosmetic drawbacks of this complication usually warrant its correction. Minor degrees of retrusion can be approached by repeating the standard MAGPI sequence. When urethral and glanular mobility are adequate, results are good. More significant regression of the ventral neourethra must be reconstructed with an onlay or perimeatal-based flap of redundant shaft skin or by tubularizing the plate in Duplay fahion (Elder, 1987b) (Fig. 16-7).

Persistent Chordee

Historically, persistent chordee usually could be attributed to its inadequate correction at prior urethroplasty.

Figure 16-7. *Significant urethral and glanular breakdown. A. Redundant shaft skin (forceps) is almost always available after these complications, and chordee is rarely present. The urethral plate has been kept intact and will be further defined to the glans tip. B. A vascularized flap can be harvested to reconstruct the neourethra using the onlay technique. (Reproduced with permission of the University of Indiana.)*

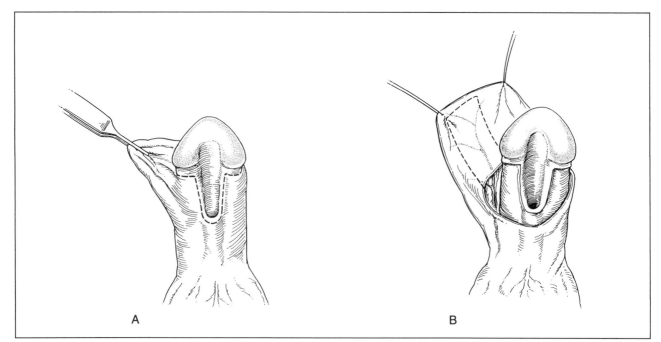

The uniform application of artificial erections should affect a significant decline in chordee as an isolated complication. Fibrosis also can be implicated, especially when other complications have occurred. Successful management follows a sequence similar to that applied to boys having chordee without hypospadias. After a circumferential incision, the penile skin is taken down to remove any superficial tethering and the artificial erection repeated. Curvature that persists is caused by either (1) deeper chordee lateral to and behind the urethra, (2) bowstringing by a fibrotic "short" urethra, or (3) intrinsic corporal scarring or corporal disproportion. For mild or moderate chordee, it is sometimes simpler and as effective to perform dorsal plications rather than more invasive measures such as dermal grafts. Otherwise, *urethral mobilization* becomes necessary to define the offending entity or what is often a combination of the three.

Mobilization with aims of urethral salvage is difficult in this setting. Urethrotomies occur in the face of scarring, and long-term viability is often jeapordized, even if the urethra can be kept intact. In many cases it is best to discard the urethra, correct the chordee, and simply start over, especially if the glanular configuration is unacceptable. In rare instances, the glans is acceptable and the urethra healthy after its mobilization. If so, the urethra can be transsected and a bridging graft or flap placed after correcting any corporal curvature that is present. The options in urethra replacement in either instance depend on the availability of genital skin, but bladder or buccal mucosal grafts are often required. When significant chordee persists and only the corpus remains as its cause, inlay grafts of dermis or tunica vaginalis are used to straighten the penis.

Urethral Hair

The best urethral substitute is non-hair-bearing skin, preferably the inner prepuce, which most closely resembles native urethra. However, we continue to encounter pubertal males who present with hair protruding from the meatus (the so-called bearded meatus) or who have dysuria or urinary tract infections from calculi that have formed on urethral hair. Cystoscopic depilation is reasonable initial management and is sometimes successful. However, excision of the involved urethra and replacement with a more suitable tissue is often necessary to resolve the problem. Avoidance is undoubtedly this complication's best solution, but the hair-bearing potential of the genital skin occasionally used in some urethroplasties is difficult to assess in the younger child.

Urethral Diverticula and Redundancy

Urethral diverticula are more common than generally supposed and have accounted for a significant number of boys referred for multiple failures of previous hypospadias repairs (Stecker, 1981). Factors implicated in their formation include excess caliber in neourethras, urinary extravasation with subsequent epithelialization of the localized urinomas, and distal obstruction leading to aneurysmal dilatation. Common presentations include decreased force of stream, urinary infections, and postvoid dribbling of urine pooled in the diverticulum. Examination frequently reveals ballooning of the urethra during voiding (Fig. 16-8), and stones that form are occasionally palpable. As a temporizing measure, the patient can be taught to "milk" the diverticulum by compressing its overlying skin. Definitive correction is done after a ventral skin incision affords ideal exposure of the involved urethra. Diverticula can be revised in a number of different ways after excising their redun-

Figure 16-8. *Urethral diverticula result in impressive degrees of urethral redundancy. In this case, the distal urethra was widely patent.*

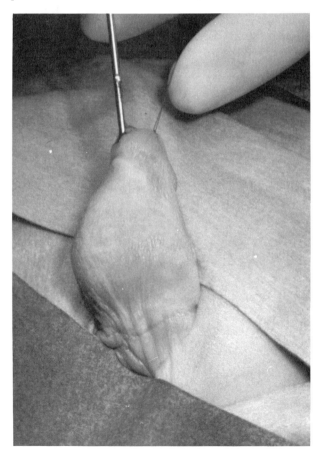

dancy and using the excess tissue to reconfigure the urethra (Winslow, 1985) (Fig. 16-9). It is necessary to correct any distal obstruction that might be present, and associated fistulas and strictures also should be ruled out and corrected when present.

The Onlay Island Principle in Failed Urethroplasties

Successful correction of failed urethroplasties is contingent on a well-conceived utilization of all "the available material." As an after-effect of many complications, excess shaft skin remains that is still in continuity with its original subcutaneous vascular pedicle. These randomly located flaps can be mobilized to serve as onlay or inlays after being tailored to fit the urethral plate, which is usually intact and well developed. We have found this approach very effective in a subgroup of patients with retrusive meatus or urethral stricture or who present with significant urethral defects between a patent glanular urethra and proximal meatus. Little or no chordee should be present in order to apply the onlay island principle effectively (Fig. 16-10).

Complex Redo Hypospadias

Patients who arrive with a combination of complications including stricture, fistula, and recurrent chordee represent the foremost challenges in the field. Histories are typically replete with a number of prior "minor" procedures, each an attempt to stem a cascade of compounded problems. Successful repairs are contingent on a thorough evaluation of the individual complications and utilization of the "available resources" in their correction. Often only an aggressive surgical approach offers a satisfactory solution. This includes replacing the scarred, unhealthy urethra. Whenever possible, genital skin should be used as a urethral replacement, but the excess shaft skin that is available is usually inadequate or unsuitably scarred, and an alternative must be sought.

Until recently, *bladder mucosal grafts* offered the primary option in replacement. The characteristics of bladder mucosa closely resemble those of the native urethra, and the tissue should not suffer from the effects of chronic exposure to urine. Disadvantages include bladder mucosa's pliability and tendency to shrink. This makes fashioning the neourethra an inexact science. The tissue also exhibits proliferative tendencies at the

Figure 16-9. *Repair of urethral diverticulum with distal stricture through ventral skin incision. A. Urethral incisions for V-Y advancement into stricture. B. After excision of redundancy, flap is advanced correcting both problems. (Adapted from Winslow et al., 1985. Reproduced with permission of the University of Indiana.)*

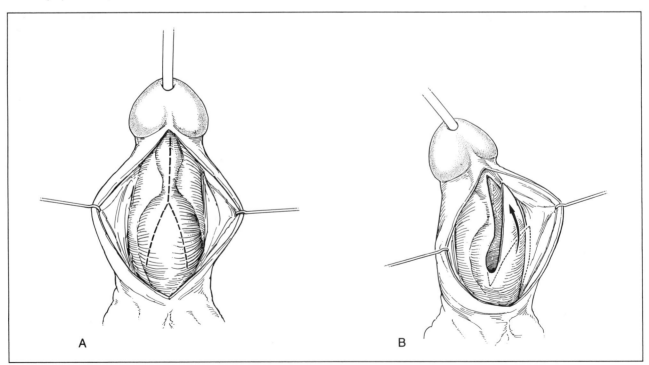

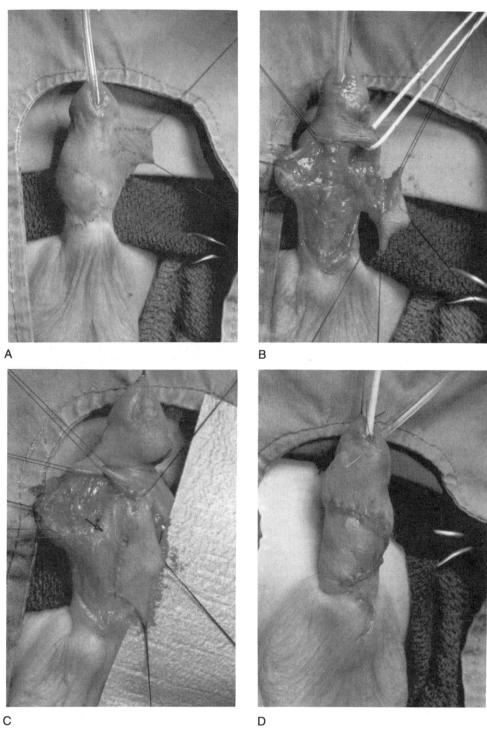

A

B

C

D

Figure 16-10. *Onlay island principle. Penis with recurrent stricture and pinpoint fistula. A. Skin marked for creation of vascularized flap from redundant distal portion and more proximal V-Y advancement coverage of repair. B. Island has been harvested and mobilized with its pedicle beneath preserved shaft skin (vessel loop) to the proximal site of the stricture. C. Stricture opened (arrow), fistula excised, and onlay flap–urethral anastomosis completed on one side. D. Final perioperative appearance.*

meatus, where it is exposed. Despite these drawbacks, the performance of bladder mucosal grafts has been commendable, especially when one considers the problems being addressed (Keating, 1990).

The introduction of *buccal mucosa* as a urethral replacement now offers another option in the management of these difficult patients (Dessanti, 1992). The tissue's thickened epithelium provides structural integrity that gives stiffness, makes it an easier tissue to work with, and may explain its avoidance of meatal protrusion. In addition, support is given to deeper layers as they go through the early tenuous stages in healing. Buccal mucosa also has a thin lamina propria that theoretically provides advantages with the establishment of neovascularity (Ewalt, 1992).

Mucosal Graft Urethroplasty

Effective application of bladder or buccal mucosa requires a logical technical sequence to maximize results (Fig. 16-11).

Preparing the Graft Bed

The bed is prepared initially so that the graft can be positioned and covered as soon as it is harvested. A circumferential incision is made proximal to the coronal sulcus, and the shaft skin is taken down to the base of the penis by defining the avascular plane between the subcutaneous tissues and corpora. This leaves the skin coverage as thick and healthy as possible. After assessing the different complications, the urethra is discarded and taken back proximally to healthy spongiosum. Distally, removal is facilitated by extending an incision in the ventral midline of the glans and circumferentially dissecting the urethra from the surrounding glans cap. In certain cases, the recipient penis and shaft skin are extensively scarred and may not provide adequate neovascularity for a free graft. When the status of the bed is questionable, we recommend a two-stage approach to maximize graft take. The penis is straightened (see recurrent chordee above), ventral shaft skin is rearranged, and a proximal urethrostomy is matured until a later date when the chances of graft take are hopefully improved.

Harvesting the Graft

After preparing the bed, the penis is wrapped in moist sponges and set aside while the graft is harvested. Bladder is exposed through a Pfannenstiel incision, and the graft is retrieved using an intra- or extravesical approach. In the former, the bladder can be entered immediately and an appropriately sized strip of mucosa sharply excised from one of its lateral walls. Alternatively, the muscularis can be incised and its plane with the underlying mucosa defined by sharp dissection, creating the so-called dome cyst. Stay sutures help define the limits of the graft before the mucosa is incised and the bladder decompressed. Additional length can be harvested by extending the dissection superiorly into and around the dome after entering the bladder (Figs. 16-12 and 16-13). Bladder mucosa should be moistened frequently and handled gently to minimize tissue trauma. Harvesting one bladder mucosal graft does not preclude the option of taking another at a later date in case of an initial failure.

Harvesting buccal mucosa from the inner cheek is done simply, although care must be taken to avoid Stensen's duct or damage to the underlying buccinator muscle. Lengths as great as 5 cm can be retrieved from one side, with compound grafts required of longer urethras. Selective cautery controls bleeding from the cheek, and suturing of the resulting defect is unnecesary in many cases. Mucosa from the inner lip also can be taken, but satisfactory graft width is difficult to obtain. Patients are fed the following day and experience amazingly little discomfort.

Tailoring the Graft

Some debate continues over the correct sizing of mucosal grafts. These grafts do contract but probably not as much as free skin grafts. Bladder mucosa is highly elastic and should be stretched gently when being measured. In adults, an ultimate no. 22 or 24 French urethra is planned by tailoring the tissue to a stretched width that is 4 or 5 mm wider. In smaller children, a 16-mm-wide graft ideally translates to a no. 12 French urethra. However, if an error is to be made in what is an understandably inexact portion of this technique, an excess is preferable to a paucity. Buccal mucosa is stiffer and may shrink less, and grafts are made only slightly larger than their intended urethral size. Grafts are tubularized over an appropriately sized red rubber catheter which is fixed to a sterile cardboard box with hypodermic needles. The mucosal surface is directed toward the lumen using a running (watertight), locking (to avert reefing) inverting polydiaxanone suture placed in the submucosal layer.

Completing the Repair

The completed graft is positioned between the generously mobilized glans wings and matured at the meatus using fine interrupted chromic sutures. Completing this portion of the repair initially allowing the graft to be

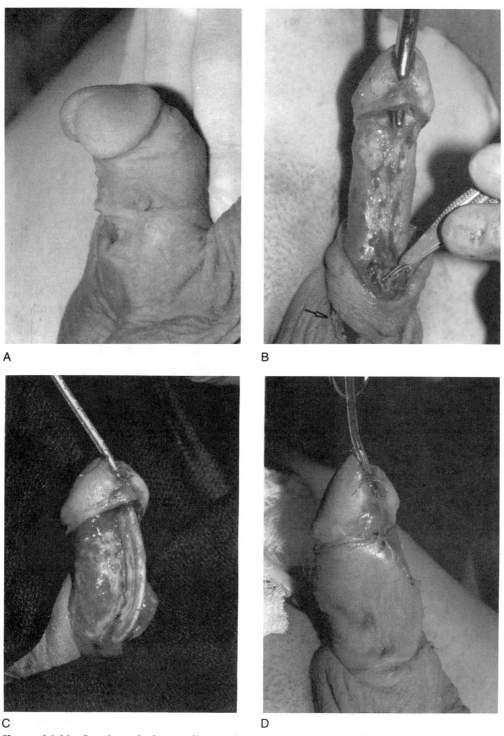

Figure 16-11. *Complex redo hypospadias. A. Preoperative assessment included chordee, proximal meatus, and paucity of shaft skin. B. Shaft skin taken down and penis straightened. Urethra (forceps) mobilized from its original position (arrow). A generous glans tunnel has been created. C. Bladder mucosa graft in place. D. Shaft skin reapproximated and repair completed.*

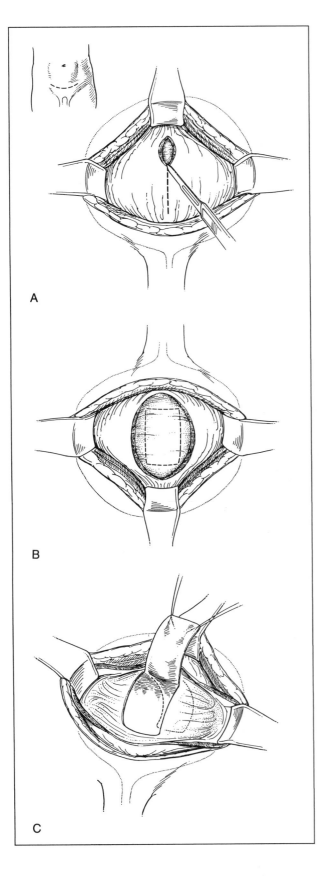

A

B

C

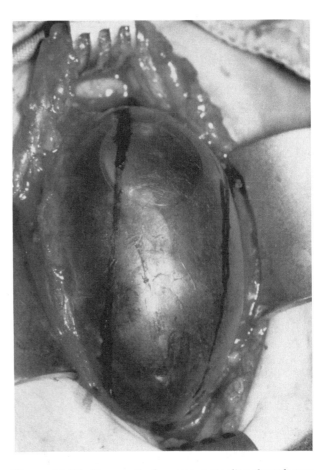

Figure 16-13. *Dome cyst of mucosa protruding through muscularis of bladder.*

stretched down to the proximal anastomosis. This serves to minimize any redundancy in length, lessening the risks of graft prolapse. Proximally, a widely spatulated anastomosis is created and a few millimeters of spongiosum are resected on the borders of the urethra to ensure a mucosal-to-mucosal anastomosis (Fig. 16-14). We also have begun to resect glans tissue from beneath the epithelium at the meatus with the hopes of minimizing stenosis (Mollard, 1989) (Fig. 16-15). Placing small skin grafts at the end of bladder mucosa grafts has not been effective in avoiding meatal problems.

Postoperative Management

A suprapubic tube provides adequate urinary drainage for these types of urethral free grafts. Subcutaneous

Figure 16-12. *Harvesting of graft. A. Bladder exposed through Pfannenstiel incision and muscularis vertically incised. B. Lateral dissections have defined plane between muscularis and the intact mucosa beneath. C. Longer grafts can be obtained by extending the dissection superiorly into and around the dome. (Reproduced with permission of the University of Indiana.)*

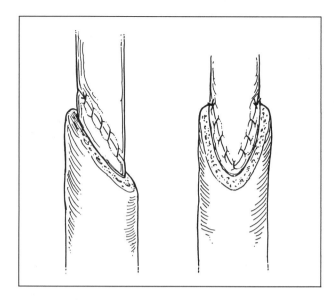

Figure 16-14. *Spongiosum is resected from the borders of the widely spatulated urethra to enable a mucosal-to-mucosal anastomosis. (Reproduced with permission of the University of Indiana.)*

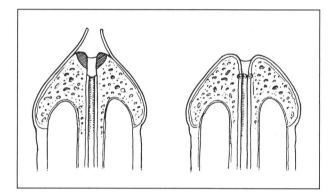

Figure 16-15. *Glans tissue is resected from beneath the meatal epithelium, recessing the bladder mucosa to minimize stenosis. (Reproduced with permission of the University of Indiana.)*

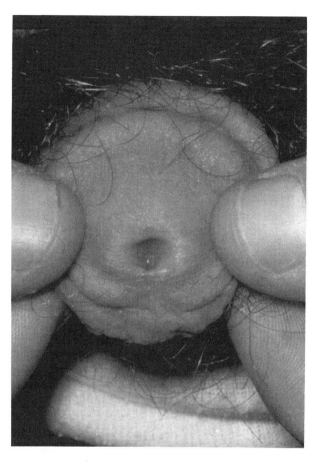

Figure 16-16. *Normal meatal appearance with bladder mucosal graft urethroplasty. Self-dilation was used postoperatively.*

drains are not used routinely. A multifenestrated no. 8 French silicone stent is placed across the graft but is positioned distal to the external sphincter to allow for the drainage of accumulated blood and secretions. Its tip is liberally coated with antibiotic ointment to prevent encrustations. If the stent is prematurely dislodged, no attempt should be made to replace it. The patient is kept at complete bed rest for 3 to 4 days to maximize immobilization of the graft and protect fragile microcapillary ingrowth. Erections pose a problem in the adult but usually can be controlled with amyl nitrate inhalers or diazepam sedation. The penile dressing is removed on the fifth postoperative day and warm soaks begun. On the tenth postoperative day, the urethral stent is re-

moved and a voiding trial given by clamping the suprapubic tube.

Results

The problems we have encountered with bladder mucosa are typical of those reported in other institutions. Bladder mucosa has been used in 11 patients with severe complications of prior hypospadias surgery. Seven patients have had excellent results, while 5 others experienced complications including graft failure (2), anastomotic stenosis (2), and meatal eversion (1). An overall 40 percent complication rate has been cited in the literature, with nearly two-thirds of these classified as minor, requiring little or no revision. Problems at the neomeatus have been by far the most common complications seen. The cause of poor performance of the tissue at this position remains unclear, but we now use meatal dilation in every patient on a daily basis for approximately 6 months after surgery (Fig. 16-16). Since incorporating dilation in the postoperative regimen, meatal stenosis or graft eversion has not been a problem. Other less common complications of bladder mucosal graft urethroplasties can be managed in a fashion similar to that described above for more standard urethroplasties.

Our experience with 12 buccal mucosa urethral reconstructions over the past 6 years has been encouraging. There have been no meatal complications and two fistulas in limited follow-up. Undoubtedly, an extended experience with the tissue will be necessary to more fully assess its value as a solution for complex redo urethroplasties. However, we strongly suspect that, at least for the time being, there will remain no perfect operation for these difficult and challenging problems.

Bibliography

Dessanti, A, et al. Autologous buccal mucosa graft for hypospadias repair: An initial report. J Urol 147:1081, 1992.

Duckett, JW. MAGPI (meatoplasty and glanuloplasty): A procedure for subcoronal hypospadias. Urol Clin North Am 8:513, 1981a.

Duckett, JW. The island flap technique for hypospadias repair. Urol Clin North Am 8:503, 1981b.

Duckett, JW, Keating, MA. Technical challenge of the megameatus intact prepuce (MIP) hypospadias variant: The pyramid procedure. J Urol 141:1407, 1989.

Duckett, JW, and Snyder, HM. The MAGPI hypospadias repair after 1000 cases: Avoidance of meatal stenosis and regression. J Urol 147:665, 1992a.

Duckett, JW. Hypospadias. In JY Gillenwater, JT Grayhack, ED Howards, and TA Stamey (eds), Campbell's Urology, 6th ed. Philadelphia: Saunders, 1992b, pp 1893–1919.

Elder, JS, Duckett, JW, and Snyder, HM. Onlay island flap in the repair of mid and distal penile hypospadias without chordee. J Urol 138:376, 1987a.

Elder, JW, and Duckett, JW. Urethral reconstruction following an unsuccessful one-stage hypospadias repair. World J Urol 5:19, 1987b.

Ewalt, DH, et al. Buccal mucosa: Rationale for use as urethral graft material (in press)

Hendren, WH, and Reda, EF. The bladder mucosal graft for urethral reconstruction. J Urol 21:189, 1986.

Hollowell, JG, et al. Preservation of the urethral plate in hypospadias repair: Extended applications and further experience with the onlay island flap urethroplasty. J Urol 143:98, 1990.

Horton, CE, and Devine, CJ, Jr. Peyronie's disease. Plast Reconstr Surg 52:503, 1973.

Johansonn, B. Reconstruction of the male urethra is stricture. Acta Chir Scand Suppl 176, 1953.

Jordan, GH: Reconstruction of the fossa navicularis. J Urol 138:102, 1987.

Kass, E, and Bolong, D. Single-stage hypospadias reconstruction without fistula. J Urol 144:520, 1990.

Keating, MA, Cartwright, PC, and Duckett, JW. Bladder mucosa in urethral reconstructions. J Urol 144:827, 1990.

Mollard, P, et al. Repair of hypospadias using bladder mucosal graft in 76 cases. J Urol 142:1548, 1989.

Noe, HN. Complications and management of childhood urethral stricture disease. Urol Clin North Am 10:531, 1983.

Retik, AB, Keating, MA, and Mandell, J. Complications of hypospadias repair. Urol Clin North Am 15:223, 1988.

Stecker, JF, Jr, et al. Hypospadias cripples. Urol Clin North Am 8:539, 1981.

Winslow, BH, Vorstman, B, and Devine, CJ, Jr. Urethroplasty using diverticular tissue. J Urol 134:552, 1985.

Complications of Neonatal Circumcision

R. LAWRENCE KROOVAND

Any surgical procedure may lend itself to errors of omission and commission. Circumcision is not immune. This chapter will address those complications occurring after circumcision which may require additional surgical intervention for remedy.

Circumcision is one of the oldest and recently most controversial surgical procedures known to humanity and represents the operation most frequently performed on neonatal males in the United States. Definitive indications for circumcision include phimosis, paraphimosis, and recurrent balanitis. None of these indications are present in the neonate. Other reasons cited by parents for circumcision include religion, a father or sibling circumcised, social custom, physical appearance, improved sexual function, and improved ease of hygiene. Neonatal circumcision is contraindicated for the sick, unstable, or premature (less than 2500 gm) baby or in the presence of any blood dyscrasia. A family history of bleeding disorder requires a thorough investigation prior to circumcision. An abnormal appearing prepuce, epispadias, hypospadias, chordee without hypospadias, penile torsion, and other penile anomalies are also contraindications to neonatal circumcision, since the prepuce may be necessary to facilitate later reconstructive procedures.

The incidence of complications following neonatal circumcision is estimated to range between 0.2 and 5 percent, varying with the method of circumcision (Gomco clamp, plastibell, free-hand sleeve resection) and the expertise of the operating surgeon. Unfortunately, neonatal circumcision frequently becomes the duty of the least experienced member of the medical team. Most complications after circumcision are inconsequential and require only local wound care for man-

agement. The more common complications after circumcision potentially requiring additional surgical management include circumcision of a penis with an unrecognized hypospadias or chordee without hypospadias, removal of excessive penile skin, denudation of the penile shaft, failure to remove an adequate amount of foreskin, and injury to the glans. Other complications potentially requiring postcircumcision intervention include slough of the penis following use of electrocautery in conjunction with the Gomco clamp, necrotizing fasciitis, skin or penile slough from too tight a dressing, urethrocutaneous fistula, and skin bridges (adhesions of shaft skin to the glans).

The key to avoiding postoperative complications rests in adequate prophylaxis. Each of the methods for circumcision has its specific advantages and disadvantages. If performed by a trained, experienced surgeon employing meticulous technique, all methods for circumcision should be relatively free from complications, making circumcision a safe surgical procedure. As outlined by Kaplan, the goal of each circumcision technique is to remove enough shaft skin and inner prepuce so that the glans is sufficiently uncovered to prevent or treat phimosis and to render the development of paraphimosis impossible. To facilitate a safe and complete circumcision, regardless of technique, the operator should observe strict aseptic technique; completely separate the inner preputial epithelium from the glans, exposing the entire coronal sulcus; adequately but not excessively excise the inner and outer preputial skin completely, exposing the coronal sulcus and glans; provide adequate hemostasis; and establish appropriate cosmesis. Electrocautery should be employed judiciously. Failure to totally separate the inner prepuce from the glanular epithelium and coronal sulcus probably represents the most common error leading to inadequate circumcision.

Complications recognized after circumcision and potentially requiring operative management may include skin bridges, inclusion cysts, removal of insufficient skin, excessive removal of skin, urethrocutaneous fistula, glanular injuries, penile necrosis, necrotizing fasciitis, and lymphedema. Each of these potential complications and their appropriate management will be discussed individually in the following sections.

Skin Bridges

Skin bridge formation (postcircumcision adhesions of the penile shaft skin to the glans) is probably the result of failure to completely separate the inner preputial epithelium from the glanular epithelium at the time of circumcision or adhesion of the circumcision scar to denuded glanular epithelium. Careful postcircumcision follow-up should permit early identification of skin bridges and manual separation of the skin bridges. More extensive skin bridges or those identified at a time remote from circumcision may require surgical incision (division). Skin bridges may be unsightly, permit accumulation of smegma under the skin bridge(s), or tether the erect penis producing penile curvature or pain during erection or sexual intercourse (Fig. 17-1). Simple hemostat crushing and surgical incision (division) provide appropriate management for skin bridges. For

Figure 17-1. *Skin bridge occurring after circumcision. Note dorsal glanular chordee even with minimal erection.*

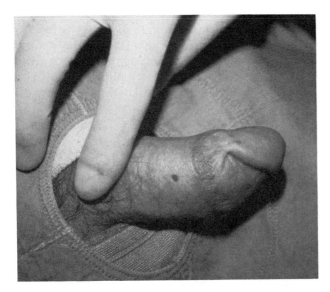

minor skin bridges, light sedation in the office and local anesthesia should permit skin bridge incision; more extensive skin bridges may require general anesthesia to permit optimal operative management.

Inclusion Cysts

Inclusion cysts along the circumcision line result from the turning in of epidermis at the time of circumcision. Inclusion cysts may become quite large and unsightly (Fig. 17-2) or even become infected. Local surgical excision (shelling out) of the entire cyst is curative. If any cyst wall is left in place, recurrence is inevitable. Large cysts that have stretched the penile skin may, in addition to cyst removal, require penile skin revision to provide appropriate cosmesis.

Insufficient Skin Removal

Removal of insufficient penile skin and inner prepuce generally is only a cosmetic problem. The boy with

Figure 17-2. *Inclusion cyst occurring after circumcision.*

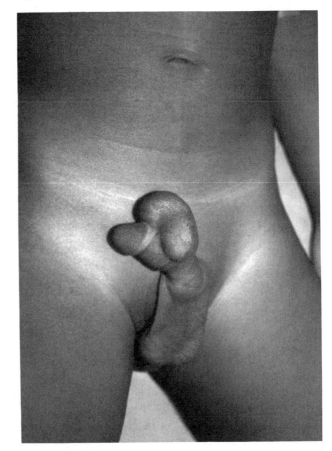

excess penile shaft skin after circumcision does not appear circumcised, a situation of little consequence, save some degree of parental consternation (Fig. 17-3). The decision to recommend additional surgical intervention versus nonintervention (observation) is controversial and beyond the scope of this discussion. If elected, recircumcision should conform to the operative standards described previously. If the circumcision scar fibroses and narrows, producing a pathologic phimosis, the boy is at risk for infection or, if the contraction is severe enough, urinary retention. Here, careful free-hand revision of the circumcision is indicated.

Excessive Skin Removal

Removal of excessive penile shaft skin may result in separation of the circumcision line, producing penile denudation or, if the circumcision scar fibroses, a buried or concealed penis. Penile denudation occurs most commonly after a Gomco or plastibell circumcision. In this situation, it is probable that too much penile shaft skin

Figure 17-3. *Removal of insufficient penile shaft skin.*

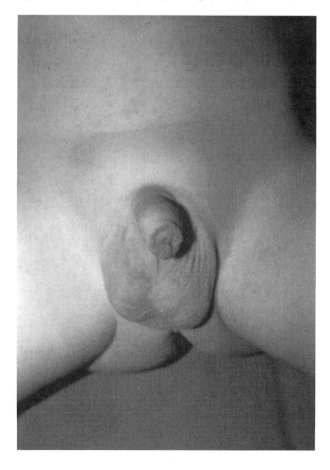

was drawn up prior to applying the Gomco clamp or plastibell. Postoperative erections may produce sufficient tension on the circumcision line that separation occurs, resulting in penile shaft denudation (Fig. 17-4).

Management of postcircumcision penile denudation is controversial. Sotolongo and associates recommend nonoperative management employing local wound care with saline- or antibiotic-soaked dressings until skin regeneration covers the denuded penis. The cosmetic results reported after such nonoperative management are excellent (Fig. 17-5). Additional options for management of penile denudation include burial of the penis under a thinned-out and stretched segment of scrotum (see Fig. 17-4B) with delayed resurrection (4 to 6 months later) (see Fig. 17-4C) employing the transferred scrotal skin to resurface the shaft of the penis (see Fig. 17-4D). The use of scrotal skin for resurfacing of the penis is not a new concept. Its advantages rest in its convenient availability and the fact that the transferred scrotal skin should remain hormonally responsive during penile growth at puberty. Potential disadvantages are that some of the transferred scrotal skin may contain hair follicles and that scrotal skin may not be cosmetically optimal. The use of a split- or full-thickness skin graft taken from non-hair-bearing epithelium is also an option. Skin grafts, split or full thickness, are felt to provide superior cosmesis; however, since such skin grafts are not hormonally responsive, they may not stretch and grow during penile growth at puberty, potentially producing secondary chordee and/or unsatisfactory cosmesis. Reapproximation of the remaining penile shaft skin to the inner prepuce is also an option for management of penile denudation but may result in a short appearance of the penis and displacement of the penile shaft into the suprapubic fat. One would think that tincture of time and normal growth and development and normal erections should permit this natural tissue expander to stretch the remaining penile skin so as to provide for appropriate penile skin coverage. Although not previously reported in this context, Silastic tissue expanders to stretch the remaining penile skin and the use of tissue culture–generated penile skin homografts are also potential salvage routes.

The boy who has had an excess of penile shaft skin removed and is further compromised by contracture and fibrosis of the circumcision scar may develop a buried (concealed) penis (Fig. 17-6A). This problem appears to be the result of excision of excessive penile shaft skin with insufficient excision of the inner prepuce. The scarring and contracture of the circumcision scar produces a secondary phimosis that displaces the penile

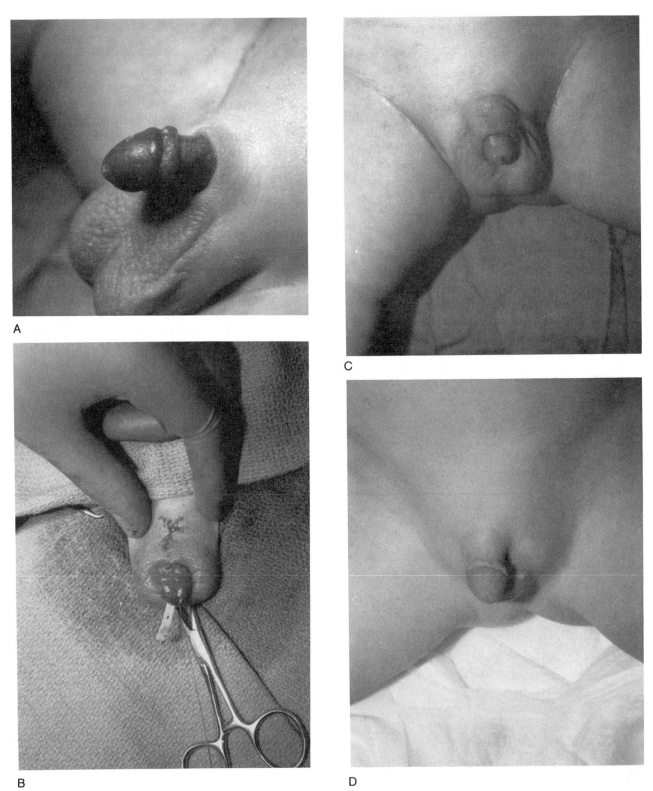

Figure 17-4. *A. Penile denudation (separation of circumcision line). B. Initial burial of penis under scrotal flap and suprapubic wound closure. C. Prior to penile resurrection. D. Cosmetic result after scrotal burial and penile resurrection.*

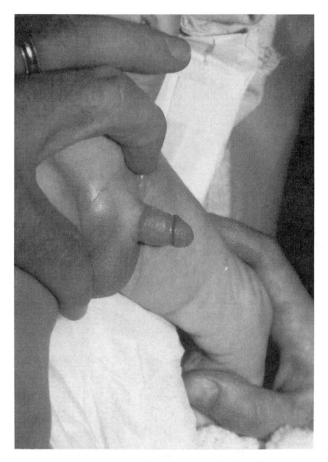

Figure 17-5. *Cosmetic outcome after management of postcircumcision penile denudation employing local wound care during epithelial regeneration.*

shaft into the suprapubic fat. If scar contracture and fibrosis are severe, urinary retention may occur (Fig. 17-7). Because there is often sufficient inner prepuce remaining to resurface the shaft of the penis, careful circumferential excision of the phimotic circumcision scar is generally preferred to a dorsal slit because circumferential excision of the circumcision scar protects the remaining shaft skin and inner prepuce, permitting their use for penile resurfacing (Fig. 17-6B, C). In situations where the excessive skin removal has involved both the shaft skin and the inner prepuce, some form of skin grafting, tissue expansion, or extensive abdominal skin-flap rotation may be required to resurface the penis.

Urethrocutaneous Fistula

Urethrocutaneous fistula may occur after circumcision. Most reported fistulas occur after circumcisions per-

formed employing either the Gomco clamp or the plastibell device. For fistula formation to occur, it must be assumed that the urethra was pulled into and crushed by the circumcising device or the urethra was incised by the scalpel blade at the time of circumcision. An additional potential etiology for postcircumcision urethrocutaneous fistula would be sutures placed in the frenular area to provide hemostasis or injury to the ventral shaft skin and urethra in a child with unrecognized hypospadias without chordee with thin ventral shaft skin and a hyposplastic urethra.

Repair of urethrocutaneous fistulas occurring after circumcision should not be attempted until all tissue healing and reaction have completely resolved (3 to 6 months after circumcision). Fistula repair is governed by the same rules of meticulous technique and non-overlying suture lines as for fistula repair after hypospadias urethroplasty. Most often a rotation flap with a vest-over-pants subcutaneous closure is curative. Further technical details and surgical options are described in standard urology texts.

Glanular Injuries

Injuries to the glans are generally preventable by performing the entire circumcision under direct vision rather than performing any aspect of the procedure blindly. Hypospadias and epispadias have both been produced after blind dorsal or ventral incision of the prepuce or while performing a circumcision on a previously unrecognized penile anomaly. If recognized at the time of circumcision, primary repair is appropriate. If unrecognized until the postoperative period, delayed repair may be indicated depending on the functional consequences of the injury and possibly the resulting cosmetic appearance. Here the principles of hypospadias and epispadias repair apply.

Laceration of the tip of the glans (Fig. 17-8) and partial or total amputation (Fig. 17-9A) of the glans have been reported when the operator has employed a blind technique for circumcision. Minor injuries may require no repair; major injuries (glanular amputation) should be managed with immediate reapproximation of the amputated glans to the remaining glanular tissue or penile shaft (Fig. 17-9B).

Glanular and/or penile necrosis and skin slough have been reported after too tight a postcircumcision dressing or after a cautery injury. Skin slough may be managed in a manner similar to that for penile denudation. Glanular and penile necrosis pose unusual and

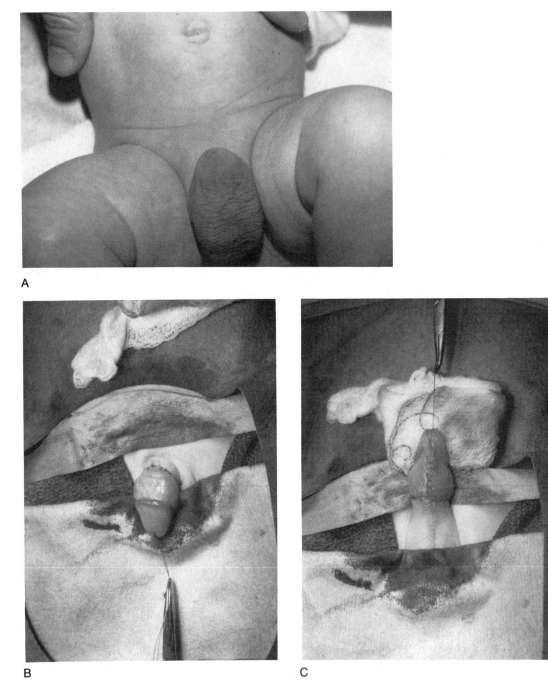

A

B   C

Figure 17-6. *A. Buried (concealed) penis after circumcision. B. Resurrection of buried penis. C. Length of inner prepuce available for penile shaft resurfacing as compared with the sparsity of penile shaft epithelium seen in part A.*

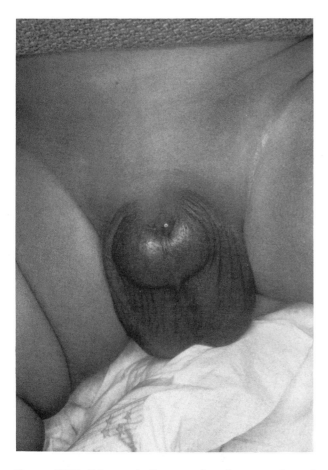

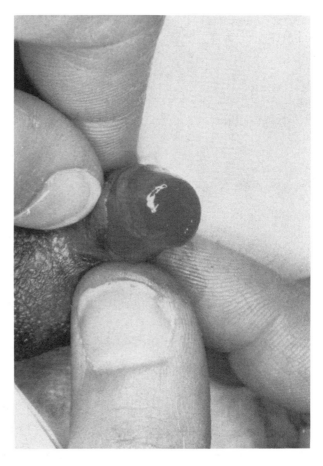

Figure 17-7. *Urinary retention occurring after severe circumcision scar contracture.*

Figure 17-8. *Glanular laceration with partial glanular amputation.*

Figure 17-9. *A. Glanular amputation—glans and foreskin. B. Cosmetic result 6 months after glanular reimplantation.*

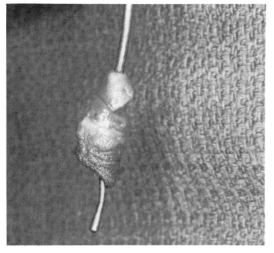

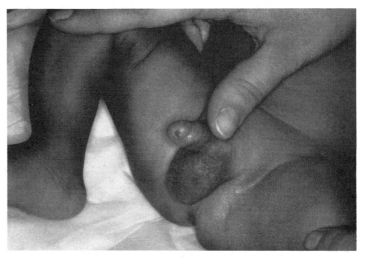

A   B

difficult situations. Major injuries with significant penile necrosis may be best managed by gender reassignment combined with gonadectomy or referral to a pediatric urologic unit with experience in total penile reconstruction. The philosophical, intellectual, and technical aspects of the management of this most unusual complication after circumcision are beyond the scope of this commentary.

Necrotizing Fasciitis Following Circumcision

Necrotizing fasciitis after circumcision represents a most uncommon and life-threatening bacterial infection producing edema, necrosis, and loss of subcutaneous fat and fascia with a reported mortality approaching 60 percent in some series. Necrotizing

Figure 17-10. *Lymphedema complicating a postcircumcision infection.*

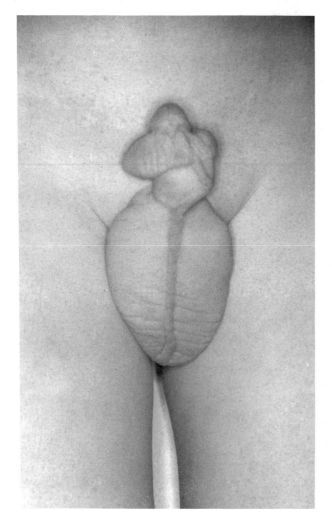

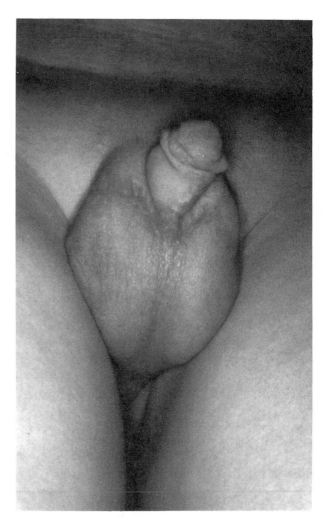

Figure 17-11. *Surgical management of lymphedema occurring after an infected circumcision (distal shaft skin and scrotal resection).*

fasciitis after circumcision occurs most frequently after the use of a plastibell device, where postcircumcision infections occur significantly more frequently than after any other methods of circumcision. Wide debridement and culture-specific antibiotic coverage offer the best chances for survival. The necessity for and extent of later reconstructive procedures are dictated by the extent of the abdominal wall defect and the nature of penile deformity remaining after resolution of the infective process.

Lymphedema

Lymphedema of the penis and scrotum may occur following circumcision, especially if the circumcision be-

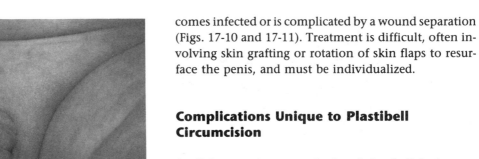

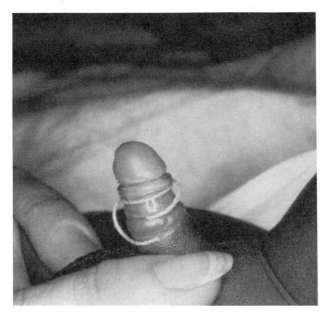

Figure 17-12. *Retained and infected plastibell.*

comes infected or is complicated by a wound separation (Figs. 17-10 and 17-11). Treatment is difficult, often involving skin grafting or rotation of skin flaps to resurface the penis, and must be individualized.

Complications Unique to Plastibell Circumcision

An ill-fitting or inaccurately placed plastibell device may migrate proximally and injure the shaft of the penis (Figs. 17-12 and 17-13*A*) or migrate distally to produce glandular injury (Fig. 17-13). Careful application of an appropriately sized plastibell device and removal of any retained plastibell rings (Fig. 17-14), using a ring cutter or bone-cutting forceps, within several days of circumcision should minimize or eliminate complications occurring after plastibell circumcision and reduce the chance for serious postcircumcision infection and necrotizing fasciitis. Glanular injuries, usually minor (Fig. 17-13*B*), generally require no additional operative

Figure 17-13. *A. Penile injury as the result of the retained and infected plastibell. B. Glanular injury after circumcision, the result of an ill-fitting or inaccurately placed plastibell device.*

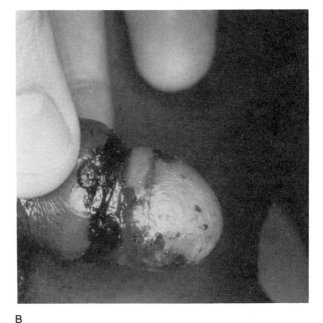

A   B

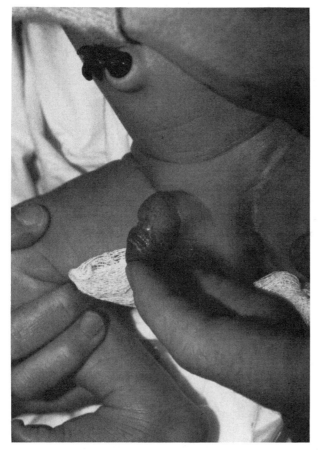

Figure 17-14. *Retained plastibell.*

management. Injuries to the penile shaft and/or urethra require debridement and skin revision or fistula repair after a period of postcircumcision healing (3 to 6 months) to permit maximum resolution of tissue reaction and to provide an optimal situation for functional and cosmetic remedy.

Bibliography

Izzidien Al-Sammarrai, AY, et al. A review of a Plastibell device in neonatal circumcision in 2000 instances: The surgeon at work. Surg Gynecol Obstet 167:341, 1988.

Kaplan, GW. Complications of circumcision: Symposium on complications of pediatric urologic surgery. Urol Clin North Am 10:543, 1983.

Kon, M. A rare complication following circumcision: The concealed penis. J Urol 130:573, 1983.

Radhakrishnan, J, and Reyes, HM. Penoplasty for buried penis secondary to "radical" circumcision. J Pediatr Surg 19: 629, 1984.

Sotolongo, JR, Jr, Hoffman, S, and Gribetz, ME. Penile denudation injuries after circumcision. J Urol 133:102, 1985.

Sterenberg, N, Golan, J, and Ben-Hur, N. Necrosis of the glans penis following neonatal circumcision. Plast Reconstr Surg 6:237, 1981.

Woodside, JR. Necrotizing fasciitis after neonatal circumcision. Am J Dis Child 134:301, 1980.

Priapism

CHESTER C. WINTER

The failure rate in the initial treatment of priapism has been reported to be as high as 50 percent. The first management may have been the injection of Neo-Synephrine with some temporary success or one of the shunting procedures (glans-cavernosa, cavernosum-spongiosum, or saphenous vein–cavernosum). In case of failure, the steps outlined in Table 18-1 and discussed below are recommended.

Ideally, the duration of priapism has been 96 hours or less from onset. First, a Doppler ultrasound study should be performed to ascertain blood flow through the penis. Then the patient is prepped and draped, and local, spinal, or general anesthesia is administered. An 18-gauge needle is inserted through the dorsal glans into one corpus cavernosum body, and an attempt is made to aspirate blood (squeezing the penis helps). If no blood can be aspirated, an operation should *not* be done, since thrombosis and/or fibrosis have already occurred, and shunting would be useless. If the blood looks very dark, this suggests venous outlet obstruction, and shunting is indicated.

If the blood has a normal hue and flows freely, this suggests that the arterial vessels are widely patent and ingress is greater than egress. Normal penile blood gases will confirm high arterial inflow, nonischemic priapism. Before any interventional procedures are done, thorough irrigation of the corpora (10 ml of saline × 10) is carried out with the needle still in place. Then 10 mg of Neo-Synephrine diluted to 500 ml of saline is prepared. The corpora are filled with this solution (5 to 10 ml), and a 30-minute wait is required to see if the priapism will resolve. This process may be repeated after 30 minutes. If no resolution is forthcoming, then inter-

nal pudendal arteriography is indicated. If a lacerated artery is found, it may be embolized; if not, ligation of one internal pudendal artery should be considered. The priapism should then resolve.

Shunting for Low-Pressure Ischemic Priapism

A glans-cavernosal shunt (Winter procedure) is performed through the same needle site by using a Travenol Tru-Cut biopsy needle, removing two cores of tunica albuginea (septum) from each cavernosal body (Fig. 18-1). If larger shunts are desired, a Kerrison rongeur may be used. This requires a scalpel to enlarge the entry site in the glans and septum. Care should be taken to ensure removal of albuginea tissue by rotating the biopsy instrument 360 degrees and tearing the piece out. The glans opening is then closed with a figure-of-eight absorbable suture. It is important after all shunting procedures to almost continuously massage or milk the penis for 12 hours to keep it detumesced. The patient can do this if he is awake and alert. Pediatric blood pressure cuffs have been used but are cumbersome and are used too infrequently (every 5 minutes). The cuff should be inflated to 200 mmHg for *only an instant*. Do not wrap the penis tightly or compromise its blood flow. Otherwise, gangrene could ensue.

An alternative to the Winter procedure is the El Ghorab operation. After anesthesia, a semicircular incision is made in the dorsal corona, and the glans is hinged back, exposing the tips of the corpora cavernosal bodies. Generous windows are made on each side, re-

Table 18-1. *Algorithm Useful in the Treatment of Priapism*

1. Doppler ultrasound study of penis.
2. Insert 18-gauge needle through glans into cavernosum body.
   a. If no blood is obtained, indicating fibrosis, *stop.*
   b. If blood is aspirated, do blood gases.
   c. If freely flowing, bright red blood is aspirated and the blood gases are normal, proceed.
3. Instill Neo-Synephrine once or twice.
   a. If the penis stays detumesced, *stop.*
   b. If priapism returns, proceed.
4. Do internal pudendal arteriography.
   a. If a lacerated artery is found, embolize.
   b. If no lacerated artery is found, unilaterally ligate.
   c. Priapism should be resolved.
5. If low-pressure ischemic priapism is seen,
   a. Do glans-cavernosal shunt.
      (1) If the penis stays detumesced, *stop.*
      (2) If priapism returns, proceed.
   b. Do corpora cavernosum-spongiosum shunt.
      (1) If the penis stays detumesced, *stop.*
      (2) If priapism returns, proceed.
   c. Do saphenous vein–corpus cavernosum shunt.
      (1) Priapism should be resolved.

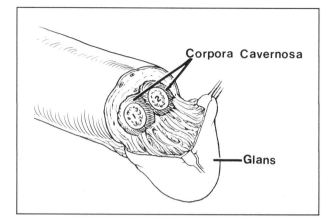

Figure 18-2. *In the El Ghorab operation, a semicircular incision is made in the corona of the penis, and the glans is hinged back. The end of each corpus cavernosum is excised.*

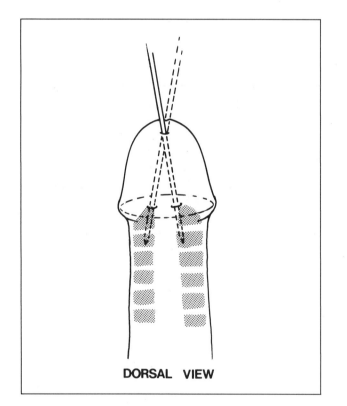

DORSAL VIEW

Figure 18-1. *The glans-cavernosa shunt is performed through a single needle aspiration site using a Travenol Tru-Cut biopsy needle.*

moving pieces of tissue (albuginea). The corona is then reapproximated (Fig. 18-2).

If one or two glans-cavernosa shunts fail, one may proceed to a spongiosum-cavernosum shunt at the base of the penis. First, a catheter is inserted to keep the urethra out of the operative field. The approach is dorsal-lateral, and the corpus cavernosum is separated from the spongiosum. The latter is flimsy and ill-defined. A button of tissue is removed from each body (albuginea and fascia), and the two bodies are anastomosed with two semicircular sutures (absorbable 4-0) so that a shunt is made. The skin incision is closed (Fig. 18-3).

If failure still ensues and blood can still be aspirated from the corpora, which can be detumesced, then one should proceed to a saphenous vein–corpus cavernosum shunt. After anesthesia, a vertical incision is made over the course of the saphenous vein, which is dissected free from its bed. It is ligated toward the knee end and brought through a subcutaneous tunnel to the base of the penis. Through a penile skin incision, a piece of tunica albuginea is removed from the corpus cavernosum and the vein anastomosed to create a shunt (Fig. 18-4).

In my experience with 107 patients, all subjects in whom blood can be aspirated and detumesced have been maintained detumescent without getting to the saphenous vein stage.

Complications

Complications of shunting are numerous. Several are discussed.

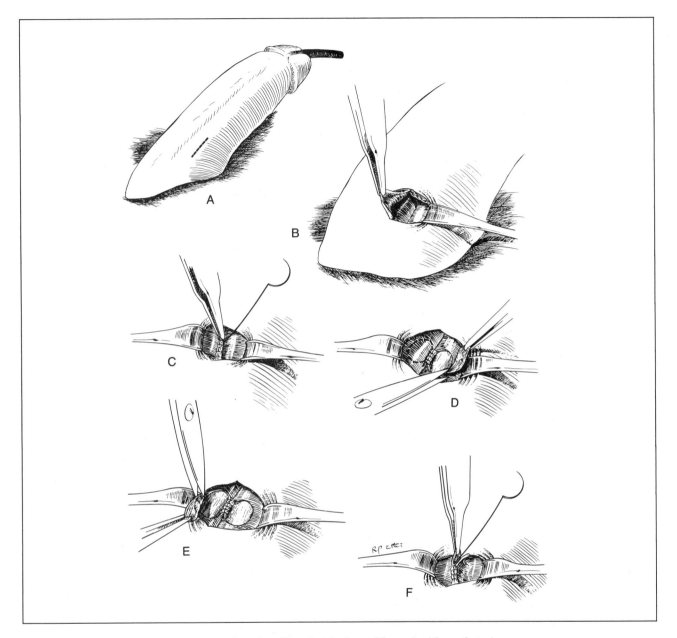

Figure 18-3. *The cavernosum-spongiosum shunt is performed at the base of the penis with a catheter in the urethra (A). The space between the flimsy spongiosum (containing catheter) and cavernosal body is developed on one side (B). A running, locking absorbable suture is commenced to form the base of the anastomosis (C). Elliptical buttons of tunica albuginea are excised from the cavernosal and spongiosal bodies (D and E). The circular anastomosis with the running suture is continued (F), creating a shunt between the spongiosum and cavernosum.*

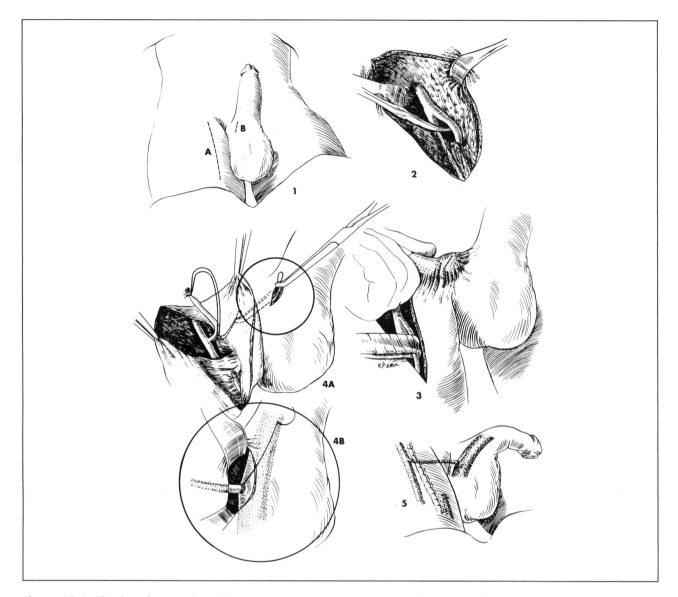

Figure 18-4. *The shunt between the saphenous vein to one corpus cavernosum is begun by making incisions in the upper medial thigh (A) and lateral base of the penis (1B). The saphenous vein is exposed and dissected for 6 inches (2) and divided proximally and the free ends ligated. A subcutaneous tunnel is made bluntly with the finger between the saphenous vein and corpus cavernosum (3). The distal saphenous vein is then passed through the tunnel to the base of the penis (4A) and sutured to the cavernosal body where a small elliptical piece of tunica albuginea has been excised (4B), completing the shunt (5).*

Chronic penile engorgement is rare and most likely due to partial egress obstruction. In most instances, nothing needs to be done, especially if the patient is potent. If aggressive treatment seems warranted, attention could be directed toward unilateral arterial ligation. Urethral fistula or diverticulum can be managed by surgical excision and primary closure. Penile gangrene and sloughing should be managed by adequate debridement

and later skin grafting or reconstructive plastic surgery. Temporary urethrostomy or suprapubic cystostomy may be useful.

Impotence can occur in up to 50 percent of patients regardless of treatment. An informed consent should be signed by the patient and/or relatives before embarking on treatment. This consent should include a statement that it is the disease and not the treatment that causes loss of potency and that the treatment is designed to try to prevent this complication. If impotence occurs after 1 year of observation, a penile prosthesis of the semi-rigid type may be placed. It may be necessary to currette out the fibrosed tissue in the cavernosal bodies. Occasionally, only one prosthesis is inserted after cutting the interseptal tissue between the two corpora cavernosal bodies.

Bibliography

Sayer, J, and Parsons, CL. Successful treatment of priapism with intracorporeal epinephrine. J Urol 140:827, 1988.

Winter, CC, and McDowell, G. Experience with 105 patients with priapism: Update review of all aspects. J Urol 140:980, 1988.

Witt, MA, et al. Traumatic laceration of intracavernosal arteries: The pathophysiology of nonischemic, high flow, arterial priapism. J Urol 143:129, 1990.

Peyronie's Disease

CHARLES J. DEVINE, JR.
GERALD H. JORDAN
STEVEN M. SCHLOSSBERG

Before considering reoperations for Peyronie's disease, the pathophysiology of Peyronie's disease must be defined and the primary surgical options must be discussed. Peyronie's disease is not rare; it may involve 1 percent of the white male population. The curvature typical of Peyronie's disease results from a scar that involves the tunica albuginea of the corpora cavernosa. This "plaque" is felt as a lump; its inelasticity limits extension of the involved aspect of the shaft, distorting the erection. A diagram of a cross section of the penis (Fig. 19-1) demonstrates the corpora cavernosa containing erectile tissue within the elastic sheath that is the tunica albuginea. At the base of the penis, the corpora are separate structures fixed to the undersurface of the pubic bones. They fuse in the shaft of the penis but are separated by a septum composed of multiple strands fixed to the midline dorsally and ventrally. The corpus spongiosum, containing the urethra, runs in the groove on the underside of the fused corpora. In the midline dorsally the deep dorsal vein runs beneath Buck's fascia with a dorsal artery on either side and the fascicles of the dorsal nerves lateral to each.

As the erectile tissue engorges with blood during tumescence, the elastic structures of the penis expand symmetrically, resulting in a straight erection. The tunica albuginea is bilaminar; the inner lamina is composed of circular fibers, and the outer is composed of longitudinal fibers. The elastic fibers of the strands of the septum fan out and are interwoven with the fibers of the inner layer of the tunica (Fig. 19-2A). During erection, the septum and tunica are stretched to the limit of their extensibility, and their configuration resembles an inflated I beam, resisting upward or downward bending and imparting to the penis its ultimate axial rigidity.

Almost without exception, the plaque of Peyronie's disease is located in the dorsal or ventral midline of the tunica where the strands of the septum are attached. When the penis is bent up or down, the attachment of the septal fibers to the tunica becomes stressed. Peyronie's disease occurs most frequently in middle-aged men and less frequently in young and older men. In a young man, the compliance of the tissues allows the elastic structures to give when buckling occurs even with vigorous intercourse. As a man ages, his tissues becomes less compliant, and such a buckling of the penis can result in trauma where the fibers of the septum are interwoven with the circular fibers of the tunica albuginea (Fig. 19-2B). Many patients have vivid memory of such buckling trauma a month or so prior to noting their plaque. In middle-aged men, intercourse often becomes less vigorous, and although the compliance of the tissues is diminished, there is not much likelihood of such an acute episode. Many will have lost some of the turgor of their erection, and despite continuing satisfactory intercourse, the shaft of the penis flexes. This action results in tissue fatigue, further reducing the compliance of the connections of the septal fibers with the tunica, over time producing multiple smaller tears in the circular fibers of the tunica (Fig. 19-2C).

In the schema proposed at our institution, Peyronie's disease results from this acute or chronic trauma. It is not an autoimmune process, nor is it caused by inflammation. With disruption of the fibers of the tunica, there is microvascular injury causing bleeding and clot formation, which result in fibrin deposition in the tissue space. With the injury there is an acute inflammatory reaction with induration. The fibrin is not cleared

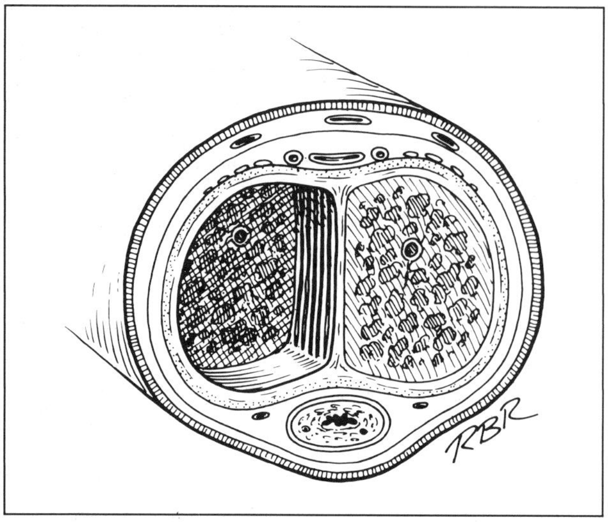

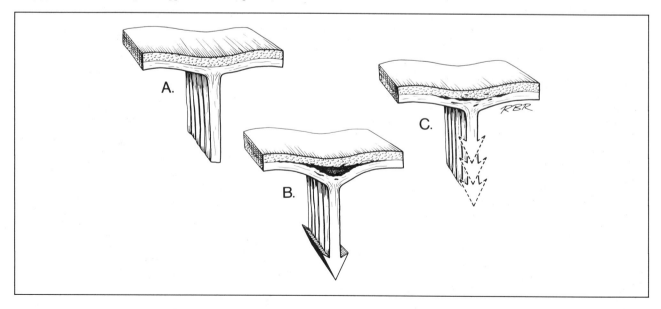

Figure 19-1. *Diagram of a cross section of the midshaft of the penis demonstrating the relationship of the septum. Note the deep dorsal vein and the dorsal arteries and nerves below Buck's fascia on the dorsal surface of the tunica albuginea and the veins lateral to the corpus spongiosum on the ventral aspect of the corpora cavernosa. (Reproduced with permission from CJ Devine, Peyronie's disease. In JF Glenn (ed),* Urologic Surgery, *4th ed. Philadelphia: Lippincott, 1991, p 865.)*

from the tunica as it would be from a more vascular tissue in the usual healing process. Retained fibrin is associated with (1) fibroblast activation and proliferation, (2) enhanced blood vessel permeability, and (3) generation of chemotactic factors for inflammatory cells (histiocytes). The lesion persists due to trapping of the fibrin or to further deposition following repeated trauma. Although collagen is not produced in excess, it is trapped, and pathologic fibrosis results; this scar is the plaque. Inflammation is the result of the process in the tunica and is present not only in the space of Smith between the tunica and erectile tissue but also between the tunica and the overlying layer of Buck's fascia.

During the acute phase of the process, this inflammation hyperstimulates the sensory and proprioceptive nerves and may cause pain during erection. Characterized as mild discomfort when the penis is flaccid, during erection and intromission it may become severe enough to produce detumescence. As the scar matures, the inflammation resolves and the pain abates, disappearing in all but a very few patients. Antihistamine medication (e.g. Seldane, 60 mg bid) may speed this process; relief of pain is *never* an indication for surgery, although a low dose of soft radiation (450 rads by the

Figure 19-2. *A. Diagram of the attachment of the septal strands with the inner circular layer of the tunica albuginea. B. Diagram illustrating the result of acute delamination of the tunica albuginea. The dark space contains a blood clot. C. Diagram illustrating chronic delamination of the tunica resulting from tissue fatigue. (Reproduced with permission from CJ Devine, Peyronie's disease. In JF Glenn (ed),* Urologic Surgery, *4th ed. Philadelphia: Lippincott, 1991, p 865.)*

beta beam of a linear accelerator) may be indicated if pain persists or is excessively troublesome.

Two presentations are observed, possibly related to the two modes of onset. Some lesions appear acutely—one erection being straight and the next bent with little or no progression. Others begin slowly with pain, then a lump in the penis, followed by progressive distortion, but eventually reaching an endpoint within 6 months to a year. With maturation of the scar, the plaque becomes somewhat more compliant; in younger men it may resolve, although it seldom disappears completely. Things will never be the same as they were before the onset of this condition. Most patients, however, can continue what they and their partner consider satisfactory intercourse despite an upward bend of 45 degrees or less or a 30-degree bend in any other direction. Less than a third of patients referred to this institution require surgery. If the plaque has been present for at least a year or is calcified and the distortion is severe enough to preclude sexual intercourse, we consider the patient to be a surgical candidate.

The plaque most frequently is on the dorsal aspect of the penis, producing an upward bend with erection; a ventral plaque will cause a downward bend. When dorsal and ventral plaques occur together, they balance each other and the penis may be almost straight but shortened with its circumference reduced in the involved area. The diminished compliance of the affected tunica limits the extension of the internal structures of the corpora. Without this internal support, the penis will be flail in the area of constriction, and the shaft distal to the constriction may not be as turgid as the portion proximal to it. This disparity is not due to a lack of blood flow beyond the lesion because the plaque involves only the tunica albuginea and does not extend into the erectile tissue. Both Doppler studies and dynamic infusion cavernosometry/cavernosography (DICC) have demonstrated unimpeded arterial flow beyond the plaque. Restoration of the compliance of the tunica by excising the scar and replacing it with elastic tissue, e.g., a dermal graft, can resolve this difficulty and restore penile function.

During evaluation, the patient is asked to bring two Polaroid photographs of his erect penis. These images define the quality of the erection and the angle of the bend. Note that the bend often increases with the turgor of the erection. A dorsal-ventral squeeze of the penis may locate the lesion, but the examination must be precise to define the extent of the scar in the tunica. The penis must be stretched so that the edges of the plaque can be palpated between the index finger and the thumb of the other hand placed laterally on the shaft. Dorsal plaques can be differentiated easily from ventral plaques that lie deep to the corpus spongiosum. The scar can reach maturity without becoming calcified, but calcification, which has been present in about 30 percent of the patients we have seen, is a sign of the end stage of the healing process. Because of this diagnostic significance, we often obtain a plain x-ray. Ultrasound also can define the plaque. It shows a thickening in the area of the tunica of the plaque and will demonstrate calcification if it is present. We have operated on several hundred patients with Peyronie's disease, and although the inflammation associated with the plaque has obliterated the space of Smith and fixed the erectile tissue against the tunica and can progress along the septal fibers, we have never observed involvement of the erectile tissue by the scar.

We use color duplex Doppler ultrasound and/or DICC to evaluate erectile function preoperatively. This is important for patients who have not had previous surgery but is essential for those who continue to have problems or who complain of impotence following a previous operation. It is not unusual to find veno-occlusive abnormalities in a Peyronie's disease patient.

Using duplex ultrasound, the caliber of the arteries in the erectile tissue and the velocity of the blood flow within them are measured before and after establishing a pharmacologic erection. Before the injection, there will be no flow during diastole. After the injection, dilation of the arteries occurs with an increase in systolic velocity, and as vascular resistance is reduced, diastolic flow will be present. Normally, when the corpora fill, internal pressure elevates, and the penis becomes turgid; the increase in systolic velocity will remain, but diastolic flow disappears. However, if venous occlusive incompetence is present, the penis never fills to rigidity, and diastolic flow persists. In these patients, we proceed to DICC to further clarify the issue.

These studies reveal an association between preoperative erectile function and postoperative results: If a patient has adequate erectile function, it is likely that he will have a good result from penile straightening and a dermal graft; if his erectile function is obviously inadequate and will not respond to a pharmacologic erection program (PEP) or be correctable by vascular surgery, he will not respond well to our surgery and should be offered penile straightening with placement of a prosthesis; if his erectile function is not adequate but also not obviously abnormal, there is a 70 percent chance that he will respond favorably to a dermal graft repair, leaving a 30 percent chance that he will have a straight but inadequately rigid penis after the surgery. He could, at a subsequent surgery, have a prosthesis placed if he

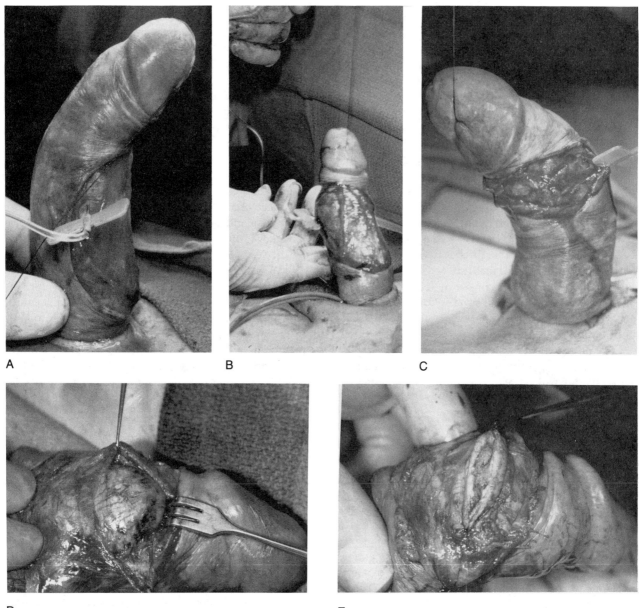

Figure 19-3. *A. Artificial erection demonstrating distortion of the penis prior to excision of a Peyronie's disease plaque and placement of a dermal graft. B. Artificial erection demonstrating straightening of the penis subsequent to the procedure. C. Artificial erection demonstrating recurrent chordee. D. Exposure of the tunica albuginea. The ellipse of tissue to be excised is marked. E. The ellipse has been excised. The tunica will be closed with interrupted and continuous sutures of PDS (polydioxanone). F. Artificial erection; the penis is straight.*

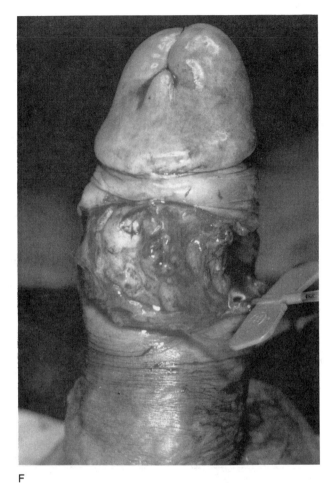

F

Figure 19-3. (*Continued*)

did not respond to a pharmacologic erection program. Note that after surgery, even in happy patients, the penis is not perfect. It may be shorter than it was before the patient developed Peyronie's disease and may still have some curvature. The goal is to provide a result that allows for resumption of satisfactory intercourse, preferably with natural erections.

A number of procedures have been described to treat Peyronie's disease. One of the oldest was to excise the plaque, releasing the curvature of the penis with the

Figure 19-4. *Diagrams illustrating excision of a dorsal plaque and placement of a dermal graft. A. the plaque is being elevated, preserving the erectile tissue. The lateral releasing incisions are shown. B. The extent of the defect on completion of the lateral incisions. The strands of the septum are seen in the midline. C. One edge of the graft is secured in place by sutures of 4-0 PDS. D. Closure of the first side has been completed with a running suture of 5-0 PDS. The midline of the graft has been marked and is being sewn to the strands of the septum with a similar suture. E. The graft has been secured and a needle inserted to repeat an artificial erection. (Reproduced with permission from CJ Devine, Jr, and CF Horton,* Bent penis. *Semin Urol 5(4):258–260, 1987.)*

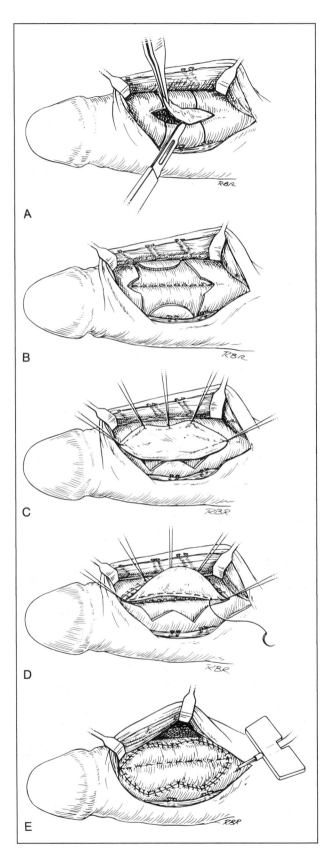

A

B

C

D

E

hope that it would remain straight. Because the defect would scar often worse than it was before, this procedure has been abandoned. Lowsley, attempting to prevent or delay recurrence of the curvature, placed a fat graft into the defect created by excising the plaque and claimed a 75 percent success rate. Horton and Devine were familiar with this work and the work of Poutasse and sought a tissue with more strength to fill the defect in the tunica. In dogs, only dermis survived as a satisfactorily elastic tissue; vein, fascia, and arterial grafts contracted and became fibrotic. The results of this work were applied to Peyronie's disease in humans, and over time in our hands this procedure has been successful. Others have had less success with the surgery and have cast about for other material to fill the defect engendered by excision or incision of the scar of the plaque: tunica vaginalis, lyophilized dura, abdominal fascia, temporalis fascia, Dexon mesh, Dacron, Gore-Tex— anything to avoid a dermal graft. Others, discouraged by

reports of failure in the application of dermal grafts, have employed the Nesbit procedure or other means of plicating the tunica opposite to the concavity of the bend to straighten the penis. Finally, many surgeons, not really understanding the pathophysiology of the disease and convinced that all patients with Peyronie's disease will become impotent or having met with failure in attempts at conservative surgery, have arrived at the conclusion that they should do something they can do well: put in a prosthesis. Many patients have sought us out because they have had a prosthesis offered to them as the "only" way to treat Peyronie's disease. Some of these patients have been able to function despite their distortion and have not needed an operation of any kind.

Complications in our patients having had a dermal graft procedure fall into two groups: (1) those in whom the graft does not become compliant to the extent that we had expected it to and who continue to have an

Figure 19-5. *A. This patient has previously had a dorsal plication. An artificial erection demonstrates the residual curvature. B. The same patient from the left side illustrating the severity of the curvature. One wonders how a surgeon could expect to correct this situation by shortening the dorsal aspect of the penis.*

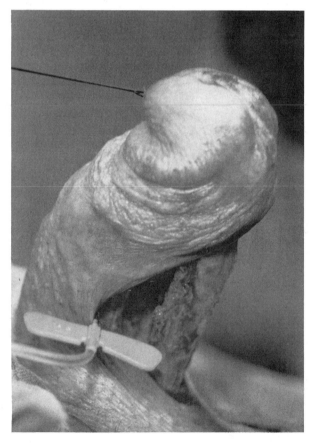

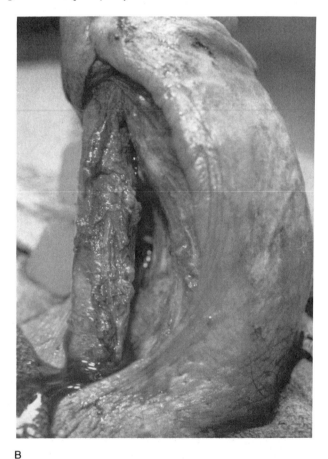

A   B

incapacitating degree of curvature after the graft has taken and matured and (2) patients who have developed impotence having a straight penis that is too flaccid for intromission. To resolve the former situation, we have used the Nesbit procedure in two cases (Fig. 19-3). In one case, the patient continued with good function. The other one was probably not successful, since he was lost to follow-up. We have used a Nesbit plication in several other patients. In two patients with extensive plaques, the penis was not completely straight at the time the artificial erection was done after a large dermal graft inlay. A tuck opposite the concavity completed the straightening. In several other patients who had residual curvature following placement of less extensive grafts, we made another incision in the tunica on the concave side and applied an additional graft. Since we have modified our dermal graft procedure, making lateral incisions into the tunica peripheral to the defect left by excision of the plaque and placing a much larger graft,

most of the problems of persistent curvature have been avoided (Fig. 19-4).

We have used plication of the long side of a bent penis to correct congenital lateral or ventral chordee. These patients have a longer than average penis, and the degree of shortening inherent in the procedure was not a significant factor in selection of the operation. In patients with Peyronie's disease, foreshortening is often already a problem, and the concept of further foreshortening is not acceptable. Papers describing the use of the Nesbit procedure are frequently illustrated with cases that show correction of minimal distortions. Many such patients in our series will offer a history of having satisfactory intercourse for themselves and their partners and by our selection criteria would not have been candidates for surgery. However, a man without a partner who has minimal distortion of a good-sized penis and cannot bring himself to reveal his distortion to a relative stranger is incapacitated and is probably an excellent

Figure 19-6. *A. Artificial erection, ventral aspect. This patient has had partial excision of a dorsal plaque and placement of too small a graft. B. The dorsal aspect further demonstrates the narrowness of the shaft. Note that the glans and superficial veins have been filled by the injected saline.*

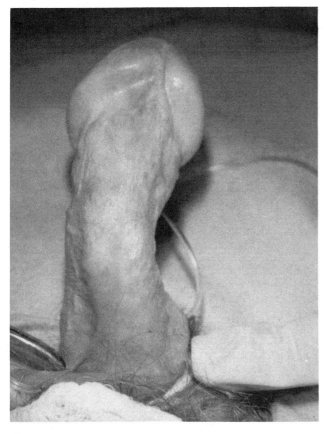

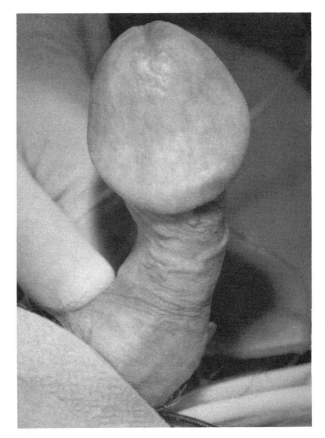

A   B

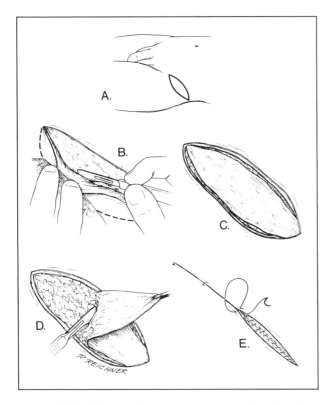

Figure 19-7. *Diagram illustrating harvest of a dermal graft. A. The donor site has been marked on the lateral surface of the abdomen over the crest of the ilium. B. The epidermis is being undermined using a no. 10 knife blade. C. The dermal graft has been incised, leaving a narrow cuff of dermis to complete closure of the skin. D. The fat is removed as the graft is elevated. E. The dermis is approximated with interrupted Vicryl sutures, and a running subcuticular 3-0 Prolene suture completes closure of the skin. (Reproduced with permission from CJ Devine, Peyronie's disease. In JF Glenn (ed), Urologic Surgery, 4th ed. Philadelphia: Lippincott, 1991, p 865.)*

candidate for this type of surgery. Secondary problems of the Nesbit procedure that we have treated have been related to the use of the procedure in patients who have marked or complex curvatures. If too much tunica has been excised, the shaft will be narrow, and despite the development of adequate turgor, an erection will not have rigidity. In these cases, the narrowed section is exposed, and the tunica is incised transversely, creating a relatively large defect that allows us to place a dermal graft.

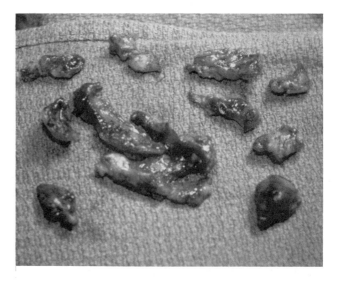

Figure 19-8. *Epidermal cyst, the result of using a full-thickness preputial graft to patch the defect in the tunica albuginea.*

When the distortion has not been corrected and the integrity of the shaft has been maintained, we have excised the plaque and applied a dermal graft as in a virgin case. The latest of these was a ventral lesion (Fig. 19-5). We made a midline ventral skin incision and released the corpus spongiosum to expose the plaque. The sutures from the previous procedure could be felt on the dorsal side, but we did not expose that aspect of the penis. We excised the plaque and applied a dermal graft. The patient has had good erections postoperatively.

Other problems with the dermal grafts include placement of a small graft (Fig. 19-6) or use of a graft from an inappropriate area. The small graft in the individual with good erectile function can be excised or incised, with a second dermal graft inlay performed. In one patient, the dermal graft had been obtained from the middle of the pubic escutcheon. When the graft was exposed through a penopubic incision, it contained multiple sebaceous cysts. The graft had been 11 cm long when placed. It had contracted, and the curve had recurred. Preoperative DICC revealed significant venous leakage into the corpus spongiosum and by way of the circumflex veins into the deep dorsal vein. We mobilized the penile shaft, and after dissecting the deep

Figure 19-9. *A. A GoreTex graft has been exposed by dissecting through the bed of the dorsal vein. Buck's fascia containing the dorsal arteries and nerves has been retracted laterally. Note the normal tunica peripheral to the graft. B. The contracted nature of the material can be seen after its removal. C. The undersurface shows the collagen clot. D. A cross section shows how contraction of the clot has distorted the GoreTex. E. A dermal graft has been applied. Note the effect of the midline sutures attaching it to the strands of the septum. F. An artificial erection shows a straight penis.*

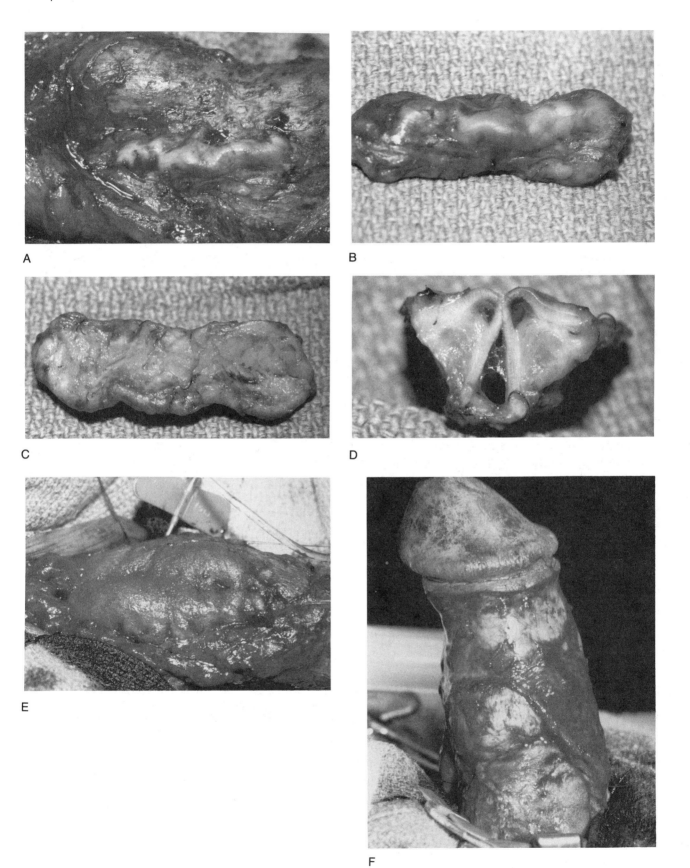

A

B

C

D

E

F

dorsal vein, it was ligated along with the crural veins at the crus of the corpora cavernosa where it joined the pampiniform plexus. As we mobilized the corpus spongiosum, venous connections to the graft were interrupted and ligated. We excised each of the cysts and made an incision in the midline of the graft, which with lateral incisions allowed us to place a 14 × 4 cm dermal graft in the defect. The patient's penis was straight, and function was restored. Subsequently, although the penis remained straight, relative impotence recurred. Another DICC revealed venous leakage to superficial veins from the region of the graft. At reexploration, these veins arose from the graft. They were removed, and function has been improved.

In our experience, the dermal graft can be reliably harvested from the area overlying or adjacent to the iliac crest. The graft is measured approximately 30 percent larger than the corporatory defect (Fig. 19-7). The epithelium is removed by undermining it free hand with a #10 knife blade or by using a dermatome. During this dissection the graft is then meticulously defatted. The donor site is closed primarily.

Other patients we have seen have had other materials placed to cover the defect after removing the plaque. Several surgeons seizing on the availability of excess skin in the foreskin of an uncircumcised patient have used that full-thickness skin as a graft. Burying the epidermis has produced a sebaceous cyst (Fig. 19-8) with a mass and inflammation. Because of the severity of the inflammatory reaction and adhesion of the tissue layers, reoperation on these patients has been difficult, requiring very tedious dissection. We have been able to get the penis straight by excising the tissue and reapplying a dermal graft. Fortunately, sensation has not been impaired, and function has persisted. We have reoperated on patients who have had tunica vaginalis applied as a graft. Usually, the plaque has been excised, but no lateral incisions have been made. The graft has matured as a very thin substance with little tensile strength, and the rim of the lesion has continued to restrict the erections. On examination of the penis, this rim has been very obvious, with the area that has been grafted feeling almost like a divot. We have exposed the defect and made lateral incisions that completed the release of the restriction and applied a new dermal graft.

Artificial material (e.g., Silastic, Gore-Tex) has been used to patch the tunica after putting in an erectile prosthesis. Others have used it to patch the tunica after excision or incision of a Peyronie's disease plaque without putting in a prosthesis. These materials are flexible but not elastic and engender a moderately severe inflammatory reaction. A collagen clot forms beneath it,

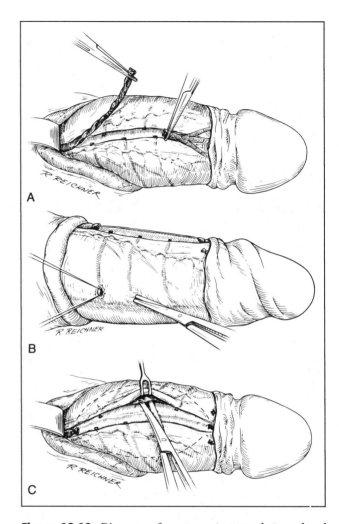

Figure 19-10. *Diagrams of our present approach to a dorsal plaque. A. A circumcising incision has been made though the scar left by the circumcision done as a newborn. The skin of the penis has been mobilized to the base of the penis. The deep dorsal vein is being resected. (Reproduced with permission from CJ Devine, Peyronie's disease. In JF Glenn (ed),* Urologic Surgery, *4th ed. Philadelphia: Lippincott, 1991, p 865.) B. The ventral termini of the encircling veins are isolated and ligated, interrupting their connection to the corpus spongiosum and the veins lateral to it. (Reproduced with permission from CJ Devine, Jr, GH Jordan, and SM Schlossberg,* Surgery of the penis and urethra. In PC Walsh, et al (eds), *Campbell's Urology, 6th ed. Philadelphia: Saunders, 1992.) C. Dissection beneath Buck's fascia exposes the plaque. Care is taken not to injure the dorsal arteries or nerves. (Reproduced with permission from CJ Devine, Peyronie's disease. In JF Glenn (ed),* Urologic Surgery, *4th ed. Philadelphia: Lippincott, 1991, p 865.)*

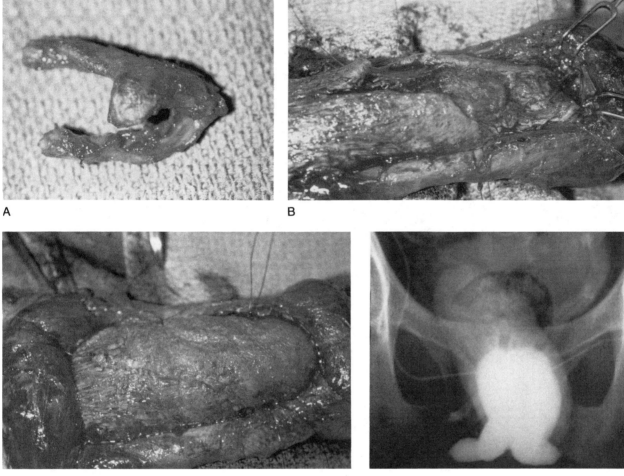

Figure 19-11. *A. Large ossified plaque removed from the distal penile shaft. B. Defect in the tunica after removal of the plaque. The glans penis is retracted by the hooks. C. A large dermal graft has been applied. D. X-ray: preoperative DICC, AP view. E. X-ray: preoperative DICC, left posterior oblique view. (Parts D and E show minimal leakage through the deep dorsal vein.) F. X-ray: postoperative DICC, AP view. G. X-ray: postoperative DICC, left posterior oblique view. (Parts F and G demonstrate filling of the circumflex veins on the right and their communication with the vein lateral to the corpus spongiosum and filling of the corpus spongiosum itself. Note that the glans penis is not illuminated.)*

and contraction of this clot regenerates the deformity (Fig. 19-9). We have been able to excise these patches and replace them with a dermal graft. The patients have continued to function sexually.

Difficulty with maintaining an adequate erection after surgery for Peyronie's disease is of continuing concern. Despite this, surveys of our patients have revealed that overall at least 75 percent have been happy with the results of their surgery, but every patient on whom we operate knows that there is a significant chance that this will happen to him. The first step in the process that

produces the tear that results in the scar of Peyronie's disease is loss of elasticity in the tunica albuginea. This is also probably the first step in the genesis of the veno-occlusive incompetence that can accompany Peyronie's disease. As noted above, we have begun to classify the erectile function of the patients that we operate on, hoping that we can identify those who are going to have trouble, and the results of these tests seem to reflect the results of the surgery. If we identify a venous leak prior to the surgery for Peyronie's disease, we undertake to mobilize and ligate the veins at the time we excise the

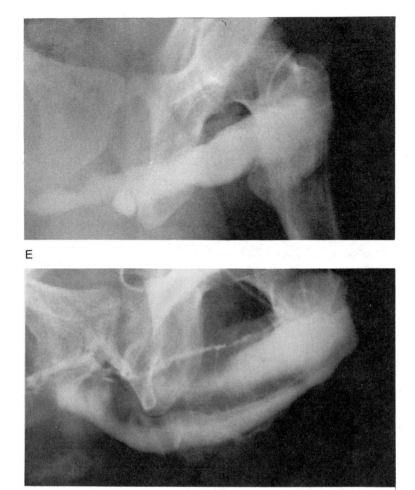

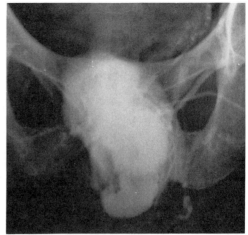

Figure 19-11. (*Continued*)

plaque and replace it with a dermal graft. However, some patients who were normal or who have had minimal venous filling evident in the DICC have developed a venous leak following placement of a dermal graft. We do not know just how this happens, but we presume that the graft is vascularized from both sides. Should a vein in the graft form an anastomosis with a vein in the erectile tissue and another in Buck's fascia, there would be an uncontrolled outlet from the erectile body. To prevent this situation occurring and functioning as a venous leak, we remove the dorsal vein and ligate its connections proximally and distally and approach the dorsal Peyronie's disease plaque through the bed of the dorsal vein (Fig. 19-10). Despite this, one patient who functioned well following application of a fairly large graft developed impotence in about 6 months. Repeat DICC showed venous leakage through the encircling veins on the right side of the penile shaft, draining into the vein

that runs lateral to the corpus spongiosum on that side and into the corpus spongiosum itself (Fig. 19-11). Fortunately, this patient has been able to attain and maintain a satisfactory erection by placing a rubber band at the base of his penis. Since this occasion, we have isolated the terminus of the encircling veins ventrally where they consolidate to form the veins lateral to the corpus spongiosum and have not seen this situation again (see Fig. 19-10*B*). Other patients who have developed impotence postoperatively have responded well to PEP or vein ligation, but we have installed erectile prostheses in others who did not.

All in all, the success of reoperations on patients who have had previous surgery for Peyronie's disease depends a lot on the type of surgery that was done before. Our overall success in restoring the ability of a patient to have sexual intercourse that he and his partner consider satisfactory runs about 50 percent, and the primary or secondary surgery that we have done has not precluded the possibility of installing a penile prosthesis if postoperative function is not satisfactory.

Bibliography

Altaffer, LF, III, and Jordan, GH. Sonographic demonstration of Peyronie's plaques. Urology 17:292, 1981.

Bailey, MJ, et al. Surgery for Peyronie's disease: A review of 200 patients. Br J Urol 57:746, 1985.

Bazeed, MA, et al. New surgical procedure for management of Peyronie's disease. Urology 21:501, 1983.

Benson, RC, Jr, and Patterson, DE. The Nesbit procedure for Peyronie's disease. J Urol 130:692, 1983.

Bruschini, H, and Mitre, AI. Peyronie's disease: Surgical treatment with muscular aponeurosis. Urology 13:505, 1979.

Bruskewitz, R, and Raz, S. Surgical considerations in the treatment of Peyronie's disease. Urology 15:134, 1989.

Carson, CC, Hodge, GB, and Anderson, EE. Penile prosthesis in Peyronie's disease. Br J Urol 35:417, 1983.

Collins, JP. Experience with lyophilized human dura for treatment of Peyronie's disease. Urology 31:379, 1988.

Coughlin, PWF, Carson, CC, III, and Paulson, DF. Surgical correction of Peyronie's disease: The Nesbit procedure. J Urol 131:282, 1984.

Das, S, and Amar, AD. Peyronie's disease: Excision of the plaque and grafting with tunica vaginalis. Urol Clin North Am 9: xxx, 1982.

Devine, CJ, Jr. Peyronie's disease. In JF Glenn (ed), Urologic Surgery, 4th ed. Philadelphia: Lippincott, 1991, pp 864, 874.

Devine, CJ, Jr, and Horton, CE. The surgical treatment of Peyronie's disease with a dermal graft. J Urol 111:44, 1974.

Devine, CJ, Jr, Jordan, GH, and Schlossberg, SM. Surgery of the penis and urethra. In PC Walsh, et al (eds), Campbell's Urology, 6th ed. Philadelphia: Saunders, 1992.

Devine, CJ, Jr, Jordan, GH, and Somers, KD. Peyronie's disease: Cause and surgical treatment. AUA Today 2:1, 1989.

Devine, CJ, Jr, et al. The surgical treatment of chordee without hypospadias in post adolescent men. J Urol (in press).

Devine, CJ, Jr, et al. A working model for the genesis of Peyronie's disease derived from its pathobiology (abstract 495). J Urol 139:286A, 1988.

Ebbehoj, J, and Metz, P. New operation of "Krummerik" (penile curvature). Urology 26:76, 1985.

El-Mahdi, AM. Personal communication, 1990.

Essed, E, and Schroeder, FH. New surgical treatment for Peyronie's disease. Urology 25:582, 1985.

Fishman, IJ. Corporeal reconstruction procedures for complicated penile implants. Urol Clin North Am 16(1):73, 1989.

Gangai, M, Rivera, LR, and Spence, CR. Peyronie's plaque: Excision and graft versus incision and stent. J Urol 127:55, 1982.

Gelbard, MK, and Hayden, B. Expanding contractures of the tunica albuginea due to Peyronie's disease with temporalis fascia free grafts. J Urol 145:772, 1991.

Goldstein, AM, and Padma-Nathan, H. The microarchitecture of the intracavernosal smooth muscle and the cavernosal fibrous skeleton. J Urol 144:1144, 1990.

Horton, CE, and Devine, CJ, Jr. Peyronie's disease. Plast Reconstr Surg 52:503, 1973.

Horton, CE, Sadove, RC, and Devine, CJ, Jr. Peyronie's disease. Ann Plast Surg 18(2):122, 1987.

Horwitz, O. Plastic operation for the relief of an incurvation of the penis. Ann Surg 5:557, 1910.

Jordan, GH. Grafts and flaps in urology. In JF Glenn (ed), Urologic Surgery, 4th ed. Philadelphia: Lippincott, 1991, pp 1085–1096.

Kodama, RT, et al. Interpretation of penile duplex ultrasound waveforms and measurements in pharmacologically induced erections (abstract 33). J Urol 143:197A, 1990.

Lowe, DH, et al: Surgical treatment of Peyronie's disease with dacron graft. Urology 19:609, 1982.

Lowsley, OS, and Gentile, A. An operation for the cure of certain cases of plastic induration (Peyronie's disease) of the penis. J Urol 57:552, 1947.

Melman, A, and Holland, TF. Evaluation of the dermal graft inlay technique for the surgical treatment of Peyronie's disease. J Urol 120:421, 1978.

Mufti, GR, et al. Corporeal plication for surgical correction of Peyronie's disease. J Urol 144:281, 1990.

Poutasse, EF. Peyronie's disease. Trans Am Assoc Genitourinary Surg 63:97, 1971.

Pryor, JP, and Fitzpatrick, JM. A new approach to the correction of the penile deformity in Peyronie's disease. J Urol 122:622, 1979.

Raz, S, DeKernion, JB, and Kaufman, JJ. Surgical treatment of Peyronie's disease. J Urol 117:598, 1977.

Schiffman, ZJ, Gursel, EO, and Laor, E. Use of Dacron graft in Peyronie's disease. Urology 25:38, 1985.

Smith, BH. Peyronie's disease. Am J Clin Pathol 45:670, 1966.

Snow, R, and Devine, CJ, Jr. The conservative management of Peyronie's disease. Unpublished Data.

Somers, KD, et al. Isolation and characterization of collagen in Peyronie's disease. J Urol 141:629, 1989.

Subrini, L. Surgical treatment of Peyronie's disease using penile implants: Survey of 69 patients. J Urol 132:47, 1984.

Wild, RM, Devine, CJ, Jr, and Horton, CE. Dermal graft repair of Peyronie's disease: Survey of 50 patients. J Urol 121:47, 1979.

Wise, HA. Gore-Tex patch graft technique for treatment of Peyronie's disease (abstract 148). J Urol 137:140A, 1987.

Failure of the Penile Prosthesis

RONALD W. LEWIS
WILLIAM R. MORGAN

Etiology

Reoperation for failure of the penile prosthesis occurs because of pain, infection, erosion, mechanical breakdown, wound problems, or a technical error in placement of the device. We recently reviewed 1358 reoperations in penile implant cases in 555 patients from March 18, 1975 to July 17, 1990, performed at the Mayo Clinic.

The mean interval from the time the primary device was placed was 42.5 months, and the mean interval between operations was 21.4 months. There was an average of 2.4 operations per patient, varying from 1 reoperation to 18. As can be seen from Table 20-1, mechanical failure was still the most common reason for reoperation. Infection and/or erosion was the etiology of reoperation in 11.5 percent in our series. This is not an infection rate, but the percentage of all reoperations in penile implants that were necessary because of infection. Reported infection rates range from 0.6 to 8.9 percent in rod prostheses and from 0.8 to 8.9 percent in inflatable prostheses.

Diagnosis

The diagnosis of failure of a penile prosthesis is not that difficult. For the most part, the simple physical evaluation of the patient is all that is needed to diagnose erosion or a technical error in placement of a component of the device (Fig. 20-1). Equally, the diagnosis of mechanical failure is simple; the device does not produce a rigid penis suitable for intercourse. A simple plain pelvic x-ray will indicate complete loss of fluid in the inflatable device if that system has been filled with diluted contrast material, break in the metal core in some semirigid devices, or malposition of components of a device. Inflate/deflate films may indicate malposition of cylinders or technical problems with cylinders. Wound problems, such as hematomas or seromas, are easily appreciated by simple palpation and inspection of the wound. Often infections will produce a fever or local drainage of purulent material—obviously no diagnostic dilemma.

Pain as a reason for reoperation of the penile implant is often a difficult complaint to deal with. It is not unusual for the patient to have a moderate amount of discomfort from the device up to 4 to 6 weeks after placement. It is often necessary to convince the patient not to have immediate removal of the device because of the pain in the early postoperative period; however, this demands a continuation of rapport that should have been developed between the implant surgeon and the patient prior to that operation. Unless the patient has other signs of infection, such as an elevated temperature, an elevated white blood cell count, or wound erythema, then he should be encouraged that the pain will probably resolve over this 4- to 6-week postoperative time period. However, prolonged discomfort in association with an implant often may be present due to infection without fever, erythema, or purulent drainage. Penile pain also can be due to inappropriate sizing of the cylinders, their being too large for the corporeal space.

Erosion is not always associated with infection. Erosion also can cause pain by producing pressure necrosis of the corpora in the subglanular region with improper cylinder sizing and in the scrotum due to pump or reservoir/pump combination.

Table 20-1. *Reason for Reoperation*

Mechanical failure or device malfunction	770	(56.7%)
Infection and/or erosion	156	(11.5%)
Unknown fluid loss	104	(7.7%)
Patient dissatisfaction or pain	86	(6.3%)
Poor position	85	(6.3%)
Staged procedure (salvage)	56	(4.1%)
Hematoma or seroma	28	(2.0%)
Encapsulation	21	(1.5%)
Could not be determined	91	(6.7%)
TOTAL	1397*	

*1357 procedures in 555 patients—more than one reason for reoperation in 39 procedures.

Patient Preparation

It is extremely important that the surgeon have a very detailed discussion with the patient who is to undergo a reoperation for a penile prosthesis problem. This discussion should center on ensuring that the patient has proper expectations from the reoperation and an understanding of common anticipated complications. This is particularly important when scarring has occurred in the corporeal tissue, in which case a replacement device will not reproduce the original cosmetic result. There is a greater chance of infection after multiple operations for a penile device; the patient should understand this. In patients who have had a prior urethral erosion or

Figure 20-1. *This is an example of an impending erosion of an inflatable penile prosthesis pump. Note the obvious swollen glistening skin in the lower portion of the right scrotum that has essentially lost normal rugae.*

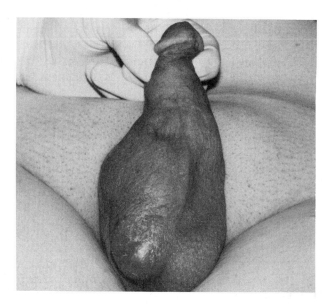

urethral tear during dilation, there should be an attempt to warn the patient of the risk of reentry into the urethra and the potential need for urinary diversion by means of a perineal urethrostomy (discussed later). For the patient in whom it is impossible to place another three-piece inflatable device, it should be stressed that the resulting erection will not be as natural as before. Any patient who has had operations on the penis, for whatever reason, including prosthetic procedures, should be told that penile shortening may occur as well as numbness of the penile shaft and particularly the glans area due to contusion or injury to the penile sensory nerves. In the case of a contusion, return of full sensation may take as long as 1 year.

Surgical Technique

Before considering specific areas of penile prosthetic reoperation, there are certain general principles applicable to all types of reoperation. In general, the choice of antibiotics prior to reoperation should be no different from those used in a primary penile implant except in certain cases, such as previous infection or when a salvage operation is being considered in the face of frank purulence. There is debate about whether diabetics have an increased risk of infection. One recent report suggests using glycosylated hemoglobin as a guide by stating that diabetics with a value of 11.5 percent or greater should be better controlled before implant surgery. In patients who have had fibrosis or wound problems in the past, we use an aminoglycoside and vancomycin given immediately preoperatively and continued until 1 day after surgery. Specific use of antibiotics in salvage techniques is addressed in one of the following sections.

If the penile shaft has to be exposed during a penile prosthetic reoperation, we recommend the use of a bipolar electrode for electrocoagulation of vessels, which results in less injury to neural and vascular structures. We actually recommend this for all penile shaft surgery. When there have been multiple approaches to the penis and scarring is present causing some concern about penile blood vessel identification, the hand-held Doppler probe is often useful.

Circumcision has been recommended by some for all patients who have placement of a penile prosthesis. On the other hand, some authors present this as an absolute contraindication because of an increased risk of infection. We do not feel that circumcision is necessary when penile-scrotal or infrapubic incisions are used; however, if a subglanular incision is performed for placement of an implant for access to the distal corpora in reoperation, circumcision is certainly indicated. In the face of balanoposthitis, circumcision should be performed at a separate procedure before penile prosthesis placement is considered.

Intraoperative technical injuries that occur during reoperation often can be managed as they are in placement of original devices. A rupture of the proximal crural corpus can occur even with careful dilation. The use of a Dacron or polytetrafluorethylene (PTFE, Gore-Tex) windsock from vascular grafts alleviates the need for a separate perineal incision and repair in that region (Fig. 20-2). This is particularly useful for semirigid or self-contained inflatable devices. If abutment against the ischium in the crural region can still be felt, we have

not found that this is necessary with any device with attached tubing, as long as there is a fixation suture in the corporotomy incision on either side of the exit tubing. The incision in the corpora must be made proximally (4 to 5 cm from the ischial tubrosity) for proper placement of this fixation suture, which will prevent later migration of the device. The patient is instructed not to use the device for 6 to 8 weeks after this type of repair. Urethral tears may be repaired directly through a circumcision incision; however, most surgeons would recommend cylinder placement only after proximal urinary diversion by catheter placed by means of a perineal urethrostomy or suprapubic catheter. It should be stressed here, however, that this type of approach

Figure 20-2. *The steps of creating of a windsock using a Dacron vascular graft to treat perforation of the proximal end of the left corpora. The windsock is fixed to the corpora with 3-0 permanent suture as shown in part D. (From IJ Fishman, Complicated implantations of inflatable penile prostheses.* Urol Clin North Am 14:217–239, 1987.)

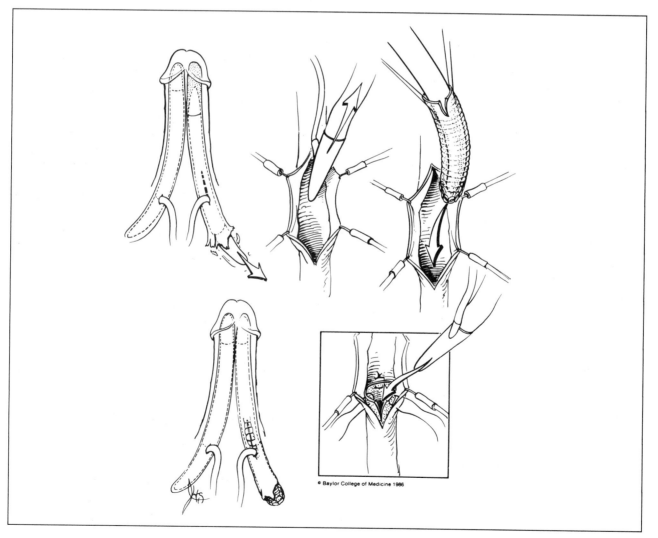

© Baylor College of Medicine 1986

should be reserved for reoperation. If an intraurethral entry occurs in a primary case, the patient is rarely prepared for urinary diversion and the increased risk of infection.

Another useful technique to remember if faced with inadequate penile skin for defect coverage is the Cecil-Culp procedure, in which the penis is buried into the midscrotum and covered by lateral flaps of scrotal skin in a second-stage procedure.

Mechanical Failures

As mentioned earlier, every effort should be made to replace a three-piece prosthesis with a similar prosthesis if possible. The patient is usually dissatisfied if this is not done. In our review of the 1358 reoperations described earlier, the etiology of mechanical failure is shown in Table 20-2. We have found that in many cases remeasurement reveals an increase in total intracorporeal length (from 1 to 3 cm). In 45 percent of cases, a longer cylinder was required. On the other hand, it was necessary to use a smaller cylinder size in only 11 percent of cases (see Table 20-3).

Since the overwhelming majority of mechanical failures in our series occurred in cylinders and tubing connected to the cylinders, bilateral removal and inspection of cylinders were necessary. This was best accomplished by dissection along the tubing and into the corpora using the electrocoagulation blade. In early mechanical failures, connector leaks are common. We usually approach connectors first, checking for security, and then, if we find no connector problems, we expose the pump and cylinders next. Modern reservoirs are usually not a source of mechanical failure except for encapsulation, which will be diagnosable on preoperative inflate/deflate films, and for the presence of the inability to fully deflate the device. Using a hand-held syringe, hydrodilation and rupture of the restricting capsule can be accomplished usually without having to expose the reservoir. All spaces explored in reoperation for component replacement are thoroughly irrigated with antibiotic solution before replacement of new components.

Position Problems

Probably the two most common position problems are an inappropriate cylinder length and a high-riding pump or reservoir/pump combination in the scrotum. If there is difficulty in replacing a pump or reservoir/pump combination into the ipsilateral scrotum, then the contralateral scrotum often can be used. The most effective way to correct an inadequate cylinder length causing a urethral glanular deformity is with the Ball procedure. In this procedure, a subcoronal transverse incision is made over the dorsum of the penis. Horizontal mattress sutures are placed through the corona and fixed to Buck's fascia or actually plicating the tunica albuginea itself, exposing the cylinders (if inflatable type) by means of incisions into the tunica albuginea. Sutures should be permanent. The skin incision is closed with a continuous subcuticular or interrupted suture technique. A difference in length between two cylinders can sometimes be addressed by a Nesbit wedge procedure on the convex side of the curvature. Improper placement of the cylinders, such as a crossover into the other corpora, can be corrected through a circumcision incision for the distal penis or a perineal incision for crossovers in the crural corpora.

Table 20-2. *Mechanical Failure or Device Malfunction*

Cylinder	524	(68.1%)
Hole	141	
Tear	97	
Input tubing wear	117	
Reinforcing rod wear	58	
Aneurysmal dilatation	111	
Tubing	137	(17.8%)
Connector	50	(6.5%)
Pump	35	(4.5%)
Reservoir	24	(3.1%)

Table 20-3. *Change of Cylinder Size with Revision*

Cylinder changes	555 pairs
Average change	0.51-cm increase
Range	−6 to +8 cm
Amount changed, cm	Changes, no.
< −3	6
−3	6
−2	10
−1	37
0	244
+1	155
+2	70
+3	23
>3	4

Erosion

As mentioned earlier, it has been shown recently in a well-documented report that erosions are for the most part salvageable. In that series, all bladder erosions were salvaged completely. It should be stressed that if a reservoir has been placed through the external ring in the inguinal area by a puncture of the transversalis fascia,

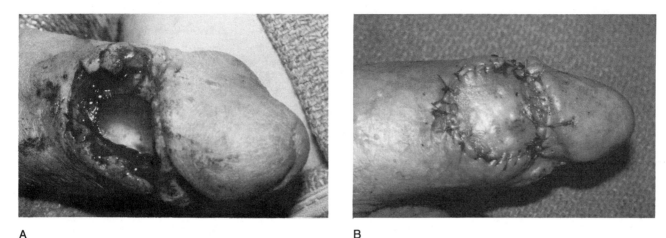

A   B

Figure 20-3. *A. A severe corporeal-cutaneous fistula in an immunocompromised patient. The device and wound were not infected. B. Successful coverage of the defect with a multilayered vascularized pedicle of scrotal tissue.*

when replacing this reservoir, a space beneath the rectus muscle in the midline should be used. This is actually the first choice for many of us who place the inflatable prosthesis through an infrapubic type of approach, since direct-vision placement is much more suitable. Of course, scrotal erosions require placement of the pump or pump/reservoir combination into the opposite scrotum. Erosions associated with infections should follow the principles outlined below. Occasionally, there may be a persistent corpora-cutaneous fistula in the penile shaft that often will require a multilayer coverage. We have been able to accomplish this with a scrotal flap with a vascular pedicle, such as that shown in Figure 20-3. These vascularized pedicle flaps can be taken from other regions near the penis, but we have found that scrotal tissue is particularly useful, and a well-vascularized pedicle usually can be created.

Recently, to decrease the erosion rate in patients who undergo intermittent self-catheterization and desire a penile implant, it was suggested that an inflatable penile prosthesis should be used with temporary proximal urinary diversion. For most cases, a perineal urethrostomy is preferable. In those unable to perform intermittent catheterization, a suprapubic tube is recommended.

Fibrosis

Reoperation in patients who have fibrosis, most often in the corporeal spaces, is probably the most difficult type of reoperation in penile implant patients. For the most part, producing a space in the corpora can be very diffi-

cult if infection or a previous implant has been present. Most surgons wait 3 to 6 months after device removal before attempting replacement. Fibrosis, unfortunately, is well established by this time. This problem has led to development of an immediate or early salvage type of procedure, which is described in the next section. Usually, in the presence of moderate to marked fibrosis, the corpora cannot be approached by one incision. Instead, a combination of incisions, such as infrapubic and circumcision-like incision, or a penile degloving with a penile-scrotal approach are made (Fig. 20-4). An invert-

Figure 20-4. *The opening of the corpora in two areas. The circumcision incision has been made, and the penis has been degloved with an opening into dense corporeal fibrotic tissue. A similar opening has been made in the proximal corpora through the infrapubic incision.*

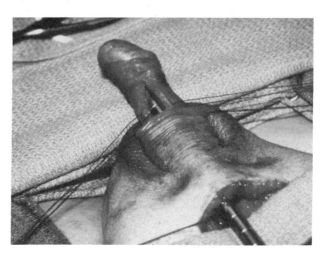

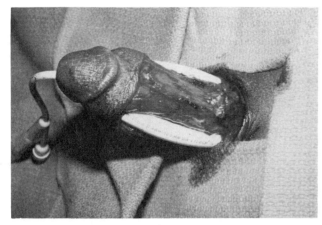

A

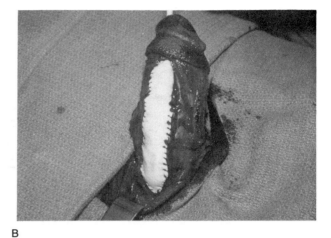

B

Figure 20-5. *A. A semirigid device placed in the corpora that have been bivalved. B. The bivalve corporal defect has been covered with a polytetrafluoroethylene (PTFE) patch.*

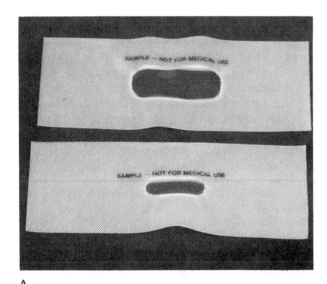

A

Figure 20-6. *A. An example of patch material that consists of a Dacron netting covered on either side by Silastic. A central window of two layers of Silastic only has been a recent modification of the patch allowing for greater elasticity. B. The approach to the dorsal corpora by elevation of the neurovascular bundle. C. Placement of the Dacron/Silastic patch material.*

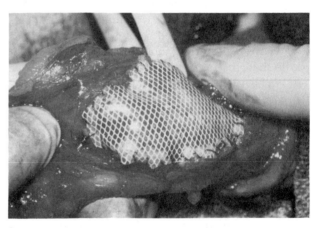

C

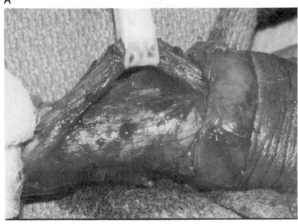

B

ing degloving technique by means of a penile-scrotal incision associated with a perineal incision may be necessary in patients with severe total corporal fibrosis. This fibrosis also can occur not only in penile implant reoperations but also in patients who have had priapism or other corporal infections that were not necessarily associated with previous implant surgery. This subject has been discussed previously in an excellent article by Dr. Irving Fishman. Certainly, multiple openings in the corpora allow for better access to dissection of the intracorporeal fibrotic tissue. Sometimes a plane between the fibrous tissue and the tunica albuginea can be developed with sharp dissection; however, in many cases, this is not possible, and a bivalving of the corpora dense fibrotic tissue may be necessary with coring out of the fibrous tissue to make a space for a penile device. The device can then be covered with some sort of patch material (Fig. 20-5).

As reported in the literature, Dacron or PTFE patches have been made from vascular graft material. We have used a specially made (Mentor Corporation, Goleta, Calif.) Dacron netting overlayed on either side by Silastic as a patch material that allows some elasticity (Fig. 20-6). This technique is most successful when used with inflatable penile prostheses. We feel that semirigid devices in these circumstances are more likely to produce erosions.

In Dr. Fishman's article, the use of a blunt brain retractor was suggested for developing a plane between the fibrous tissue and the tunica albuginea to core out the fibrous tissue (Fig. 20-7). We have not found this to be applicable in many cases of significant fibrosis. There also has been a boring type of tool described for removal of this dense fibrous tissue, but use of this type of device is recommended only for very experienced surgeons,

Figure 20-7. *One method of removal of the dense fibrous core in the right corpora for placement of a penile device in a patient with severe fibrosis. (From IJ Fishman, Complicated implantations of inflatable penile prostheses.* Urol Clin North Am *14:217–239, 1987.)*

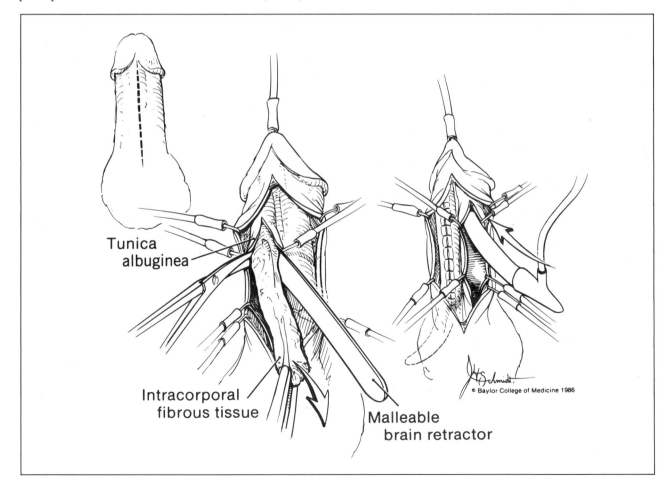

since urethral injury or neurovascular injuries are certainly at greater risk with this type of approach.

Infection

In the face of infection associated with a penile prosthesis, previous dogma has advised immediate removal of the penile implant. We concur when there is frank purulent material present around a penile prosthesis and would recommend removal of the device with one caveat. We suggest that under these circumstances, a tubular fenestrated suction drain be placed into the corporal spaces and irrigated with an antibiotic solution every 4 to 8 hours for 7 days. We recommend Dab's solution, containing 500 mg neomycin, 80 mg gentamicin, and 100 mg polymyxin in 1000 cc isotonic saline. This decreases the amount of dense fibrous tissue when reoperation is performed. We more recently have recommended salvage procedures in infections not associated with frank purulent material or when only one portion of the penile implant, such as the pump in the scrotum, is involved with purulent drainage. Under most conditions, we would still recommend removal of the entire device and replacement of all components of the device along with concomitant fenestrated tubular suction drains. In the presence of infection when immediate salvage is performed, we recommend that the cylinders be placed into the corpora with a Furlow introducer along with the drain (attached to the suture of the tip of the prosthesis by passage through one of the fenestrations in the tubular drain) at the same passage. The original pump site is drained with a tubular fenestrated suction drain. The new pump site, usually in the opposite scrotum, is also drained. Finally, the reservoir space, whether new or in the same place, is similarly drained. All the tubular drains exit from separate stab wounds, are irrigated with Dab's solution every 4 to 6 hours, and are kept to grenade suction at other times (Fig. 20-8).

It should be stressed that the use of antibiotics in the presence of infection is not prophylactic but therapeutic. Therefore, the types of antibiotics used in a salvage procedure should be different. We recommend an aminoglycoside and vancomycin in the first 24 to 48 hours, beginning in the immediate preoperative period and continuing until the offending organism can be identified. At that time, we then select the most appropriate antibiotic based on culture and sensitivities for continued parenteral therapy during the antibiotic irrigation salvage time, which is usually 7 to 10 days in the hospi-

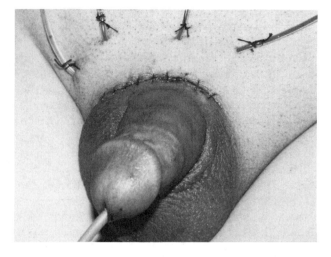

Figure 20-8. *Four fenestrated tubular suction drains in a salvage reoperation of an infected penile prosthesis draining each of the corpora and the pump and reservoir sites.*

tal. We have reported the results of this type of radical salvage procedure in selected cases. A similar type of procedure has been presented by Fishman in the past. It is important to stress that in most cases the entire device should be removed, particularly in the presence of certain organisms, since a bacterial biofilm can result in persistent prosthesis-associated infections.

In the patient who has had a history of multiple infections and who is not diabetic or immunosuppressed, the physician should suspect unusual conditions such as methicillin-resistant *Staphylococcus*. We had such a patient who had a disasterous outcome after an attempted salvage reoperation and was later discovered to be a nasal carrier of methicillin-resistant *Staphylococcus*. In patients who have a history of unexplained infections, a preoperative culture of the nasal pharynx is recommended.

Results of Intervention

For the most part, reoperation in the patient with penile prosthetics can be very successful, particularly in cases of erosion without infection, mechanical failures, and position problems. The patients who should be prepared for a high risk of failure are those with corporeal fibrosis. By adhering to some of the technical recommendations described here, in particular, planning for urinary diversion in the face of urethral tears, many patients can have a very successful outcome. The reoperation of patients with infection continues to be a major problem. It is less controversial to remove the whole device and reoperate 3 to 6 months later; however, this usually results in dense corporeal scarring. For this reason, there is a growing experience of salvage penile reoperation procedures that require a longer hospitalization associated with the use of local antibiotic irrigation and parenteral antibiotic therapy. In our hands, this has been quite successful in over 80 percent of patients.

Bibliography

Ball, TP. Surgical repair of penile "SST" deformity. Urology 15:603, 1980.

Bishop, JR, et al. Use of glycosylated hemoglobin to identify diabetics at high risk for penile periprosthetic infections. J Urol 147:386, 1992.

Carson, CC. Infections in genitourinary prosthesis. Urol Clin North Am 16:139, 1989.

Finney, RP. Coring fibrotic corpora for penile implants. Urology 24:73, 1984.

Fishman, IJ. Corporeal reconstruction procedures for complicated penile implants. Urol Clin North Am 16:73, 1989.

Fishman, IJ, Scott, FB, and Selim, AM. Rescue procedure: An alternative to complete removal for treatment of infected penile prosthesis (abstract 396). J Urol 137:202A, 1987.

Furlow, WL, and Goldwasser, B. Salvage of the eroded inflatable penile prosthesis: A new concept. J Urol 138:318, 1987.

Lewis, RW, and McLaren, R. Reoperation for penile prosthesis implantation. In C Carson (ed), Problems in Urology— Prosthetics in Urology. Philadelphia: Lippincott, 1993, pp 382–402.

Morgan, WR, and Lewis, RW. Salvage of the complicated infected urinary prosthesis with aggressive management (abstract 878). J Urol 143:408A, 1990.

Mulcahy, JJ. A technique of maintaining penile prosthesis position to prevent proximal migration. J Urol 137:294, 1987.

Nickel, JC, et al. Bacterial biofilm in persistent penile prosthesis-associated infection. J Urol 135:586, 1986.

Roberts, JA, Fussell, EN, and Lewis, RW. Bacterial adherence to penile prostheses. Int J Impotence Res 1:167, 1989.

Steidle, CP, and Mulcahy, JJ. Erosion of penile prosthesis: The complication of urethral catheterization. J Urol 142:736, 1989.

The Failed Vasovasostomy/ Vasoepididymostomy

ARNOLD M. BELKER

Fourteen percent of men who undergo bilateral micro-surgical vasovasostomy are azoospermic postoperatively. A survey of 107 bilateral microsurgical vaso-epididymostomies performed by me, Dr. Ira Sharlip (San Francisco), Dr. Anthony J. Thomas, Jr. (Cleveland), and Dr. Marc Goldstein (New York City) revealed that 43 (40 percent) of the patients were azoospermic post-operatively. With increasing numbers of men undergoing vasectomy reversal procedures, it becomes important for the surgeon to be prepared to properly advise patients about the management of failed procedures.

Although reoperation may be offered after a failed first vasectomy reversal procedure, my experience has been that most men do not undergo a second procedure for several reasons. The financial burden of a second procedure may be prohibitive. Hospital and anesthesiologist fees and the loss of income while the patient remains away from work postoperatively may be too large of a financial burden. Many insurance carriers do not cover other expenses for vasectomy reversals, even if the surgeon charges a reduced fee or no fee for a reoperative procedure when the surgeon's original procedure failed. Also, the patient's motivation affects his decision to undergo a second procedure. The majority of men who have a vasectomy reversal have had children by a previous marriage and undergo the reversal so that they may have a child with a new wife who has not had children. Some of these men really may not be eager to have another child but have had the reversal performed primarily to please the new wife. When faced with the need to undergo a second operative procedure to restore fertility, few men ultimately do so. Finally, the decision to undergo a second reversal procedure may depend on the couple's perception of the success rate of reoperative procedures. This perception will depend on information given to them by the surgeon.

Definition of Failure

If sperm do not appear in the semen within 3 to 6 months of bilateral vasovasostomy, then the operation has failed. However, it may take 6 to 12 and occasionally 18 months after bilateral vasoepididymostomy for sperm to appear in the semen. Reasons for such long delays until the appearance of sperm in the semen after vasoepididymostomy are not understood.

It is less easy to determine if the operation is a technical failure when sperm are present in the semen postoperatively but their motility is poor. Reduced sperm motility after vasovasostomy or vasoepididymostomy may result from either antisperm antibodies, which are present in 50 to 70 percent of men after vasectomy, or epididymal dysfunction resulting from prolonged obstruction, genital tract infection, or anastomotic strictures. After vasoepididymostomy performed at a relatively high epididymal level (upper corpus or caput), reduced sperm motility is not uncommon and occurs because sperm do not pass through a sufficient length of the epididymal tubule to acquire their full motility and/or fertilization potential.

When encountering a patient who has had good sperm concentration but consistently reduced sperm motility after vasovasostomy or vasoepididymostomy, I first obtain sperm antibody studies. If the patient has high sperm antibody levels by whatever method of measurement, then I believe that his chance for a conception is poor. Such patients do not seem to have their

245

fertility improved by any available therapy. They therefore would be poor candidates for reoperative procedures. Unfortunately, preoperative sperm antibody test results before a first reversal cannot predict if the patient's fertility will be impaired by the presence of sperm antibodies postoperatively. Men who have high levels of sperm antibodies regularly achieve pregnancies in their wives after first vasectomy reversal procedures. In fact, of 132 patients in whom I have measured serum sperm antibody levels before a first reversal, the man with the highest level of sperm antibodies achieved a conception (unpublished data). A high sperm antibody level seems to have adverse prognostic significance only for the patient who has good sperm concentration with poor sperm motility after a first reversal.

If genital tract infection is present, it should be treated. However, I never have seen a patient whose reduced sperm motility after a vasectomy reversal procedure resulted from infection. Unfortunately, no test is available to determine if reduced sperm motility after reversal procedures results from epididymal dysfunction.

Reduced sperm motility after vasovasostomy may occur in patients who have developed anastomotic strictures. Their sperm concentrations may be high at times but usually fluctuate considerably from high levels to severely oligospermic levels, often finally becoming azoospermic. I have illustrated the serial semen analysis results in such a patient, who subsequently had persistently good sperm motility and achieved a conception after a repeat vasovasostomy.

Reasons for Failure

The old adage that an ounce of prevention is worth a pound of cure certainly applies to techniques used during the original reversal procedure. When an original vasectomy reversal is performed, the surgeon must be certain that he has resected the old scarred portions of the vas completely (Fig. 21-1). Anastomosis of scarred ends obviously will result in failure.

When bleeding is controlled on the vas, only bipolar cautery should be used. The surgeon should *never* cauterize bleeders on the surface of the transected end of the vas (Fig. 21-2).

Another cause of failure is anastomotic tension. Anastomotic suturing should not begin until the surgeon is certain that there will not be tension on the anastomosis. When exploring failed vasovasostomies, I sometimes find that the old anastomosed ends are separated by a distance of 1 to 2 cm because anastomotic tension was present during the first procedure. The use of an infrapubic incision enables the surgeon to mobilize a sufficient length of the abdominal end of the vas to perform vasovasostomy or vasoepididymostomy without tension even when long portions of the vas were resected during the vasectomy. Tension during vasovasostomy may be prevented by approximating the spermatic fascia at the base of the isolated ends of the vas (Fig. 21-3). Tension during vasoepididymostomy may be prevented as illustrated in Figure 21-4.

The surgeon must be careful not to devascularize the ends of the vas when they are isolated. It is better to leave perivasal tissue intact than to strip the perivasal tissue away from the end of the vas (Fig. 21-5). If a leakproof anastomosis is not created, then the resulting anastomotic sperm granuloma may cause anastomotic obstruction. The detrimental effect of an anastomotic sperm granuloma was shown by Hagan and Coffey, although Carey and colleagues found that anastomotic sperm granulomas did not seem to have such a detrimental effect.

Figure 21-1. *The surgeon must be certain to resect the entire scarred portions along each side of the old vas anastomosis before performing the repeat vasovasostomy procedure.*

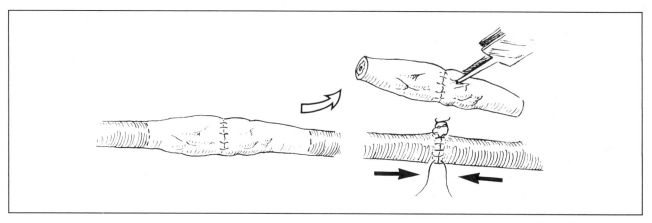

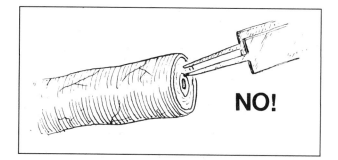

Figure 21-2. *Never cauterize bleeders on the transected surface of the vas. Cautery in this location will produce cicatricial reaction.*

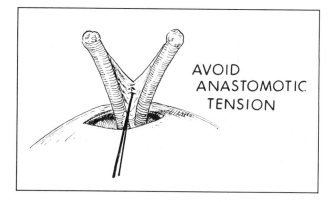

Figure 21-3. *To avoid anastomotic tension during vasovasostomy, spermatic fascia at the base of the isolated ends of the vas is approximated with absorbable sutures.*

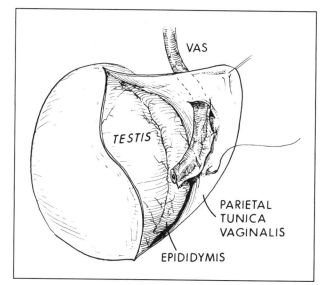

Figure 21-4. *During vasoepididymostomy, tension on the anastomosis may be prevented by suturing the perivasal tissue to the parietal tunica vaginalis. The vas is brought out through a stab opening in the parietal tunica. Perivasal tissue is sutured to the parietal tunica at the point of entry of the vas into the cavity of the tunica and at lower levels along the vas with interrupted 6-0 nylon. To prevent unintended occlusion of the epididymal tubule above the level of the vasoepididymal anastomosis, these sutures should not be placed on the surface of the epididymis.*

Finally, a back pressure–induced rupture of the epididymal tubule and the resulting epididymal sperm granuloma that may occur after vasectomy will be a cause for failure of vasovasostomy even when the anastomosis is patent. Whether the surgeon should perform vasovasostomy or vasoepididymostomy when sperm are absent from the intraoperative vas fluid during vasectomy reversal procedures depends on several factors. It is possible to have normal semen parameters after bilateral vasovasostomy even when sperm were absent from the intraoperative vas fluid bilaterally. Most patients whose intraoperative vas fluid does not contain sperm bilaterally but resembles water (clear, colorless, and transparent) have good results after bilateral vasovasostomy.

During the original vasoepididymostomy, the surgeon must be sure that the anastomosis is performed at a level above the epididymal obstruction. This is ascertained by verifying through microscopic examination of the epididymal tubular fluid that the fluid contains sperm. If the anastomosis is not performed at a level in the epididymal tubule at which sperm are present, then the epididymal obstruction still will be superior to the vasoepididymal anastomosis.

Assessing the Feasibility of a Reoperative Reversal

Review of the operative note of the first reversal may help in planning a reoperative procedure. To perform the repeat anastomosis, it usually is necessary to resect a several centimeter length of vas above and below the old anastomosis in order to obtain vasal ends free of scarring. If an anastomosis was difficult to perform during the first reversal because a long length of vas had been resected during the vasectomy, it is possible that a repeat procedure on that side cannot be accomplished. Review of the initial reversal operative note may tell the surgeon if sperm were present in the vas fluid during the initial procedure. If sperm were absent from the vas fluid during the initial procedure, vasoepididymostomy probably will be required for the repeat reversal.

While it almost always is possible to perform a repeat vasovasostomy, it may not be possible to perform a repeat vasoepididymostomy if an initial vasoepidi-

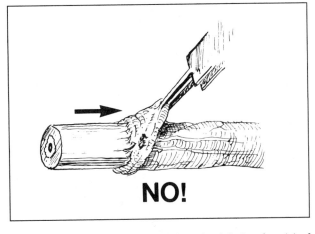

Figure 21-5. *When the vas ends are isolated during the original or reoperative procedure, the surgeon should take care not to strip the perivasal tissue containing nutrient vessels away from the transected end of the vas. Excessive stripping of the perivasal tissue away from the end of the vas may result in devascularization and scar formation.*

dymostomy failed. The scarring that results from an initial vasoepididymostomy may cause complete obliteration of the cavity of the tunica vaginalis. In such instances, it may not be possible to expose the epididymis without jeopardizing the testicular arterial supply.

Operative Techniques

Although I perform most initial vasectomy reversals with local anesthesia, I prefer epidural regional anesthesia for reoperative procedures. The scarring that results from the initial reversal makes it necessary to perform more dissection in repeat than in initial reversal procedures. Also, vasoepididymostomy is more likely to be required for a repeat than for an initial reversal. The patient often becomes restless during a vasoepididymostomy procedure performed with local anesthesia due to the longer time required to perform vasoepididymostomy.

When performing a repeat vasectomy reversal, I first isolate the vas below the old anastomosis and perform a microsurgical cutdown into the lumen of the vas at that level. The cutdown is performed with a microsurgical scalpel, and care is taken to avoid incising the posterior wall of the mucosa. Vas fluid is obtained from the cutdown site and is examined microscopically for sperm content. If sperm are present in the vas fluid in a patient who is azoospermic after the first reversal, then the old anastomosis is obstructed. In such a situation, I

then resect the old anastomosis and subsequently anastomose the new vas ends microsurgically. The two-layer microsurgical vasovasostomy technique that I use is the same as that used for the initial reversal procedure. This technique has been well illustrated diagrammatically and with operative photographs.

If sperm are absent from the fluid obtained from the vas cutdown site, then vasoepididymostomy will be required in order to bypass an epididymal obstruction. However, the old vas anastomosis also may be obstructed. I test patency of the old anastomosis by instilling Ringer's solution through a 24-gauge blunt-tipped needle inserted into the vas lumen through the cutdown. If the Ringer's solution flows freely, the old anastomosis is patent. If much pressure is required to instill the Ringer's solution, then the old anastomosis is narrowed and should be excised before vasoepididymostomy is performed. If the Ringer's solution cannot be instilled at all, then the old anastomosis is completely obstructed. The surgeon may prefer to perform a vasogram through the cutdown site to determine patency of the old anastomosis.

If vasoepididymostomy is required, the anastomosis is performed using the vas at the level of the cutdown or above the old vasovasostomy site (depending on whether or not the old anastomosis is patent). The technique of vasoepididymostomy for a repeat procedure is no different than that used for a first procedure, and I have illustrated that technique previously.

Complications

Because more dissection is required for reoperative reversals than for first reversals due to scarring after the first procedure, hemorrhage and infection theoretically are more likely after reoperative than after first reversals. However, I have not observed a more increased rate of either of these complications after reoperative reversals compared to the rate after first reversals. As a consequence of the meticulous hemostasis required for microsurgical procedures, I do not use drains after either first or repeat vasectomy reversals.

Postoperative Care

The care after repeat reversals is the same as after first reversals. Patients are advised to remain at home for 1 week postoperatively and to avoid intercourse for 2 weeks postoperatively. For 4 weeks after operation, the patient is advised to use a scrotal support and avoid heavy physical activity.

Results

Results of repeat vasectomy reversals are not as good as the results after first reversals. The Vasovasostomy Study Group found patency and pregnancy rates after 1247 first reversals to be 86 and 52 percent, respectively, while the rates after repeat reversals were 75 and 43 percent, respectively.

I have performed 76 repeat vasectomy reversals. Of 69 second reversals, I had performed the first reversal in 28. Seven of the 76 were third reversals; the second reversal had been performed by me in 4 of the 7. Of 55 repeat reversal patients who had postoperative semen analyses performed, 18 (33 percent) were azoospermic. This is a considerably higher postoperative rate of azoospermia than the rate of 14 percent that occurs after first reversals.

When calculating pregnancy rates after vasectomy reversal procedures, one must remember that the average time to conception after a reversal is 12 months and that it takes 24 months for the majority of conceptions to occur. Sixteen (44 percent) of my 36 repeat reversal patients who were eligible for pregnancy rate calculations achieved a pregnancy. Twenty-six patients were characterized as lost to pregnancy follow-up because they were followed less than 24 months postoperatively. Only patients known to have sperm in the semen postoperatively were so characterized. All azoospermic patients were characterized as failing to achieve a pregnancy regardless of the duration of their follow-up. Of seven third-time reversals that I have performed, two were lost to follow-up immediately postoperatively, two were azoospermic postoperatively, and the wives of three became pregnant.

Conclusions

Reoperative vasectomy reversal usually is more difficult than a first reversal and occasionally may be very difficult due to the presence of a large amount of scar tissue resulting from the original procedure. Information contained in the original reversal operative report may help in planning a reoperative procedure. My approach to reoperative procedures is based on findings when a microsurgical cutdown into the vas lumen is performed below the level of the old anastomosis. The vas fluid sperm content at this level and observations regarding patency of the old vas anastomosis when instilling Ringer's solution through it determine whether vasovasostomy or vasoepididymostomy is required at the time of a reoperative procedure. The importance of resecting all scarred portions of the vas before performing a repeat anastomosis is emphasized. While the results of reoperative vasectomy reversals are not as good as the results of original procedures, some couples will feel that the results of reoperative procedures are sufficiently good enough to justify the discomfort, expense, and time away from work that are associated with a repeat reversal.

Bibliography

Ansbacher, R, Keung-Yeung, K, and Wurster, JC. Sperm antibodies in vasectomized men. Fertil Steril 23:640, 1972.

Belker, AM. Microsurgery for the urologist. AUA Update Series, vol 3, lesson 2. Houston: American Urological Association, Inc., Office of Education, 1984.

Belker, AM. Microsurgical two-layer vasovasostomy: Simplified technique using hinged folding-approximating clamp. Urology 16:376, 1980.

Belker, AM. Vasovasostomy. In MI Resnick (ed), Current Trends in Urology, vol 1. Baltimore: Williams & Wilkins, 1981, pp 20–41.

Belker, AM. Vasovasostomy and vasoepididymostomy. AUA Update Series, vol 1, lesson 2. Houston: American Urological Association, Inc., Office of Education, 1981.

Belker, AM. Microscopic vasovasostomy. In Male Infertility, Urology Today Videotape Series, vol 4, no 1. Norwich, NY: Norwich Eaton Audiovisual Library, 1985.

Belker, AM. Microsurgical repair of obstructive causes of male infertility. Semin Urol 2:91, 1984.

Belker, AM. Microsurgical vasectomy reversal. In B Lytton, et al (eds), Advances in Urology, vol 1. Chicago: Year Book Medical Publishers, 1988, pp 193–230.

Belker, AM. Infrapubic incision for specific vasectomy reversal situations. Urology 32:413, 1988.

Belker, AM, et al. Results of 1469 microsurgical vasectomy reversals by the Vasovasostomy Study Group. J Urol 145:505, 1991.

Carey, PO, et al. Effects of granuloma formation at site of vasovasostomy. J Urol 139:853, 1988.

Hagan, KF, and Coffey, DS. The adverse effects of sperm during vasovasostomy. J Urol 118:269, 1977.

Silber, SJ. Epididymal extravasation following vasectomy as a cause for failure of vasectomy reversal. Fertil Steril 31:309, 1979.

The Failed Orchiopexy

JACK S. ELDER

Cryptorchidism is the most common disorder of male sexual differentiation and affects approximately 0.8 percent of 1-year-old male infants. Long-term sequelae of cryptorchidism include infertility and testicular tumor. By light microscopy, the undescended testis shows a diminished number of germ cells, diminished seminiferous tubular size, and peritubular hyalinization and fibrosis by 18 months of age, and abnormalities are evident by electron microscopy at 1 year of age. Consequently, orchiopexy generally is recommended at 12 to 18 months to maximize chances for fertility.

The location of the cryptorchid testis may be classified as (1) canalicular, lying within the inguinal canal between the internal and external inguinal rings, (2) ectopic, located outside the normal pathway of descent, usually superficial to the external oblique fascia, or (3) intraabdominal, located inside the internal inguinal ring. Some boys with suspected cryptorchidism have a retractile testis, in which the cremasteric reflex pulls the testis back into the groin during stimulation.

Approximately 20 percent of undescended testes are impalpable, and more than 50 percent of impalpable testes are atrophic or "vanishing" (Elder, 1993). A vanishing testis usually results from testicular torsion in utero. In these patients, surgical exploration reveals a vas and testicular artery terminating in an atrophic testis or a small nubbin of tissue that may contain a few seminiferous tubules and deposits of hemosiderin. In other cases, the vas and vessels end blindly. Inexplicably, testicular torsion in utero occurs on the left side in 80 percent of cases.

Surgical Anatomy

Three arteries provide the vascular supply to the testis. The major vessel is the testicular artery, which originates from the aorta on each side. Normally, the testicular artery penetrates the tunica albuginea on the posterior aspect of the testicle, travels just deep to the tunica albuginea medial or lateral to the midline toward the anterior surface of the testicle, and divides into multiple arteries that penetrate the substance of the testis. The vasal and cremasteric arteries are minor vessels that provide multiple branches over the surface of the testis. The vasal artery, a branch of the inferior vesical artery, courses through the spermatic cord attached to the vas deferens. The cremasteric artery, a branch of the inferior epigastric artery, is present superficially in the cremasteric fascia and tunica vaginalis. There are multiple anastomotic communications between the testicular and vasal arteries in 90 percent of patients. Furthermore, in 50 percent of cases there are anastomotic connections between the cremasteric artery and either the testicular or vasal artery (Jarow, 1990). The intratesticular blood supply is variable, but the areas of the testis most likely to contain a major superficial arterial branch are the medial, anterior, and lateral surfaces of the lower pole. The areas of the testis least likely to contain a major arterial branch are the medial and lateral aspects of the upper pole (Lee et al., 1984). These factors are important in the placement of traction sutures through the testis.

In the undescended testis, epididymal anomalies are common and affect 50 to 80 percent of boys with an undescended testis (Elder, 1992a). In some cases, the epididymis may be twice as long as the testis and not have a normal attachment to the lower pole of the testis, and on rare occasion, it may be atretic. In some patients with an intraabdominal testis, the vas deferens may loop distally for a variable distance through the inguinal canal, termed a long-looping vas. Recognition of these anomalies is important in order to minimize the likelihood of trauma to the delicate epididymis and vas.

Several factors must be addressed in performing an orchiopexy. First, in the undescended testis, the testicular artery is short. In addition, the testicular artery normally assumes a triangular course through the internal inguinal ring. In 85 percent of cases there is an associated hernia sac that is adherent to the spermatic cord (Elder, 1992a). Finally, there are external spermatic fibers lateral to the spermatic cord near the internal inguinal ring that restrict testicular mobility. A strong understanding of the concepts applicable to a standard orchiopexy facilitates the approach to the failed orchiopexy.

Technique of Standard Orchiopexy

In most cases, an orchiopexy may be performed on an ambulatory basis, even if an intraabdominal dissection is necessary. Bupivicaine may be infiltrated into the inguinal incision for postoperative analgesia, or a caudal or inguinal block may be performed.

A 3.5- to 4.5-cm incision is made in the inguinal skin crease, and the external oblique fascia is identified (Fig. 22-1). The external oblique fascia is opened through the external ring, and the ilioinguinal nerve is protected by retracting it medially over the fascia. The longitudinal cremasteric fibers are then separated bluntly to expose the testis and spermatic cord. In many cases, compression of the abdomen allows the testis to be manipulated beyond the external ring, enveloped by the processus vaginalis. If the testis is ectopic in the superficial inguinal pouch, it needs to be mobilized before opening the external oblique fasica.

The processus vaginalis is then incised sharply to expose the testis, with great care not to cut the testis or epididymis. Next, a 4-0 polyglycolic acid (PGA) stitch is placed through the gubernaculum, the distal aspect of the processus, or the testis itself. A traction stitch through the testis should be placed through the middle of the bulk of the testis in its upper half, and the capsular vessels should be avoided. Such a stitch is unlikely to result in significant damage to the testis (Jarow, 1990; Lee et al., 1984). However, throughout the dissection,

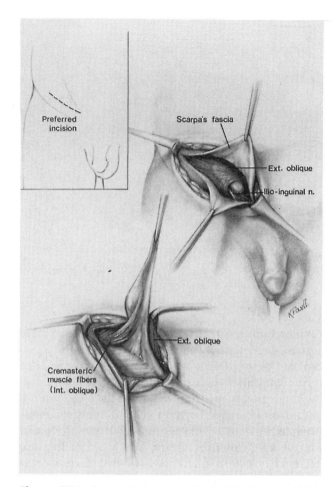

Figure 22-1. *See insert: transverse skin incision in inguinal skin crease. Scarpa's fascia is opened. The external oblique fascia is opened, avoiding the ilioinguinal nerve, and the testis is identified. (From FF Marshall and JS Elder,* Cryptorchidism and Related Anomalies. *New York: Praeger, 1982.)*

moistened gauze should be used to grasp the testis rather than using the traction stitch itself to pull on the testis. At this point it is important to examine the epididymis for abnormalities and identify the vas deferens, because either of these may loop down several centimeters toward the scrotum. The distal gubernacular attachments are then transected, being careful to achieve hemostasis and avoid epididymal/vasal injury. Next, the testis, processus vaginalis, and vessels, surrounded by external spermatic fibers, can be mobilized proximally to the internal inguinal ring.

In almost all cases, there is a patent processus vaginalis. The processus is usually thin and extremely adherent to the vas. In general, it is easier to mobilize the sac from the spermatic cord near the internal ring than from where the sac is opened (Fig. 22-2). Some have suggested injecting a small amount of saline under the

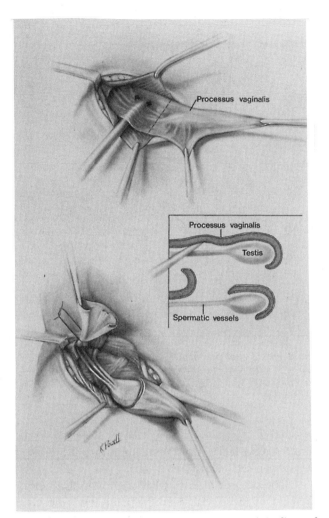

Figure 22-2. *The processus vaginalis (hernia sac) is dissected from the remainder of the spermatic cord and ligated. Opening of the hernia sac may facilitate dissection. (From FF Marshall and JS Elder,* Cryptorchidism and Related Anomalies. *New York: Praeger, 1982.)*

sac to facilitate the dissection, but usually this maneuver is unnecessary. A fine mosquito clamp is used to separate the sac bluntly from the spermatic cord. After the sac has been separated from the vas and cord, it is bluntly dissected proximally to the internal ring. Minimal sharp dissection is necessary. The surgeon must be extremely careful not to grasp the vas or spermatic vessels during this dissection, because they are extremely fragile structures and are injured easily. A high ligation of the sac is performed with two 3-0 PGA suture ligatures. At this point, the testis should be sufficiently mobilized to be near the scrotum.

Inferomedial traction is then placed on the testis with the gauze sponge, and the cremasteric and external spermatic fibers that are attached to the spermatic cord are cut. Transection of the fibers lateral to the cord allows the greatest mobilization of the testis. The dissection is carried into the retroperitoneum beyond the point where the testicular artery and vas diverge. A small Deaver retracter aids in separation of the peritoneum from the spermatic vessels and vas. In most cases, the testis should reach the scrotum without tension following these maneuvers. However, if the testis still does not reach the scrotum easily, then a Prentiss maneuver is performed (Fig. 22-3). This maneuver is performed by incising the transversalis fascia, which forms the floor of the inguinal canal, and ligating and dividing the inferior epigastric artery and vein. Further mobilization of the vas and testicular vessels in the retroperitoneum also is performed in order to allow the testicular vessels to assume a more direct course to the scrotum.

The testis may then be placed in a pouch in the scrotal wall between the skin and dartos (Fig. 22-4). A transverse incision through the skin is made in the inferior aspect of the scrotum, and a generous pouch is made by blunt dissection inferiorly and superiorly initially with a small mosquito clamp followed by a standard mosquito clamp. A clamp is then passed through this retrograde incision to the inguinal canal, and the traction stitch through the testis is grasped. The testis is brought through the scrotal incision, and the neck of the scrotum is closed with a 4-0 PGA stitch to prevent retraction of the testis. The testis is placed into the dartos pouch, and the incisions are closed. An external fixation stitch is rarely necessary and may irreversibly traumatize the testis by injuring the capsular vessels (Jarow, 1990).

If the testis is not identified in the inguinal canal, then the peritoneal cavity must be opened to locate the testis. In almost all cases, if the testis is present, it is just inside the internal inguinal ring. In most patients with an intraabdominal testis, the testis cannot be brought down to the scrotum in a single stage by the technique described, and mobilization of the testis to the scrotum represents an operative challenge. One option is a Fowler-Stephens procedure, in which the testicular artery is divided, in the hope that the testis will retain sufficient vascularity from collateral blood flow through the deferential and cremasteric arteries (Elder, 1989). Success with this technique requires early intraoperative recognition of the potential need for this procedure, since the peritoneal attachment to the vas deferens must be preserved. In 20 to 30 percent of cases, testicular atrophy results secondary to inadequate collateral arterial flow, generally because of transection of the differential artery or arterial spasm during mobilization of the testis. In order to improve the potential success of the

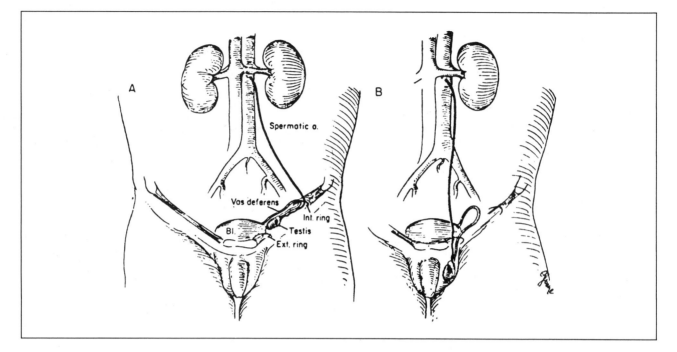

Figure 22-3. *The Prentiss maneuver. A. The floor of the inguinal canal is incised, and the inferior epigastric vessels are divided. B. The testis and spermatic cord are brought down in a straight line into the scrotum. (Reproduced from EW Fonkalsrud, The undescended testis.* Curr Probl Surg *15:1, 1978.)*

procedure, a newer approach, termed a *staged* Fowler-Stephens procedure, may be performed, in which the testicular artery is simply ligated in situ to allow the collateral blood supply to develop without mobilizing the testis itself (Elder, 1992b). Between 6 and 12 months later, a standard Fowler-Stephens orchiopexy is performed. The testis and vas are mobilized together with a strip of peritoneum at least 3 cm wide.

Another approach in patients with an intraabdominal testis is a planned two-stage orchiopexy. In this procedure, the testis is mobilized and brought into the inguinal canal as far as possible. The testis and spermatic cord may be wrapped with a silicone sheath to prevent adhesions to the testis, which would increase the risk of vascular injury during a second operation. The second stage is performed approximately 1 year later. The success rate with this technique has been 70 to 80 percent.

Another surgical option for the correction of a high undescended testis is testicular autotransplantation. In general, this procedure is anticipated preoperatively and is not performed until at least 2 to 4 years of age. The testicular artery and internal spermatic vein are divided and anastomosed to the inferior epigastric artery and vein, respectively, in the inguinal canal. There has been

limited experience with this technique, but the results have been satisfactory.

In 4 percent of boys with cryptorchidism and 50 percent of those with a nonpalpable testis, no viable testis is identified. To make the diagnosis of vanishing testis, the vas deferens and testicular vessels should be identified not only grossly but microscopically. It is insufficient to identify only the vas deferens, because the epididymis and vas may be completely separated from the testis itself. Some patients with an intraabdominal testis have a vas deferens that loops down the inguinal canal. Therefore, if an inguinal dissection reveals the vas deferens to end in a nubbin of tissue at the external ring or scrotum, the peritoneum should be opened to be absolutely certain that there is not a testis associated with a long-looping vas.

Results of Standard Orchiopexy

Generally, an orchiopexy is extremely successful. In a series of 295 patients reported by Moul and Belman (1988), there was a complication rate of 12 percent. The most common problem was a high-riding testis in the scrotum (10 patients, 3.4 percent), and 3 patients

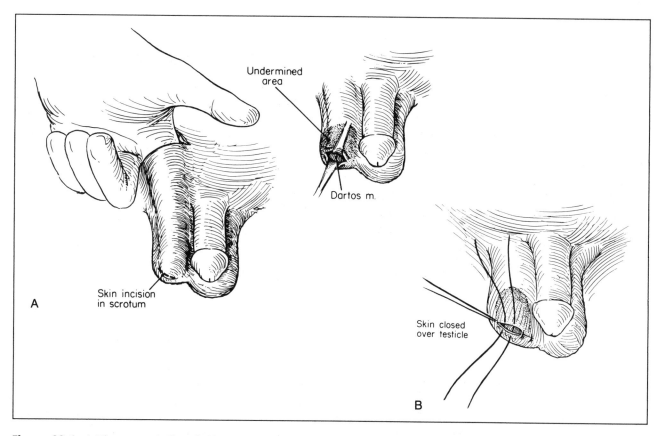

Figure 22-4. *A. The scrotum is distended by the surgeon's index finger, and a small incision is made in the most dependent portion of the ipsilateral scrotal skin. The dartos and underlying fascia are dissected free from the scrotal skin to form a subcutaneous pouch. B. The scrotal skin is closed over the testis with absorbable suture. (From EW Fonkalsrud, The undescended testis.* Curr Probl Surg 15:1, 1978.)

(1 percent) required reoperation because of unsatisfactory placement. None of the patients with a palpable testis developed testicular atrophy. One patient experienced inadvertent transection of the vas deferens, and in one patient the testicular artery was transected. In another series of 175 orchiopexies, 8 (4.6 percent) required a secondary orchiopexy because of unsatisfactory placement of the testis during the first orchiopexy (Evans et al., 1978).

The Failed Orchiopexy

Failure of the testis to be in a satisfactory position may result in a significant therapeutic dilemma. The scrotal location of the testis is essential for normal spermatogenesis and epididymal function, since it is 1.5 to 2.0°C cooler than body temperature. Furthermore, although most think that an orchiopexy does not diminish the risk for the development of a testicular tumor, recent studies have indicated that seminoma is much more common in nonoperated cryptorchid testes, whereas nonseminomatous tumors are more common in undescended testes that have been brought down to the scrotum (Abratt et al., 1993; Halme et al., 1989).

The failed orchiopexy may be divided into three situations. The most common group is composed of patients who have undergone an orchiopexy but in whom the testis is in an unsatisfactory position. Included in this group should be children who have undergone previous inguinal herniorrhaphies in whom the testis has retracted into the groin, presumably from scar tissue, failure to return the testis to a satisfactory scrotal location at the end of the procedure, or those in whom the testis was undescended in the first place and in whom an orchiopexy was not performed. The second group is composed of children who have undergone an orchiopexy who experience testicular atrophy, in whom the residual testicular tissue is impalpable. The third group includes children who have undergone an incomplete exploration for an impalpable testis, in whom an intraabdominal testis may be present, with or without a long-looping vas deferens.

Patient Evaluation

Although boys often have a brisk cremasteric reflex, the technique of orchiopexy often denervates this reflex. Consequently, following an orchiopexy, the exact location of the testis generally is easy to appreciate. The child should be examined in both the supine and sitting positions. One hand should be placed at the level of the anterosuperior iliac spine, which is superolateral to the internal inguinal ring. The hand should then be swept firmly down the inguinal canal, while the other hand is positioned at the scrotum. In most cases the testis is easily palpated, although in boys with obesity it may be extremely difficult to locate the testis unless it is in the scrotum or beyond the pubic tubercle. However, when boys are sitting, the testis often drops a few millimeters and facilitates examination.

Undescended Testis Following Previous Orchiopexy or Herniorrhaphy

Ideally, the surgeon should wait 12 months before reoperating on an undescended testis in order to allow the tissues to soften and make the dissection slightly easier. Strong consideration should be given to administering human chorionic gonadotropin (HCG) 3000 IU weekly for 4 weeks immediately before the secondary orchiopexy, which should increase local blood flow to the testis and increase the size of the testis, presumably rendering it less susceptible to damage from reoperative surgery. The use of HCG in this situation is theoretical, since there are no data that the success rate is improved. Although HCG has been used to try to induce testicular descent in boys with primary cryptorchidism, the urologist should not expect the position of the testis to change if the child has had previous inguinal surgery. Ideally, the previous operative report should be obtained and reviewed carefully to assess the steps that were performed during the previous inguinal surgery. Specifically, if the child has had a previous orchiopexy, it is important to ascertain whether a patent processus vaginalis was present, whether it was ligated, whether a Prentiss maneuver was performed, and so forth. The parents of the child should be aware that because the surgery is reoperative, there is significant risk of injuring the testis and/or its vascular supply.

On the day of surgery, the child is not allowed to ingest solids, formula, or milk after midnight but is allowed to take clear liquids ad libitum until 2 to 3 hours before the scheduled surgery.

The previous incision is entered and is lengthened by 1 cm. Scarpa's fascia generally is not a distinct structure, and sharp dissection is necessary to identify the external oblique fascia. It is useful to identify the fascia in a location that was dissected out previously and then work one's way toward the inguinal canal and external ring. By careful dissection, the external oblique over the inguinal canal is dissected out. The external inguinal ring is then opened in the direction of the fascial fibers. In reoperative situations, it is usually difficult to identify the ilioinguinal nerve. The spermatic cord and testis are then identified. One should mobilize the entire spermatic cord and place a small Penrose drain around it, isolating the cord from the remainder of the inguinal canal.

The testis itself should not be dissected out as one would in a primary orchiopexy unless the testis still resides within the tunica vaginalis, because there is a significant risk of damaging either the testis itself or the epididymis. Next, a 4-0 PGA traction stitch is placed through the middle of the upper aspect of the testis. By careful sharp dissection, the distal attachments of scar tissue to the testis are severed. After placing traction on the testis with a moistened gauze sponge, the spermatic cord is sharply dissected free from the inguinal canal up to the level of the internal ring. At this point, it is important to assess which of the pertinent anatomic factors had prevented the testis from being placed in the scrotum during the previous operative procedure. At the internal ring, it is helpful to dissect even further proximally, since it is likely that there will be less scar tissue. The peritoneum should be identified, and one should ascertain whether there is a persistent patent processus vaginalis. If there is a small hernia sac, it should be dissected away carefully from the vas and the remainder of the spermatic cord as described in the preceding section. Once the sac is dissected out, a high ligation is performed with two 3-0 PGA suture ligatures. One may then recheck the position of the testis to ascertain whether it has been mobilized sufficiently to reach the scrotum. If not, then the lateral external spermatic fascial fibers and lateral scar tissue should be incised. During the dissection, if there is bleeding along the spermatic cord, it is important to ground the testis by letting it rest in the wound during electrocautery in order to prevent transmission of the current superiorly along the spermatic cord, which could result in testicular artery thrombosis. During this part of the procedure, it is important not to do too much dissection within the spermatic cord itself, since the vas or testicular artery could be damaged. If the testis still does not reach the scrotum, then the peritoneal cavity should be opened widely, and a Prentiss maneuver can be performed as described in the preceding section. These maneuvers should allow the testis to reach the scrotum or at least reach the upper aspect of the scrotum. In the latter situation, further superior dissection may be accomplished after one lengthens the incision, which affords better access to the retroperitoneum.

If the child has begun to undergo pubertal changes, the testis should be biopsied to be certain that there is no evidence of malignancy. Changes of carcinoma in situ generally are present throughout the testis rather than existing in a focal manner. If malignant changes are present, an orchiectomy should be performed.

If the testicular artery appears to have been injured during the procedure, then it should be observed a bit longer before deciding whether to remove the testis or perform an orchiopexy. If one decides to remove the testis, then consideration should be given to placement of a testicular prosthesis (see below).

The testis is then placed in the dartos pouch. As with a standard orchiopexy, placement of an external fixation suture rarely is necessary. The incision may then be closed with absorbable sutures. Ideally, the patient should stay relatively inactive for at least 1 to 2 weeks following reoperative surgery, in order to maximize the likelihood of the testis remaining in a satisfactory scrotal position.

Results of Reoperative Surgery

There are few data on the results of secondary orchiopexy. Maizels et al. (1983) reported a series of 36 boys who underwent secondary orchiopexy, which comprised approximately 10 percent of the total number of patients undergoing an orchiopexy during that period of time. Preoperatively, it was apparent that 20 testes (55 percent) were distal to the external inguinal ring, and the remainder were in the inguinal canal. The extent of surgical mobilization of the testis and spermatic cord varied. In 16 patients, it was necessary to perform extensive dissection in the inguinal canal and retroperitoneum, as well as the Prentiss maneuver. In 12 patients, dissection of the inguinal canal and superficial inguinal pouch with creation of a dartos pouch was the only techniques necessary for a successful result. Overall, 16 (44 percent) underwent the Prentiss maneuver with extensive retroperitoneal dissection, 5 (14 percent) required inguinal and retroperitoneal mobilization, 13 (36 percent) underwent inguinal mobilization alone, and 2 (6 percent) underwent an orchiectomy. In the series by Moul and Belman (1988), 6 had undergone

a previous orchiopexy and 17 had undergone a previous inguinal herniorrhaphy. There were no reports of testicular atrophy in either of these series. In contrast, in a report by Evans et al. (1978), at the 5-year examination, 6 of the 8 testes subjected to secondary orchiopexy had atrophied and one patient was not available for follow-up. Obviously, the success of the reoperative procedure depends on numerous factors, including the position of the testis and experience of the surgeon (Table 22-1).

Management of the Child Who Has Undergone Previous Orchiopexy Who Has an Impalpable Testis

If the child has undergone a previous orchiopexy, the testis may be present but may be retracted into the inguinal canal, or it may have undergone atrophy. If the urologist has been able to palpate the testis during serial examinations and has subsequently determined that it is atrophic, then no further intervention is necessary. However, if there is significant concern that there was a relatively normal testis that now cannot be palpated because of significant retraction into the inguinal canal and/or because the child is obese or difficult to examine, then a secondary orchiopexy should be considered.

The technique of exploration is identical to the one described in the preceding section. If the testis is identified, it should be mobilized in the usual manner and placed in a dartos pouch. However, if the testis is an atrophic nubbin, then consideration should be given to inserting a testicular prosthesis. In these cases, the child should be given broad-spectrum antibiotics intravenously preoperatively as well as postoperatively. Because of concern regarding the safety of gel-filled silicone prostheses, the American Urological Association currently recommends that these not be inserted (Elder, 1989). However, a solid silicone polymer testicular prosthesis may be appropriate. In these cases, the child should be given broad-spectrum antibiotics intravenously preoperatively and postoperatively.

Table 22-1. *Results of Reoperative Orchiopexy*

Series	No. of Patients	No. of Successful Outcomes
Evans et al., 1978	7	1
Maizels et al., 1983	36	36
Moul and Belman, 1988	23	23
Livne et al., 1990	34	34
Cartwright et al., 1993	25	25
TOTAL	125	119 (95%)

Previous Inadequate Exploration for an Impalpable Testis

In some patients with an intraabdominal testis, the vas deferens travels through the inguinal canal, sometimes as far as the scrotum, before it courses back up to the internal ring. In such a patient, if a standard low inguinal exploration is performed, the vas and its associated deferential artery, as well as small collateral vessels, might be misidentified as the vas deferens and testicular artery. If the surgeon then followed these structures down to their apparent "termination" near the external ring, the gubernacular remnant might resemble an atrophic nubbin, and one might assume that they represent the remnants of intrauterine testicular torsion and remove these structures, when in reality the testis was intraabdominal. Consequently, in a child with an impalpable testis who seems to have an atrophic nubbin or testis in the canal or scrotum, exploration of the abdomen is mandatory to be absolutely certain that there is not an intraabdominal testis. Laparoscopy is an ideal method of evaluating these patients (Elder, 1988, 1993). Although radiologic imaging techniques such as ultrasound, CT scan, and magnetic reasonance imaging have been used to try to localize an impalpable testis, surgical visualization of the peritoneal cavity and inguinal canal is the only definitive method of determining whether the testis is present. In a series by Boddy et al. (1985), of 13 patients with a previous inguinal exploration for an undescended testis, 5 were found to have an intraabdominal testis.

Technique of Laparoscopy

Relatively few instruments are needed for laparoscopy (Fig. 22-5). At the beginning of the procedure the bladder is drained with a small catheter. The Verres needle is used to create a pneumoperitoneum (Fig. 22-6). This needle has an outer sleeve with a sharp tip, inside of which is a blunt rounded needle mounted on a spring. When the needle is inserted, the pressure against the abdominal wall or peritoneum causes the blunt inner needle to retract, leaving the sharp outer sleeve unguarded to penetrate the abdominal layers. However, once the needle has entered the peritoneal cavity, resistance is overcome and the inner blunt needle springs out, preventing any damage by the sharp edge to the intraabdominal viscera. One must be certain that the spring works well before using this needle. After the needle has been inserted into what is thought to be the peritoneal cavity, one must ascertain that its tip is intraperitoneal. The most reliable method of assessing this is by performing the saline aspiration test, in which 5 cc of injectable

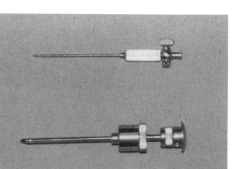

Figure 22-5. *Equipment for laparoscopy. (Above)* Verres needle. *(Center)* A 5-mm cannula with trocar. *(Below)* Pediatric cystoscope lens with adapter (sheath) for a laparoscope. (Reproduced from JS Elder, Laparoscopy and the Fowler-Stephens orchiopexy in the management of the impalpable testis. Urol Clin North Am 16:399, 1989.)

saline is injected through the needle, and aspiration is performed. If the needle is in the correct position, no saline will be aspirated. If, however, the needle is extraperitoneal, then some of the fluid can be aspirated. If the needle has inadvertently entered the bowel, stained saline will be returned.

After the Verres needle is inserted, the insufflation tubing is attached to the needle. The insufflator is set on the low or manual position, and CO_2 insufflation is started. The abdomen is filled with CO_2 until it is mildly tense, when the intraperitoneal pressure is approximately 15 mm Hg. Most children require 1 to 1.5 liters, and it takes approximately 30 to 60 seconds for the peritoneal cavity to fill. Overdistension can result in difficulties in ventilation.

Next, the surgeon inserts the trocar/cannula. The path of insertion is essentially identical to that traversed by the Verres needle. The nondominant hand tenses the anterior abdominal wall, and the trocar is inserted at an angle of 45 degrees toward the hollow of the sacrum. Usually one feels a single distinct pop as the trocar is inserted. The trocar is then removed from the cannula sheath, and the lens is inserted. The insufflator is set on the low/automatic or maintain position, and the laparoscope is attached to a high-intensity light source.

At this point it is helpful to place the patient in a 15- to 20-degree Trendelenburg position, which raises the pelvis and allows the bowel to retract cephalad. The

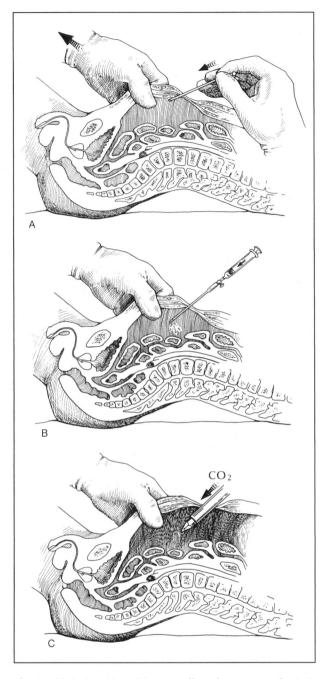

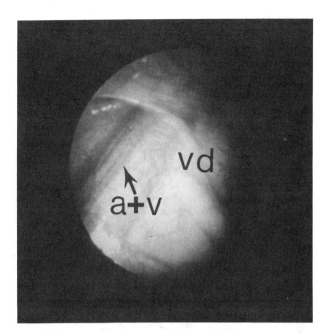

Figure 22-7. *Laparoscopic view of left internal inguinal ring. Note the vas deferens (VD) joining the testicular vessels (A + V) at the internal ring. (Reproduced from JS Elder, Laparoscopy and the Fowler-Stephens orchiopexy in the management of the impalpable testis. Urol Clin North Am 16:399, 1989.)*

Figure 22-6. *Insertion of Verres needle and trocar cannula. A. As the needle passes through the fascial layer, the inner round-ended needle (not shown) retracts into the sharp outer sleeve. Note that the insufflation port is directed toward the abdomen. B. Then 5 to 10 ml of saline is injected, which one should not be able to aspirate if the needle is in the appropriate position. C. After the peritoneal cavity has been filled with carbon dioxide, the trocar and cannula are inserted. (Reproduced from JS Elder, Laparoscopy and the Fowler-Stephens orchiopexy in the management of the impalpable testis. Urol Clin North Am 16:399, 1989.)*

peritoneal cavity can be inspected with a 0- or 30-degree lens. An antifog agent should be applied to the lens and eyepiece before inspection.

One should identify the internal inguinal rings, which have a crescentic medial margin. In general, it is helpful to examine the normal side first. The vessels lie vertically in the retroperitoneum, while the vas deferens is identified as a small white cord that rises out of the pelvis and joins the gonadal vessels at a 60- to 90-degree angle just proximal to the internal ring (Fig. 22-7). If one sees the vessels and vas entering the internal ring, then no further evaluation is necessary. If a testis is identified, then either a Fowler-Stephens orchiopexy should be performed or orchiectomy considered. If neither testis nor vessels are identified, then an intraabdominal exploration is necessary.

Summary

The standard orchiopexy is successful in approximately 98 percent of cases. When one is performing a secondary orchiopexy, the success rate generally is good, and one should follow essentially the same principles as those utilized for a primary orchiopexy.

Bibliography

Abratt, RP, Reddi, VB, and Sarembock, LA. Testicular cancer and cryptorchidism. Br J Urol 70:656, 1993.

Boddy, S-AM, Corkey, JJ, and Gornall, P. The place of laparoscopy in the management of the impalpable testis. Br J Surg 72:918, 1985.

Cartwright, PC, et al. A surgical approach to reoperative orchiopexy. J Urol 149:817, 1993.

Elder, JS. Laparoscopy and Fowler-Stephens orchiopexy in the management of the impalpable testis. Urol Clin North Am 16:399, 1989

Elder, JS. Laparoscopy for the impalpable testis. Semin Pediatr Surg (in press)

Elder, JS. Epididymal anomalies associated with hydrocele/hernia and cryptordism: Implications regarding testicular descent. J Urol 148:624, 1992a.

Elder, JS. Two-stage Fowler-Stephens orchiopexy in the management of intraabdominal testes. J Urol 149:1239, 1992b.

Elder, JS. The undescended testis: Hormonal and surgical management. Surg Clin North Am 68:983, 1988.

Elder, JS, Keating, MA, and Duckett, JW. Infant testicular prostheses. J Urol 141:1413, 1989.

Evans, JP, Rutherford, JH, and Bagshaw, PF. Orchiopexy in prepubertal boys: Five-year survey. Urology 12:509, 1978.

Fonkalsrud, EW. The undescended testis. Curr Prob Surg 15:1, 1978.

Holme, A, et al. Morphology of testicular germ cell tumours in treated and untreated cryptorchidism. Br J Urol 64:78, 1989.

Jarow, JP. Intratesticular arterial anatomy. J Androl 11:255, 1990.

Lee, LM, Johnson, HW, and McLoughlin, MG. Microdissection and radiographic studies of the arterial vasculature of the human testes. J Pediatr Surg 19:297, 1984.

Livne, PM, Savir, A, and Servadio, C. Re-orchiopexy: Advantages and disadvantages. Eur Urol 18:137, 1990.

Maizels, M, Gomez, F, and Firlit, CF. Surgical correction of the failed orchiopexy. J Urol 130:955, 1983.

Marshall, FF, and Elder, JS. Complications of orchiopexy. In FF Marshall (ed), Urologic Complications, 2d ed. St Louis: Mosby–Year Book, 1990, p 545.

Marshall, FF, and Elder, JS. Cryptorchidism and Related Anomalies. New York: Praeger, 1982.

Moul, JW, and Belman, AB. A review of surgical treatment of undescended testes with emphasis on anatomical position. J Urol 140:125, 1988.

Sheldon, CA. Undescended testis and testicular torsion. Surg Clin North Am 65:1303, 1985.

Residual Lymphadenopathy after Surgery, Chemotherapy, or Radiation Therapy

RICHARD S. FOSTER
JOHN P. DONOHUE

Retroperitoneal lymph node dissection in non-seminomatous testis cancer is utilized in both low- and high-stage disease. The use of retroperitoneal lymph node dissection in both low- and high-stage disease is twofold. After radical orchiectomy, retroperitoneal lymph node dissection in clinical stage I patients will identify the 30 percent who indeed are pathologic stage II patients. In addition, retroperitoneal lymph node dissection in these pathologic stage II patients may be therapeutic, eliminating the need for subsequent chemotherapy. In high-stage disease after chemotherapy, full bilateral retroperitoneal lymph node dissection identifies the minority who have persistent carcinoma in the retroperitoneum. These patients have not had a complete response to chemotherapy and are therefore given two more courses of platinum-based chemotherapy postoperatively. Additionally, postchemotherapy retroperitoneal lymph node dissection is therapeutic in the 40 to 45 percent of patients who have teratoma remaining after initial chemotherapy.

Full bilateral retroperitoneal lymph node dissection is an effective procedure to control retroperitoneal disease. The Indiana University experience indicates an overall local recurrence rate of only 1 percent after primary retroperitoneal lymph node dissection performed effectively. Nonetheless, reoperation is more often required after postchemotherapy retroperitoneal lymph node dissection where regional recurrence may be seen. Reoperation in this setting requires a commitment from the surgeon, in that these operations are sometimes long and intensive. The urologic surgeon embarking on a procedure of this type should be prepared to use his or her entire armamentarium, including techniques of vascular control.

Indications for Surgery

Four basic categories of patients are candidates for reoperation or operation after chemotherapy in nonseminomatous testis cancer. These categories include patients who have had a laparotomy for initial diagnosis followed by chemotherapy and subsequent retroperitoneal lymph node dissection, patients who have experienced a partial remission after chemotherapy and are subsequently candidates for retroperitoneal lymph node dissection, patients who have experienced a recurrence of teratoma after retroperitoneal lymph node dissection, and finally, patients with localized retroperitoneal chemoresistant disease who have exhausted all chemotherapeutic options. Each of these categories will be discussed separately.

Some patients unfortunately have had the diagnosis of retroperitoneal nonseminomatous testis cancer made by laparotomy instead of radical orchiectomy. These patients usually present initially with back pain and a retroperitoneal mass. The testicular primary may be too small to be felt or may be neglected. After the frozen-section diagnosis of high-volume germ cell cancer is made at laparotomy, the abdomen is closed, and chemotherapy is given. Approximately 30 percent of these patients will not experience a complete remission and are therefore candidates for retroperitoneal lymph node dissection. Reoperation in this setting is not extremely difficult, although we have seen intraperitoneal seeding, probably secondary to the biopsy at laparotomy done for diagnosis. If the pathology at retroperitoneal lymph node dissection reveals teratoma, all these areas of intraperitoneal seeding must be removed in order to decrease the chance of recurrence.

The second category of patients are those who have presented initially with high-volume nonseminomatous testis cancer, have undergone standard first-line chemotherapy, and have persistent radiographic disease after chemotherapy with normalization of serum alpha-fetoprotein and beta human chorionic gonadotropin (Fig. 23-1). These patients are therefore candidates for standard postchemotherapy retroperitoneal lymph node dissection. The technique of postchemotherapy retroperitoneal lymph node dissection is well described, involving mobilization of the aorta and vena cava and resection of lymphatic tissue from the crus of the diaphragm to the bifurcation of the common iliacs, the lateral borders being the ureters (Fig. 23-2). The pathology of the resected material will show fibrosis/scar 45 percent of the time, teratoma 45 percent of the time, and persistent cancer approximately 10 percent of the time in the primary treatment group and about 50 percent of the time in the postchemotherapy group. These procedures may be relatively straightforward with preservation of normal tissue planes or may be extremely difficult. Chemotherapy has an unpredictable effect on retroperitoneal germ cell cancer, and the surgeon embarking on this type of procedure must make a commitment in terms of time and effort. Techniques of vascular control, bowel resection, nephrectomy, and caval resection are sometimes required. It is extremely difficult to prospectively identify preoperatively which patients will require any of these varied techniques. The appearance of retroperitoneal tumor on the CT scan may not be helpful in predicting the amount of desmoplastic reaction and obliteration of tissue planes. Therefore, the surgeon must be versatile and capable of altering his or her approach if necessary.

Figure 23-1. *Residual disease after primary chemotherapy. Alpha-fetoprotein and beta human chorionic gonadotropin were normal.*

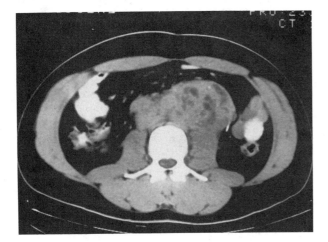

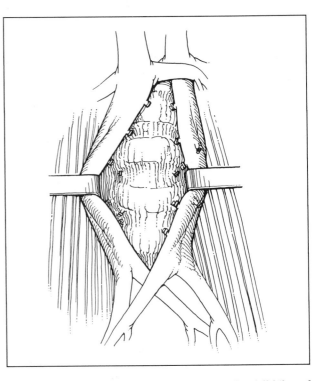

Figure 23-2. *Appearance of retroperitoneum after full bilateral postchemotherapy retroperitoneal lymph node dissection. Note division of lumbar arteries and veins.*

The third indication for complicated testis cancer surgery is the patient who has undergone previous retroperitoneal lymph node dissection and experiences a retroperitoneal, pelvic, or retrocrural recurrence of teratoma (Fig. 23-3). Patients who initially undergo postchemotherapy retroperitoneal lymph node dissection and have high volumes of teratoma removed at the initial procedure are at increased risk for subsequent recurrence of teratoma. Typically, these recurrences are at the edge of the previous operative field, but occasionally, recurrences within the operative field are seen. These procedures may require varied surgical techniques, as will be discussed subsequently.

Finally, the patient who has exhausted all chemotherapeutic options and who has persistent elevation of serum markers indicating the presence of carcinoma is a candidate for salvage surgery. These highly selected patients have localized retroperitoneal disease as the only apparent source of the elevation in serum markers. Full bilateral retroperitoneal lymph node dissection in this situation can be extremely difficult and demanding, since these patients have usually had previous attempts at retroperitoneal lymph node dissection. Additionally, all have been heavily treated with chemotherapy.

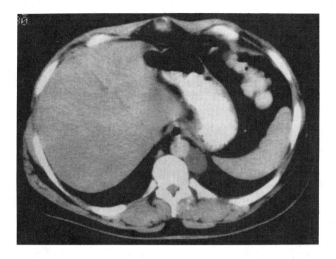

Figure 23-3. *Retrocrural recurrence of teratoma. The patient was negative at time of initial retroperitoneal lymph node dissection.*

Patient Preparation

Most patients presenting for retroperitoneal lymph node dissection after chemotherapy have been administered bleomycin. Bleomycin has known pulmonary toxicity that may relate to a capillary leak phenomenon. Therefore, patients are administered intravenous colloid the day before surgery in a effort to diminish the large amount of fluid given intravenously at the time of anesthetic induction. A type and crossmatch for 2 to 4 units of blood is performed routinely in these patients. If the procedure is a redo procedure, a full bowel preparation is sometimes administered. The dehydration that may occur during full bowel preparation further necessitates the use of preoperative intravenous colloid administration. Vascular instruments are routinely available for postchemotherapy retroperitoneal lymph node dissection. Additionally, if a thoracoabdominal exposure is necessary, thoracic instruments are available.

Technique

Patients who have experienced a partial remission after initial chemotherapy for high-volume testis cancer are candidates for postchemotherapy retroperitoneal lymph node dissection. The serum markers have normalized in these patients, but persistent radiographic disease remains. Standard full bilateral retroperitoneal lymph node dissection with mobilization of the great vessels and resection of lymphatic tissue from the crus of the diaphragm to the bifurcation of the iliacs from ureter to ureter is performed in these patients (see Fig. 23-2).

In patients who have not been operated previously, this is a relatively straightforward procedure. However, as mentioned previously, the amount of desmoplastic response in the retroperitoneum secondary to tumor and chemotherapy cannot be predicted reliably. Normal tissue planes may or may not be preserved.

Special mention should be made in this situation of the necessity for preservation of the adventitia of the aorta. Dissecting in a subadventitial plane sometimes is easier, but removal of this adventitial layer dramatically weakens the wall of the aorta. Attempting to repair the aorta in this situation is exceedingly difficult, since sutures do not hold well in the absence of the adventitia. Indeed, an inability to preserve the adventitial layer may be an indication for aortic replacement.

Aortic replacement has been performed 10 times during retroperitoneal lymph node dissection at Indiana University. Most were done emergently. An inability to preserve the adventitial layer with resultant aortic weakening was the indication for replacement. Currently, 7 of the 10 patients are alive and free of disease.

Reoperation for recurrent teratoma or operation in the patient who has exhausted all chemotherapeutic options and has elevated markers requires special considerations. First, after completion of full bilateral retroperitoneal lymph node dissection, care should be taken to reperitonealize the small bowel mesentery (Fig. 23-4). We have performed redo retroperitoneal lymph node dissection on several patients who did not undergo reperitonealization at the time of the prior procedure, and recurrent tumor was extremely adherent to bowel, ne-

Figure 23-4. *At the completion of retroperitoneal lymph node dissection, the posterior peritoneum should be restored to its normal anatomy.*

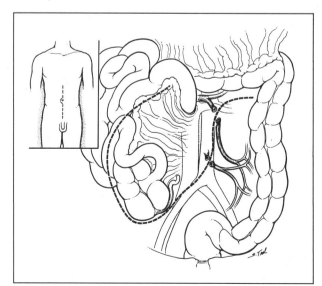

cessitating bowel resection. With reperitonealization at the completion of the first procedure, bowel resection probably would not have been necessary.

Reoperation for teratoma or the salvage patient requires the surgeon to develop a preoperative strategy. If the previous procedure was transabdominal, a thoracoabdominal incision is sometimes chosen for the redo procedure in order to gain early vascular control (Fig. 23-5). Although we do not routinely gain early control of the aorta and vena cava during standard retroperitoneal lymph node dissection, this is sometimes necessary in the more complicated redo procedures. Usually, the aorta may be encircled slightly distal to the superior mesenteric artery but superior to the origin of the renal arteries bilaterally. Characteristically, no lumbar arteries are present in this area, and the previous procedure has typically not included the aorta at this level. If this approach is not available transabdominally, a thoracoabdominal incision will allow control of the aorta at a higher level. Distally, control of the iliacs is usually attained without difficulty.

Attaining early vascular control of the vena cava is sometimes more difficult. Although characteristically lumbar veins are not present immediately superior to the junction of the renal veins with the vena cava, the anatomy of lumbar veins is not as predictable as that of the lumbar arteries. Various vascular control techniques may be necessary, including vessel loops, Romel tourniquets, vascular clamps, and sponge sticks. We do not hesitate to perform resection of the vena cava if neces-

sary for tumor clearance, since in the long term these patients do very well in terms of developing collateral venous drainage. The technique of resection of the vena cava is not difficult. Control is developed superiorly distal to the renal veins and caudad at the level of the distal vena cava or proximal iliacs. Lumbar veins are divided, after which either vascular staples or clamps and running monofilament suture are used to secure the cut ends. In some cases, division of the distal vena cava is necessary prior to lumbar vein division. The tumor mass and vena cava are then mobilized off the anterior spinous ligament, exposing lumbar veins, which are then divided.

Vena caval resection has been performed in 42 instances during retroperitoneal lymph node dissection at Indiana University. The indications for resection have included a venal caval thrombus in 20 patients, tumor clearance in 16, and scar occlusion in 6 (Table 23-1).

Lumbar arteries and veins have sometimes not been divided during the previous retroperitoneal lymph node dissection. These vessels must be divided to perform a complete and adequate retroperitoneal lymph node dissection. Division of these lumbar vessels is sometimes

Table 23-1. *Short-Term Complications of Vena Caval Resection, 42 Patients*

Leg edema	8
Ascites	8
Venous thrombosis	1
Renal insufficiency	6

Figure 23-5. *A. Left thoracoabdominal approach yields good exposure of crus, suprahilar area, and upper aorta. B. Appearance after division of crus, division of lumbar (intercostal) arteries, and removal of retrocrural tumor.*

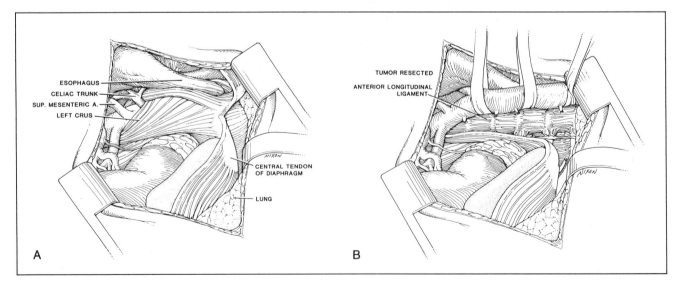

exceedingly difficult due to the fibrous reaction from tumor, chemotherapy, and previous surgery. In lieu of simple division of the lumbars in this situation, suture ligation is sometimes necessary. This, then, is another reason to preserve the adventitial layer, since the sutures ligatures sometimes will not hold without the benefit of the adventitia.

Drains are not used routinely after retroperitoneal lymph node dissection or reoperative retroperitoneal lymph node dissection. One instance, however, in which drains are used is after pancreatic resection or injury. If partial pancreatectomy has been performed, or if pancreatic injury is suspected, a closed suction drain is left near the area of the pancreas in the retroperitoneum. An amylase determination from the drain usually will establish the presence of a pancreatic leak. Fortunately, most leaks resolve with continued drainage and alimentation.

The urologic surgeon embarking on these difficult procedures must be prepared to perform bowel resection. In redo operations, especially involving the left side of the retroperitoneum, a large amount of mesentery of the left colon may be sacrificed. This, coupled with the fact that the inferior mesenteric artery has been divided at the previous retroperitoneal lymph node dissection, may embarrass the blood supply of the left colon. Fortunately, the marginal artery of Drummond usually compensates for resection of some of this mesentery, but we have noted loss of left colon vascular supply in a small number of patients. If a full bowel preparation has been performed, colonic resection in this situation may be necessary.

A severe fibrous scarring reaction sometimes is seen in the area of the retroperitoneal duodenum. Rarely, this may require partial duodenal resection in order to clear all tumor. In this situation, the duodenum is closed in two layers, and a retroperitoneal drain is left. Proximal diversion of gastrointestinal contents is attained by nasogastric tube, gastrostomy tube, or duodenostomy tube. Occasionally, an omental pedicle is fashioned and placed between the duodenum and the aorta in this situation to deter fistula formation or aortic leak.

Conclusion

Postchemotherapy retroperitoneal lymph node dissection and reoperative retroperitoneal lymph node dissection are time-consuming, demanding procedures. It should be emphasized that it is extremely hard to predict how difficult the procedure will be based on the preoperative appearance of the CT scan of the abdomen and chest. Therefore, the surgeon embarking on these types of procedures must be willing to make a large time investment and have the flexibility to alter the surgical strategy should this be necessary.

Bibliography

Bihrle, R, Donohue, JP, and Foster, RS. Complications of retroperitoneal lymph node dissection. Urol Clin North Am 15:2, 1988.

Donohue, JP, et al. Transabdominal retroperitoneal lymph node dissection. In DJ Skinner and G Lieskovsky (eds), Diagnosis and Management of Genitourinary Cancer. Philadelphia: Saunders, 1988, pp 802–816.

Prostatectomy for Benign Disease

RUSSELL K. LAWSON

Reoperation for benign prostate disease can be divided into four time periods: a few hours to a few days, 2 to 4 weeks, 1 to 12 months, and 1 or more years following the original surgery. The reason for reoperation can be divided into three categories: persistent bleeding, obstructing residual tissue, or regrowth of benign prostatic hypertrophy. There is little reliable information in the literature regarding the reasons for a repeat operation if postoperative bleeding is excluded as a factor. Holtgrewe and Valk analyzed the results of transurethral resection of the prostate in 2015 patients over a 5½-year period and found a "recurrence" rate of 3 percent in patients treated for benign prostatic hypertrophy and 9 percent in those treated for bladder neck obstruction. A similar study by Chilton et al. over a 4-year period found a recurrence rate of 5.1 percent following transurethral resection of the prostate for benign disease. However, in both these studies, nearly half the patients with recurrence required repeat operation within 6 months of the original procedure. These data strongly suggest that many patients who require reoperation have obstructing residual tissue rather than regrowth of benign prostatic hypertrophy. There are well-documented cases of regrowth of benign prostatic hypertrophy many years after open prostatectomy, but these cases are uncommon. A more recent study by Wennberg using claims data suggests a recurrence rate of 2.5 percent per year following transurethral resection of the prostate and 1.3 percent per year following open prostatectomy for benign prostatic hypertrophy. The rate reported by Wennberg is considerably higher than previously reported and is very likely due to flaws in study design.

Patients with excessive bleeding immediately following prostatectomy who do not respond to conservative measures must be returned to the operating room on an urgent basis to stop the bleeding. Patients who have had either an open prostatectomy or a transurethral resection of the prostate and require more than 2 units of blood postoperatively should be strongly considered for reoperation. Such patients may be hypervolemic because of frequent vigorous irrigation of the Foley catheter or rapid continuous bladder irrigation through a three-way catheter. Absorption of irrigant also may result in electrolyte imbalance depending on the composition of the irrigating fluid. Blood loss may have substantially reduced the hematocrit, adding to the operative risk in these urgent cases. Patients who exhibit excessive bleeding following prostatectomy should undergo laboratory investigation for a bleeding disorder. Coagulation problems may not have been apparent prior to the first procedure or may be acquired through blood transfusions or sepsis. Every effort should be made to correct any fluid and electrolyte abnormalities, deficiency in oxygen-carrying capacity, and bleeding disorders prior to returning the patient to the operating room. Depending on the severity of the hemorrhage and the urgency of the case, transurethral fulguration of bleeding points or an immediate open procedure may be selected.

The operative technique for transurethral fulguration is important to ensure the best chance of controlling the hemorrhage. The first and most important step is vigorous and thorough irrigation with an Ellik evacuator or Toumy syringe through a large-bore resectoscope sheath to remove clots from the bladder and prostatic fossa. Arterial bleeders beneath blood clots cannot be seen and fulgurated. Often, despite vigorous irrigation, clots remain on the wall of the prostatic fossa and must be scraped off with the resectoscope loop. The operator should adopt a systematic plan to completely remove clots and closely inspect the underlying tissue for bleeding points throughout the entire prostatic fossa. Particular attention should be directed to the bladder neck, where arterial bleeders may be found "around the corner" pumping away from the operator into the bladder. Bleeding from small to midsized veins is often better controlled by placing the resectoscope loop adjacent to the open vein in four quadrants with heavy coagulation of the tissue. This maneuver is usually more successful than attempts to directly coagulate open veins. Flaps of tissue may cover bleeding points, and additional resection of such flaps or small amounts of residual tissue may be necessary to visualize the underlying bleeding points. When bleeding is severe and clots form that rapidly obscures vision, the irrigant may be changed from glycine to water. Visualization is better with water irrigation and can be used safely if Mannitol is given intravenously. Thus 500 ml of water with 20% Mannitol should be started when water irrigation is started and infused over 40 to 60 minutes. If the patient's blood pressure has fallen because of blood loss, the bleeding points causing the problem may not be evident. The blood pressure should be brought back into the patient's normal range before concluding that the bleeding has been controlled adequately.

Following fulguration of the bleeding vessels, a standard Foley catheter or three-way catheter should be inserted over a catheter guide. Mild traction (up to 1 pound) on the catheter and/or continuous bladder irrigation are useful adjuvant measures in the postoperative period. Traction on the catheter should be maintained for no more than 1 to 2 hours because of the risk of postoperative incontinence that can be caused by prolonged heavy traction. The patient should be maintained on broad-spectrum antibiotic therapy postoperatively because of the increased risk of urinary tract infection resulting from the almost inevitable breaks in sterile technique during preoperative bladder irrigation. The catheter can be removed on the second or third day after reoperation, providing the urine is clearing and there are no fresh blood clots present.

Life-threatening hemorrhage or bleeding that cannot be controlled by transurethral fulguration requires immediate open surgery. Reoperation following transurethral resection of the prostate or suprapubic prostatectomy should be carried out through an anterior bladder wall incision down to but not through the bladder neck, whereas bleeding following a retropubic pros-

tatectomy is usually best managed by reopening the prostatic capsule suture line. I have found that with rare exception, direct visualization of the bleeding vessels with fulguration and/or suture ligature of the bleeding points will stop the bleeding. However, following a transurethral resection of the prostate or suprapubic prostatectomy, it is often difficult to visualize bleeding points in the distal prostatic fossa. Placement of a Mallamet suture around the bladder neck is an excellent method to control postprostatectomy bleeding when the bleeding points are difficult to find (Fig. 24-1). I use a number 1 monofilament nylon for the suture. This suture material is usually available in the operating room as prepacked retention sutures. Any large monofilament suture will suffice. The suture should be loaded on a large curved, tapered needle and placed around the bladder neck as a purse string. The suture is placed inside the bladder neck, and each end should exit through the anterior bladder wall. The ends of the suture are then crossed and placed through the abdominal wall on a long Keith needle, exiting to the left and the right of the midline. A Foley catheter with a 30-cc balloon is then inserted so that the balloon is proximal to the purse-string suture, and the balloon is inflated with 10 cc of water. The operator should then pull up on the Malamet suture to determine if the suture will slide easily around the bladder neck so that it can be removed later without difficulty. It is also important to be certain that when the suture is pulled up the prostatic fossa is completely excluded from the bladder by the purse string. The bladder and abdominal incisions are then closed in a standard fashion. The Malamet suture is passed through a short segment of rubber tubing and tied on the anterior abdominal wall. The Malamet suture is very useful for

Figure 24-1. *Placement of Mallemat suture around the bladder neck to control postprostatectomy bleeding.*

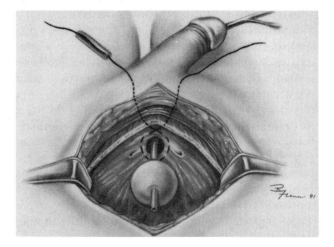

controlling postprostatectomy bleeding and has almost completely eliminated the need to pack the prostatic fossa regardless of the cause of the bleeding. Occasionally, some bleeding will occur from the urethral meatus, which has tracked down the outside of the catheter. Blood loss from this site is almost always minimal, and no attempts should be made to stop the bleeding by meatal or glanular compression because of the risk of causing glanular necrosis. The Malamet suture should be removed on the second or third postoperative day. The Foley catheter balloon should be filled with additional fluid to an appropriate volume before removing the suture.

Delayed bleeding, following prostatectomy, is an infrequent cause for reoperation. The phenomenon of delayed bleeding does not correlate with the extent of bleeding following the original procedure. The patient usually presents between the second and fourth week postoperatively in urinary retention from blood clots. If the usual measures for removal of blood clots by irrigation, traction on the Foley catheter, and continuous bladder irrigation do not control the bleeding, then reoperation is necessary. Persistent delayed bleeding is usually easily controlled with transurethral fulguration of the bleeding points.

Reoperation for obstructive voiding problems is usually carried out 1 to 2 weeks postoperatively in patients with significant residual tissue. Regrowth of benign prostatic hypertrophy with recurrence of obstructive voiding symptoms may be seen years after the original procedure and requires a repeat prostatectomy. In either case, the procedure is almost always carried out by the transurethral route.

Difficulty voiding following prostatectomy is obviously not always due to incomplete resection of benign prostatic hypertrophy or retained tissue following open prostatectomy. Factors such as a myogenic/neurogenic bladder from long-standing obstruction with high residual urine or massive distension following urinary retention may be the primary cause for difficulty voiding following prostatectomy. Urocholine use to increase detrusor contraction or an alpha$_1$ blocker to decrease prostatic capsule smooth muscle tone may be of help in patients who continue to have difficulty voiding following prostatectomy. Reoperation to resect additional apical tissue should be undertaken with great care because of the risk of rendering the patient permanently incontinent. Patients who exhibit prolonged detrusor dysfunction following urinary retention are better managed with intermittent self-catheterization than facing the difficult problem of severe stress incontinence that may follow repeat transurethral resection of apical tissue.

Regrowth of benign prostatic hypertrophy can result in recurrence of obstructive voiding symptoms. Such patients should be placed on an alpha$_1$ blocker before considering reoperation. I have found that 5 to 10 mg of terazosin per day often will remarkably improve flow rates in patients with recurrent benign prostatic hypertrophy. Those patients who have not responded to pharmacologic management require transurethral resection of the obstructing tissue.

A final mid- to long-term complication of prostatectomy that may require reoperation is bladder neck contracture. This problem occurs almost exclusively following transurethral resection of the prostate. The bladder neck contracts down as a rigid scar and may cause severe obstructive voiding symptoms. A bladder neck contracture should not be resected throughout its circumference with a resectoscope because it will very likely recur. This problem is best managed by carrying out two incisions through the bladder neck at 3 and 9 o'clock

Figure 24-2. *Transurethral incision of bladder neck, at 9:00 and 3:00 position, for bladder neck contracture.*

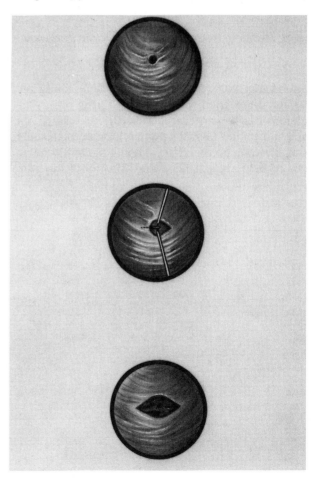

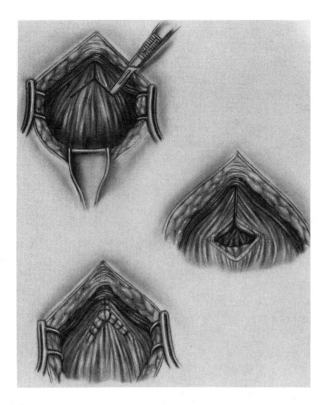

Figure 24-3. *Y-V plasty of bladder neck for bladder neck contracture.*

countered a few patients with extensive bladder neck scarring who do not improve with transurethral incision (TUI) of the bladder neck and require a V-Y plasty to correct the problem. This procedure should only be carried out when transurethral incision has failed. A Y-shaped incision across the bladder neck with the two upper limbs extending onto the anterior bladder wall is made (Fig. 24-3). The apex of the two upper bladder incisions is then brought down to the bottom of the Y incision, converting the suture lines to a V shape. The pliable, well-vascularized bladder segment that is interposed into the scarred bladder neck prevents recurrence of the contracture. The suture lines are completed in two layers. The first is a running locked 2-0 chromic catgut suture, followed by interrupted bolstering sutures of the same material. A Foley catheter is inserted, and a drain is placed in the operative site. The catheter should be left in place for 5 to 7 days following the procedure.

Bibliography

Chilton, CP, et al. A critical evaluation of the results of transurethral resection of the prostate. Br J Urol 50:542, 1978.

Holtgrew, HL, and Valk, WL. Late results of transurethral prostatectomy. J Urol 92:51, 1964.

Lehman, TH, et al. Intravenous mannitol during transurethral prostatectomy using distilled water as an irrigating medium. J Urol 95:396, 1966.

Malament, M. Maximal hemostasis in suprapubic prostatectomy. Surg Gynecol Obstet 120:1307, 1965.

Wennberg, JE, et al. Use of claims data systems to evaluate health care outcomes: Mortality and reoperation following prostatectomy. JAMA 257:933, 1987.

position (Fig. 24-2). The incisions release the contracted scar and allow the bladder neck to spring open. The incisions can be carried out with either a cold or hot knife and should be made deeply through the bladder neck. Bleeding points, if any, should be lightly fulgurated to help prevent new scar formation. I have en-

Radical Prostatectomy

J. EDSON PONTES

The last 10 to 15 years have seen a progressive increase in the number of radical prostatectomies being used as a primary treatment for localized prostatic cancer. This mode of treatment has been influenced by technical improvements in surgical procedures and by the evidence that a number of patients will continue to exhibit positive biopsy after curative radiation therapy. Among the advances in surgical techniques, understanding of the anatomy of the pelvis and the relationship of the prostate and its vascular surroundings, and the recognition and preservation of the neurovascular erectile bundle have allowed for progressive decrease in morbidity that traditionally had been associated with this procedure. Indeed, in large centers, the percentage of intraoperative and postoperative complications has decreased to insignificant levels. As an increasing number of prostatectomies are done, intraoperative and postoperative complications will arise that necessitate surgical reoperation. I will describe herein the most common problems associated with this surgical procedure that necessitate reoperation. Surgery for urinary incontinence will not be discussed here.

Intraoperative and Immediately Postoperative Problems Necessitating Reoperation

Uncontrollable Bleeding

No problems in this surgical procedure have intimidated novice surgeons more than the threat of "uncontrollable" bleeding. I believe that most of the time this fear occurs because of a lack of understanding of some basic anatomic principles. It is difficult, if not impossible, to coagulate some of the profuse bleeding coming from the pelvis. Most of that bleeding is accentuated by upward traction of the prostate. Bleeding from the dorsal vein complex can be controlled by figure-of-eight sutures placed horizontally in the area of bleeding. Some surgeons have proposed temporary clamping of the internal iliac arteries in an attempt to decrease intraoperative bleeding. According to published reports, the blood saving is modest at best. I only utilize such procedures in patients who are unable to receive blood transfusions for religious reasons. In my experience, the most troublesome bleeding is that caused by disruption and tearing of the skeletal muscle fibers that intertwine with the apex of the prostate. Attempts to coagulate such bleedings usually lead to deeper lesions in the pelvic floor with profuse hemorrhaging. When such bleeding develops intraoperatively, or when patients need reoperation in the immediate postoperative period, the best way to control the bleeding is with nonabsorbable (3-0 silk) suture with a long needle using a figure-of-eight pattern and, if needed, over Oxicell (Fig. 25-1). Other intraoperative vascular injuries associated with the venous part of the node dissection can be controlled by vascular sutures.

Rectal Injuries

Rectal injuries have been reported in between 0 and 6 percent of radical prostatectomies. It is believed by most modern urologists with large experience with this procedure that most rectal injuries can be repaired primarily without temporary colostomy. In most centers,

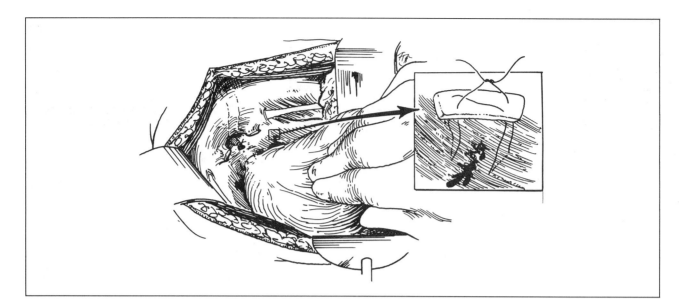

Figure 25-1. *Illustrated in this figure is a tear on the pelvic floor with profuse bleeding. In general attempts of fulguration fail. A figure-of-eight suture is being tied over a roll of Oxicell.*

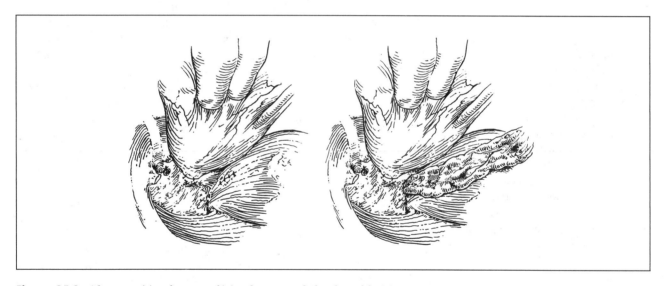

Figure 25-2. *After recognition that a rectal injury has occurred, the edges of the injury are resected, and a two-layer closure is accomplished with a running 4-0 polyglycol and a second layer using a 4-0 silk.*

preoperative bowel preparation with hypertonic solution and antibiotic therapy ensures a clear bowel lumen. Conditions that predispose to rectal injury include previous multiple transrectal biopsies, extensive transurethral resection, or repeated bouts of prostatitis. The most important factor for a successful outcome of a rectal injury is recognition of the injury. In my experience, the use of right-angle scissors to dissect between the prostate and rectum and good hemostasis to allow

good visualization help to prevent bowel injury. When rectal injury occurs, excision of the edges and closure in two layers using a 4-0 polyglycol in the mucosa and a 4-0 silk in the muscularis are sufficient (Fig. 25-2A). Postoperatively, anal dilatation, intravenous antibiotics, and parenteral nutrition for 10 days will, in most cases, lead to a successful outcome. Some authors have proposed the immediate use of omentum to be interposed between the vesicourethral anastomosis and the rectum

(Fig. 25-2B). I do not utilize this procedure routinely for the initial rectal injury.

Ureteral Injuries

Ureteral injuries have been reported to occur in less than 1 percent of operations. In my experience, such an injury occurred in only 1 case among over 400 radical prostatectomies. Ureteral injuries occur as part of pelvic lymphadenectomy, as part of wide excision of the bladder neck, or from inadvertent dissection of the posterior bladder neck. Treatment of such injuries, once recognized during surgery, includes stenting of the ureter, end-to-end anastomosis with 4-0 polyglycol if the injury is high, or reimplantation of the ureter. In the adult patient, reimplantation of the ureter without an antireflux procedure is sufficient.

Other Problems

Rarely, injury to the obturator nerve occurs during pelvic lymphadenectomy. When recognized, an intraoperative consult with a neurosurgeon is advisable. When an intraoperative consultant is not available, an end-to-end anastomosis utilizing 7-0 or 8-0 nonabsorbable sutures to approximate the nerve sheath will give the best results.

Late or Secondary Problems

Unrecognized rectal or ureteral injuries will present late as fistulas. Ureterocutaneous fistulas are usually associated with hydronephrosis and in modern urology can be approached endoscopically by internal stenting with or without percutaneous nephrostomies. In cases of complete ureteral disruption, an initial percutaneous nephrotomy can be placed to provide drainage and preservation of renal function followed by secondary repair. Rectourinary fistulas are best treated by an initial diverting colostomy, since the usually high intestinal pressure will prevent spontaneous closure. If after the initial diverting colostomy and urinary drainage the fistula does not close, surgical reexploration with omentum interposition is indicated (see Fig. 25-2).

Vesicourethral Stenosis

Stenosis of the vesicourethral anastomosis occurs in 2 to 20 percent of cases in different series. Prevention of bladder neck stricture can be accomplished by inverting the bladder neck mucosa and employing a tensionless watertight anastomosis. In most series, when bladder neck contracture occurs, it is corrected by internal urethrotomy. Usually, after a short period of incontinence, all patients regain urinary control. In recent years, with

Figure 25-3. *A combined perineal and abdominal approach is utilized. Perineally, the bulbous urethra is mobilized and transected at the urogenital diaphragm. Abdominally, the bladder neck is freed from the previous anastomosis and the edges resected. The urethra is pulled through the pelvic floor and anastomosed with the bladder neck.*

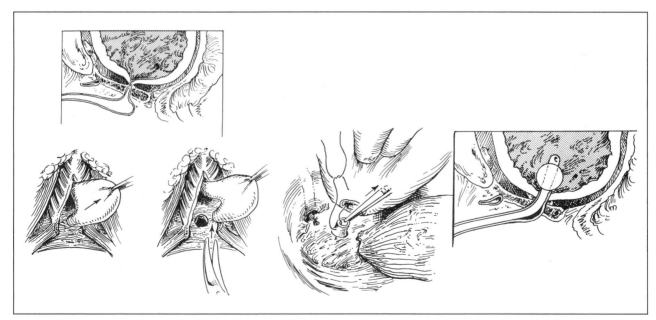

an increased number of radical prostatectomy done by less experienced surgeons, I have been referred patients who never developed a patent anastomosis after the initial surgery. I believe that this is the result of lack of completion of the anastomosis during the surgery or complete disruption of the vesicourethral anastomosis. These patients do not have epithelialization of the anastomotic areas, and removal of the Foley catheter will lead to restricture. Technically, the surgical approach to such problems poses a significant challenge. In the last few years, I have approached these cases with a combined perineal and abdominal approach (Fig. 25-3). Perineally, the urethra is completely separated from the urogenital diaphragm. An abdominal approach will identify the bladder neck at the point of stricture, and excision of the scarred area is done. The previously transected urethra is brought down through the pelvic floor and reanastomosed to the bladder. All these patients are informed in advanced of the high likelihood of urinary incontinence, which can be treated at a later date.

Recognition of basic principles of anatomy and surgical technique will prevent most problems discussed in this chapter. When problems develop, early recognition and repair are essential for a favorable outcome.

Bibliography

Ackermann, R, and Frohmuller, HGW. Complications and morbidity following radical prostatectomy. World J Urol 1:62, 1983.

Igel, TC, et al. Perioperative and postoperative complications from bilateral pelvic lymphadenectomy and radical retropubic prostatectomy. J Urol 137:1189, 1987.

Kavoussi, LR, Myers, JA, and Catalona, WJ. Effect of temporary occlusion of hypogastric arteries on blood loss during radical retropubic prostatectomy. J Urol 146:362, 1991.

Lange, PH, and Reddy, PK. Technical nuances and surgical results of radical retropubic prostatectomy in 150 patients. J Urol 138:348, 1987.

Scardino, PT, and Wheeler, TM. Local control of prostate cancer with radiotherapy frequency and prognostic significance of positive results of postirradiation prostate biopsy. Natl Cancer Inst Monogr 7:95, 1988.

Walsh, PC, and Donker, PJ. Impotence following radical prostatectomy: Insight into etiology and prevention. J Urol 128:492, 1982.

Complications Associated with Ileal and Colon Conduits

THOMAS W. COLEMAN
JOHN A. LIBERTINO

Extirpation of pelvic malignancies is the most common indication for the creation of an ileal or colon urinary conduit. After difficult and time-consuming radical procedures, meticulous surgical precision is required for proper construction of a urinary conduit. Occasionally, imperfect technique is responsible for postoperative complications associated with high morbidity and mortality. These complications require precise, timely diagnoses and a comprehensive plan for management, as detailed in our original report (Eyre et al., 1982). In the absence of sepsis and shock, temporizing measures can be performed to diagnose the problem accurately and to implement adequate trials of conservative treatment. Recent radiologic advances have permitted successful percutaneous treatment of serious urinary and bowel complications. However, some complications still require reoperation for resolution. The indications, diagnosis, and treatment of these problems are the focus of this chapter.

Types of Complications

Common complications associated with major operations in elderly patients include myocardial infarction, pulmonary embolism, stroke, pneumonia, and upper gastrointestinal tract bleeding. In addition to these complications, patients undergoing radical pelvic extirpative procedures and urinary intestinal conduit formation are at risk for bowel or ureterointestinal anastomotic complications or both in the early postoperative period. Stoma-related problems, ureterointestinal strictures, and small bowel obstruction are the most com-

mon late complications. The cornerstone of therapy in the management of both early and late complications is reliance on conservative therapy unless the development of sepsis or clinical deterioration mandates the use of surgical intervention.

Preoperative Assessment

The preoperative nutritional status of a patient can have a significant impact on the occurrence of postoperative complications. Delayed hypersensitivity to intradermal antigens, a history of weight loss, and depressed serum protein levels and total lymphocyte count portend poor wound healing and predispose the patient to anastomotic complications. If nutritional incompetence is diagnosed, high protein and calorie nutritional supplements can be administered orally or by means of a small no. 8 French Silastic feeding tube when the gut is functional. Infrequently, total parenteral nutrition is necessary to establish nutritional competence before major operation. The standard 1-day bowel preparation in which high-volume osmotic cathartics are used can lead to electrolyte imbalance and dehydration preoperatively. Therefore, routine intravenous hydration with correction of hypokalemia is employed.

Long-term patient acceptance of urinary diversion is dependent on the ease of stomal care. Consequently, every effort should be made to ensure adequate visibility of the stoma and a watertight seal of the appliance. An enterostomal therapist is invaluable in marking the optimal site of the stoma along with an alternative site, which will ensure that these requirements are met. However, the surgeon must be confident that the stoma site

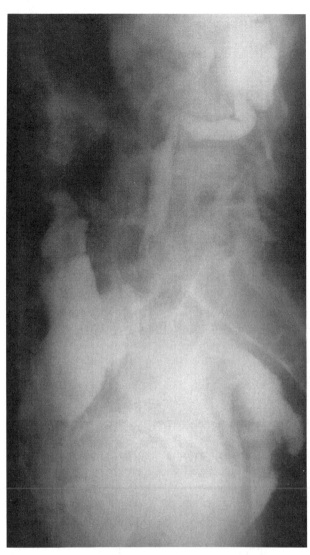

A

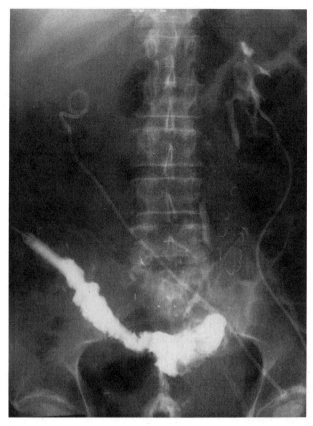

B

Figure 26-1. *A. Loopogram demonstrates fistula between sigmoid colon loop and Hartmann's pouch in a male patient after cystectomy for pelvic leiomyosarcoma with end transverse colostomy and sigmoid colon urinary conduit. B. Loopogram shows decreased fistula output after placement of bilateral nephrostomy tubes and rectal tube decompression. C. Three weeks of upper tract decompression allowed spontaneous closure of fistula. D. Note faint opacification on nondilated right kidney.*

ultimately selected avoids compromising blood flow to the intestinal segment.

Surgical Technique

Successful construction of a urinary conduit requires adherence to several important principles. The length of ureter available for anastomosis to the bowel is dictated by lack of malignant involvement, determined by frozen-section examination of the distal ureter. In construction of an ileal conduit, the left ureter must be brought under the sigmoid colon mesentery and across the midline for anastomosis. Therefore, it is of paramount importance to divide the ureter at the lowest safe

level and to dissect it proximally with careful preservation of blood supply to allow an adequate length for a tension-free anastomosis to the bowel. Improper mobilization of the ureter leads to kinking at the level of the sigmoid mesentery or, worse, skeletonization of the ureter with resultant devascularization. When the length of left ureter is limited, the butt end of the conduit can be brought under the sigmoid colon to the ureter for a tension-free anastomosis. With adequate ureteral length, isolation of a 15- to 20-cm ileal segment approximately 15 cm from the ileocecal valve is performed. Division of the proximal mesentery can be short, but the distal mesentery must be divided far enough from the mesenteric border of the bowel to allow easy placement through the abdominal wall without vascular compro-

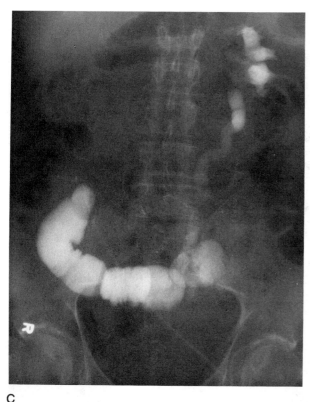

C

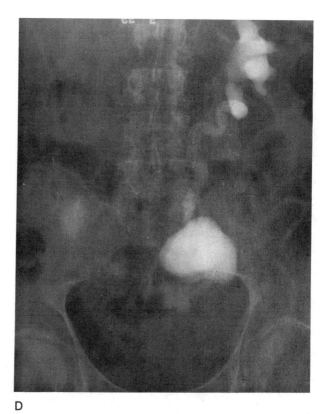

D

Figure 26-1. *(Continued)*

mise. Reconstruction of the gastrointestinal tract by means of a hand-sewn technique or the use of stapler devices incurs approximately the same complication rate. The surgeon's preference dictates the choice.

Creation of an everting rosebud stoma with a straight path through the abdominal wall is the goal. A cruciate incision in both the anterior and posterior rectus fascia should allow passage of two fingers through the opening. To avoid staggering these incisions, tension is applied on the midline fascia with two Kocher clamps, simulating the closed fascia.

Meticulous handling of the bowel and ureter in an atraumatic fashion is imperative during creation of the ureterointestinal anastomosis. A spatulated left ureteral anastomosis to the butt end of the conduit and a standard Bricker right ureteral anastomosis are performed over single-J Silastic ureteral stents. In addition to internal stenting of the ureterointestinal anastomosis, we routinely provide external drainage with either Penrose or Jackson-Pratt closed continuous suction drains. This ensures evacuation of small urine collections often encountered in the first few days after operation. To further promote adequate conduit drainage, a small no. 14 French red rubber catheter is inserted through the stoma

to just below the fascial level for 4 to 5 days. Avoidance of relative stomal stenosis secondary to postoperative edema can decrease the chances of early persistent ureterointestinal anastomotic urinary leakage.

Early Urinary Leakage

Minor urinary leakage from the ureterointestinal anastomosis in the first few days after operation is not problematic, provided external drainage is adequate. Without external drainage, diagnosis of persistent leakage must rely on the documentation of decreased urinary output in a well-hydrated patient, a high blood urea nitrogen (BUN) to creatinine ratio, and an elevated serum ammonia level. With adequate external drainage, the diagnosis is made easily by measuring the BUN and creatinine concentrations in the draining fluid. Any persistent drainage beyond 3 to 4 days requires placement of a red rubber catheter in the stoma to treat occult stomal stenosis, which can lead to high intraluminal pressure transmitted to the ureterointestinal anastomosis. If high residual urine is discovered, this maneuver is frequently both diagnostic and therapeutic because it

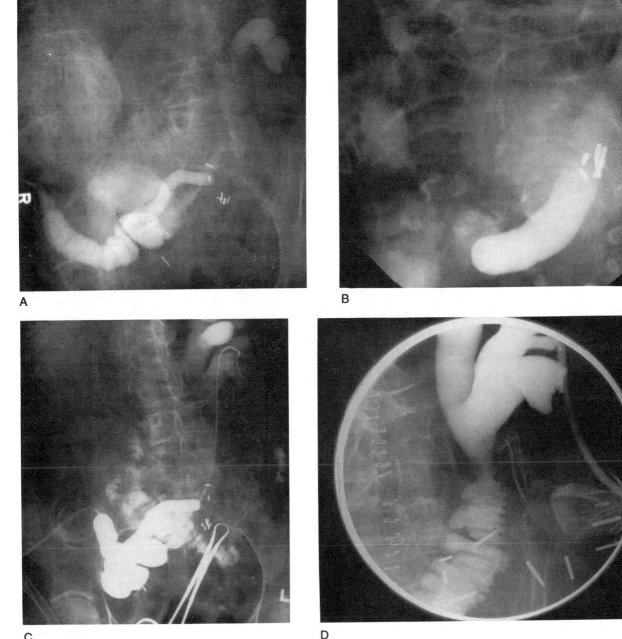

Figure 26-2. *A. Loopogram of a patient referred after unsuccessful left balloon dilation and subsequent ileal loop revision demonstrates right ureteral obstruction and migrated stent through leaking left ureteroileal anastomosis. Left percutaneous nephrostomy was performed, followed by antegrade placement of a ureteral stent. B. After removal of the stent, azotemia developed, and left percutaneous nephrostomy with antegrade pyelography demonstrated distal left ureteral obstruction with extravasation. C. Antegrade stenting attempts were unsuccessful. A combined nephrostogram and loopogram demonstrated a small bowel fistula from the left ureter and distal right ureteral obstruction. D. Resection of the small bowel fistula and revision of ileal loop were performed with left pyeloileal anastomosis for an ischemic left ureter and right distal ureteral obstruction. E. Loopogram demonstrates no leak or obstruction.*

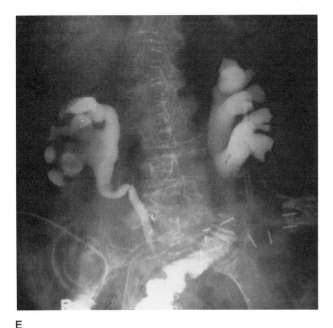

E

Figure 26-2. *(Continued)*

decompresses the loop and allows egress of urine externally rather than across the anastomosis.

The most common serious early complication of intestinal urinary diversion is prolonged ureterointestinal anastomotic leakage. The reported incidence of this complication ranges from 1.9 to 5.5 percent, with mortality rates as high as 48 percent in patients without primary external drainage. When anastomotic leakage is identified on a loopography and excretory urography, proximal decompression with percutaneous nephrostomy should be performed, reserving open nephrostomy for failed percutaneous attempts. If ureteral stents have been removed or were not used primarily, antegrade stent placement across the anastomosis and site of leakage should be performed. If the leakage is from the butt end of the conduit away from the ureterointestinal anastomoses, only proximal decompression is necessary. Occasionally, anastomotic leakage may continue from wide-caliber unobstructed ureters despite percutaneous nephrostomy drainage. Needle-vented suction through the nephrostomy tube may be successful in diverting the urine from the anastomosis long enough to allow complete healing (Fig. 26-1).

Hyperalimentation and proximal decompression with anastomotic stenting are pursued for a minimum of 3 weeks before surgical intervention is contemplated. Enteral feedings are preferable if the intestine is functional. Otherwise, total parenteral nutrition by means of a subclavian vein catheter is administered to optimize wound healing and to support adequate immune competence. Our recent experience at the Lahey Clinic included successful treatment by percutaneous techniques of 7 of 10 referred patients with urinary leakage; 3 patients required open revision.

Numerous surgical procedures are available for the treatment of urinary leakage not successfully managed conservatively. Frequently, revision of the ureteroileal anastomosis over a stent is possible. Careful inspection of the distal ureters in addition to frozen-section assessment is necessary to determine viability. When ureteral loss is excessive, the surgeon must be prepared to perform an add-on ileal segment or an ileal ureter interposition (Fig. 26-2). Indications for transverse colon conduits include prior radiotherapy and the presence of pelvic sepsis, because the new ureterocolonic anastomoses are out of the radiotherapeutic field and away from the pelvis.

Nephrectomy is a viable option in the patient with normal contralateral function who cannot afford to lose additional bowel or in whom major reconstructive surgery is not possible because of poor medical condition and increased surgical risk. Difficult reconstructive procedures are undertaken only when the nutritional status is optimized or in the presence of ongoing sepsis (Fig. 26-3).

Early Bowel Complications

The incidence of bowel complications does not differ between hand-sewn and stapled anastomoses. Meticulous technique is necessary to reconstitute the gastrointestinal tract successfully with either ileal or colon conduits. The acute presentation of sepsis with leakage of bowel contents through the wound or drainage site requires prompt establishment of adequate external drainage and proximal decompression by means of a nasogastric tube or long intestinal tube. The site of extravasation can then be localized with a Gastrografin upper gastrointestinal series in conjunction with an ultrasonography or computed tomographic (CT) scan to identify undrained collections of fluid.

Complete anastomotic breakdown, sepsis secondary to undrained leakage, and persistent anastomotic obstruction are indications for early surgical intervention. However, well-controlled fistulas often can be managed successfully with total parenteral nutrition and proximal decompression alone. When the fistula fails to close after 4 to 6 weeks of conservative management, surgical therapy is indicated. The most common surgical procedure performed is resection with entero-

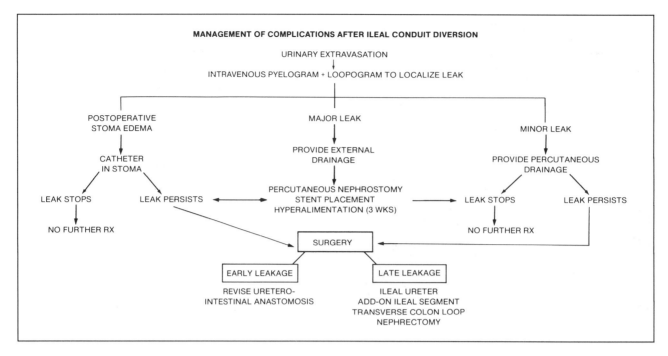

Figure 26-3. *Management of urinary leakage after ileal conduit diversion. (From JA Libertino and RC Eyre, Plan for management of complications after ileal conduit diversion. In TP Ball Jr (ed), AUA Update Series, lesson 7, vol III. Houston: American Urological Association, Inc, 1984, p 3, with permission.)*

enterostomy. However, terminal ileostomy, colostomy, or fistula bypass may be required in the presence of intense adhesions surrounding the site of extravasation. We have treated three patients successfully with total parenteral nutrition and proximal decompression with long tubes. Four patients required either primary resection or fistula bypass to restore gastrointestinal tract continuity successfully (Fig. 26-4).

Loop Infarction

An inadequate blood supply to the ileal loop can result in infarction and necrosis of the loop. Venous congestion with a dusky appearance of the stoma is normal for the first few days after operation. Persistence of this ischemic appearance warrants flexible endoscopy of the remainder of the loop to assess mucosal viability. If sloughing of the mucosa is evident, immediate reoperation with construction of a new ileal or colon conduit is indicated.

Ischemia can result from ligation of the blood supply, mesenteric hematoma, or excessive stretch on the vascular pedicle. Arterial insufficiency secondary to a ligated blood supply usually leads to a prompt diagnosis.

However, venous occlusion with compression of arterial inflow follows an indolent course marked by stomal deterioration with resultant loop atrophy and stenosis. This situation also requires revision with a new ileal or colon conduit.

Wound Infections

Cystectomy creates a pelvic space that becomes filled by bowel with a fresh anastomosis, ureterointestinal anastomoses, and serous fluid. Consequently, the incidence of pelvic abscess formation ranges from 4 to 8 percent. When there is no ongoing urinary or bowel leakage, percutaneous attempts at draining these abscesses are reasonable. If adequate drainage is not feasible, operative debridement is necessary, and drainage must be established.

Ureterointestinal Anastomotic Strictures

The presentation of ureterointestinal anastomotic strictures varies widely. Patients may have asymptomatic hydronephrosis on routine screening, flank pain, or re-

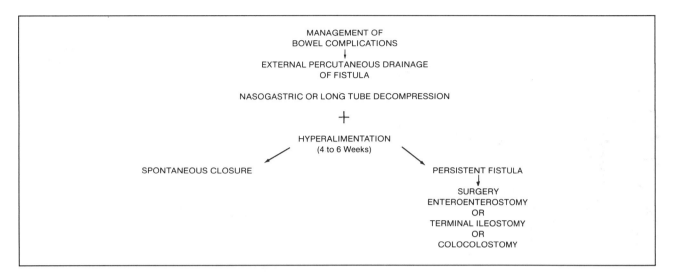

Figure 26-4. *Management of bowel complications after ileal conduit diversion. (From JA Libertino and RD Eyre, Plan for management of complications after ileal conduit diversion. In TP Ball Jr (ed), AUA Update Series, lesson 7, vol III. Houston: American Urological Association, Inc, 1984, p 5, with permission.)*

nal failure. An excretory urogram and loopogram usually delineate the site and length of the stricture. However, patients with nonfunctioning renal units or renal insufficiency require antegrade pyelography. Short distal strictures are amenable to percutaneous antegrade stenting with or without balloon dilation of the stricture. We have treated 17 patients with 20 obstructed units with antegrade stent placement. Six of these patients also have undergone balloon dilation of the strictures. However, eventual open surgical revision was avoided in only 5 of the 17 patients at maximum follow-up of 4 years (Fig. 26-5).

Longer strictures can be managed temporarily with placement of an antegrade stent to permit correction of renal insufficiency secondary to obstruction. Options for open surgical revision include add-on ileal segments, ileal ureters, transverse colon loops, and nephrectomy for nonfunctioning kidneys.

Combined Urinary and Bowel Complications

The most challenging and difficult complications to treat result from concomitant urinary and bowel complications. Predisposing factors include pelvic irradiation and reoperation for anastomotic bowel or urinary leaks, which can result in more bowel or conduit injury. Bowel fistulas to another segment of bowel with extension to the pelvis or skin along with urinary leakage or obstruction constitute the usual scenario. A loopography and antegrade pyelography will usually localize the

site of urinary leakage, whereas the precise location of bowel leakage is often difficult with upper gastrointestinal studies. Adequate external drainage and proximal decompression of the gastrointestinal and urinary tracts are established while nutritional competence is restored. Patience with conservative therapy is the cornerstone of treatment.

Surgical intervention is indicated with ongoing sepsis or after a failed 4- to 6-week trial of conservative therapy. Resection of the fistula with primary enteroenterostomy is the most common operation performed for bowel fistulas and should be performed first if a staged reconstruction is undertaken. We prefer to manage concomitant urinary and bowel complications with a primary bowel and urinary reconstruction with creation of a transverse colon conduit because it removes the ureterointestinal anastomosis from the field of radiation and pelvic sepsis (Table 26-1).

Surgical Techniques of Repair

If ureterointestinal leakage does not abate with conservative measures, reexploration and a reconstructive procedure are required. A Foley catheter is inserted into the loop to just below the fascial level, and the balloon is filled with only 3 ml of saline to avoid pressure necrosis. This will facilitate identification of the loop when the abdomen is entered. Preoperatively, a stent should be placed through the percutaneous nephrostomy tube to

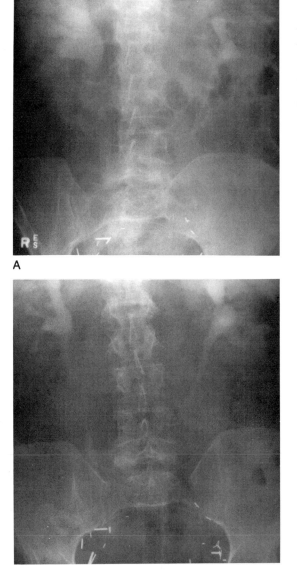

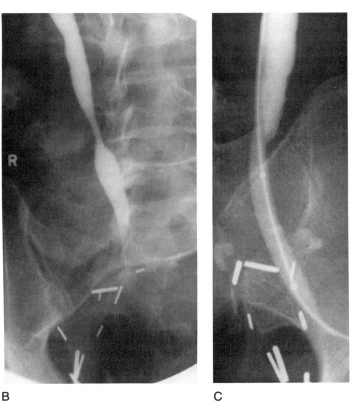

Figure 26-5. *A. Intravenous pyelogram obtained after cystectomy demonstrates right hydroureteronephrosis. B. Antegrade pyelogram shows right ureterectasis above short ureteroileal stricture. C. Balloon dilation of ureteroileal stricture. D. Postdilation intravenous pyelogram with resolution of obstruction.*

facilitate ureteral identification at the time of the procedure. Methylene blue contrast material also can be injected into the nephrostomy tube to help identify the site of the ureterointestinal anastomotic leakage.

When the site of leakage is identified, the ureterointestinal anastomosis may be revised. An add-on ileal segment, a transureteroureterostomy, or a transverse colon conduit may be used to reconstruct the urinary tract. A transverse colon conduit is resorted to in the presence of concomitant urinary and bowel complications. Nephrectomy is performed when the patient's medical condition precludes a reconstructive procedure in the presence of a normal contralateral kidney.

Ureterointestinal Revision

The leaking ureterointestinal anastomosis is identified and exposed. The ureter is transected 2 to 4 cm above the original ureterointestinal anastomosis and is observed. Bleeding from the distal ureter is noted. A frozen-section specimen is obtained to assess ureteral viability if the patient has had prior radiotherapy. The ureter is resected until healthy ureter is reached. A stented anastomosis in the same or another portion of the loop is carried out in standard Bricker fashion for the right ureter and in an end-to-side fashion for revision of the left ureterointestinal anastomosis (Fig. 26-6). The stents are sutured to the bowel mucosa at the anastomotic site and to the stoma with 4-0 chromic sutures.

Transureteroureterostomy

If the left ureter is devascularized for a significant length, it is mobilized (Fig. 26-7). The right ureter is exposed 5 to

Table 26-1. *Complications of Ileal and Colon Conduits and Their Management*

Complications and Treatment	No. of Patients	Outcome	
		Success	Failure
Urinary leakage	10		
Percutaneous therapy	10	7 (70%)	3 (30%)
Open revisions	3	3 (100%)	
Bowel leakage	7		
TPN* and proximal decompression	6	3 (50%)	3 (50%)
Resection and entero-enterostomy	4	2 (50%)	2† (50%)
Ureterointestinal strictures	20		
Percutaneous stenting	11	3 (27%)	8 (73%)
Balloon dilation	6	2 (33%)	4 (66%)
Combined percutaneous treatment	17	5 (29%)	12 (71%)
Open revisions	11	11 (100%)	

*TPN = total parenteral nutrition
†Operative mortality.

6 cm above the right ureterointestinal anastomosis, which is sufficient length to permit anastomosis without mobilizing the ureter from its bed. The left ureter is then passed above or below the inferior mesenteric artery, depending on the length of ureter remaining. The ureter must not wedge under the inferior mesenteric artery, be angulated, or be under tension. The left ureter is trimmed obliquely and spatulated to provide a 1.5-cm

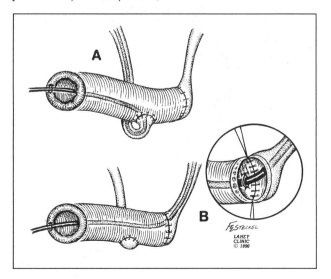

Figure 26-6. *Ureterointestinal revision. A. Right ureteroileal anastomosis. B. Left ureteroileal anastomosis is made to the butt end of the loop with a deeply spatulated ureter. (Reproduced with permission of the Lahey Clinic.)*

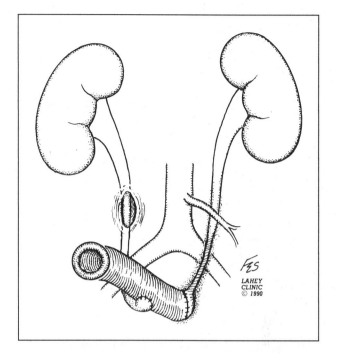

Figure 26-7. *Devascularization of the left distal ureter requires proximal mobilization with anterior exposure of the right ureter 5 to 6 cm above the ureteroileal anastomosis. (Reproduced with permission of the Lahey Clinic.)*

anastomosis (Fig. 26-8). The medial wall of the recipient right ureter is opened with hooked blade and Potts scissors for a distance slightly longer than the opening in the donor left ureter. The ureter should not be inserted on the anterior wall of the right ureter to avoid angulation. The senior author (JAL) prefers interrupted 4-0 chromic sutures to create the anastomosis over a 90-cm single-J stent, which is anchored at the stoma exit site. Omentum may be tacked around the transuretero-ureterostomy to enhance wound healing. The stent is left in place for 10 days, at which time a stentogram is obtained. When complete healing is demonstrated and no extravasation exists, the stent and the Penrose or Jackson-Pratt drain at the anastomotic site are removed.

Add-On Ileal Segment

If revision of the anastomosis or transureteroureterostomy is not possible because of a long segment of devascularized ureter or tension on the anastomosis, an add-on ileal segment is used. The length of ileum needed depends on how much ureter is to be replaced. The sites of bowel transection are chosen so that the cuts in the mesentery are deep enough to allow the upper end of the ileum to reach the renal pelvis. On the left side, a segment of descending colon may be used as an alterna-

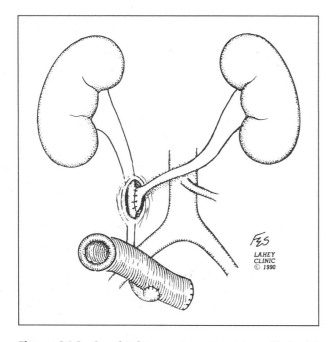

Figure 26-8. *Completed transureteroureterostomy with the left ureter crossing above the inferior mesenteric artery. (Reproduced with permission of the Lahey Clinic.)*

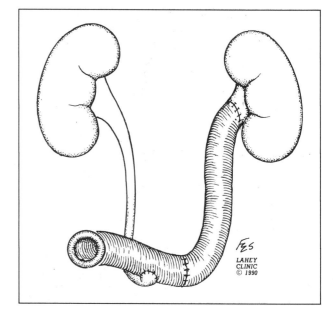

Figure 26-9. *Add-on ileal segment. Extensive loss of the left ureter requires ileal interposition from the renal pelvis to the butt end of the loop. (Reproduced with permission of the Lahey Clinic.)*

tive to ileum. The segment of bowel should be placed in an isoperistaltic direction. The length of the segment of bowel to be used can be approximated by using an umbilical tape to measure the length of the defect from the renal pelvis or distal ureter to the existing ileal conduit. Bowel continuity is restored in the usual fashion. The ileum is then widely spatulated for anastomosis to the renal pelvis with 2-0 interrupted chromic sutures. The distal end of the ileal add-on ureter is anastomosed end-to-end with the ileal conduit, again using 2-0 interrupted chromic sutures (Fig. 26-9).

If a shorter segment of ileum is required, the ureter is spatulated and reimplanted into the posterior surface of the add-on ileal segment with 3-0 interrupted chromic sutures. The butt end of the add-on segment is closed in two layers: the mucosa with 2-0 interrupted chromic sutures and the seromuscular layer with 4-0 Ti-Cron. Add-on ileal segments are stented with a 90-cm single-J stent and drained retroperitoneally (Fig. 26-10).

Transverse Colon Conduit

When ureterointestinal revision or add-on ileal segments have been attempted unsuccessfully or the surgeon is confronted with concomitant bowel and urinary complications in a previously irradiated pelvis, the transverse colon conduit is the reconstructive procedure

Figure 26-10. *Shorter segments of ileum can be interposed with anastomosis of the spatulated ureter to the posterior surface of the ileum. (Reproduced with permission of the Lahey Clinic.)*

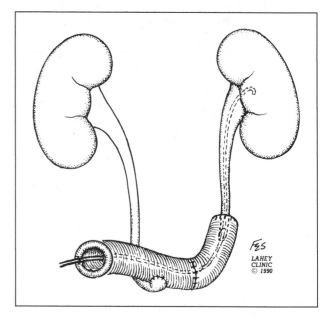

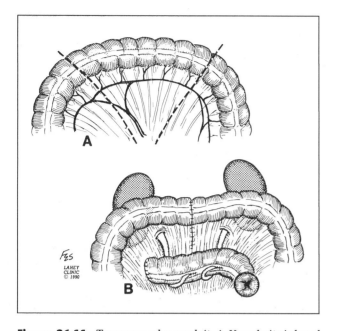

Figure 26-11. *Transverse colon conduit. A. Vascularity is based on the middle colic artery. B. Ureterocolic anastomoses are made in an antirefluxing fashion into the taenia coli. (Reproduced with permission of the Lahey Clinic.)*

of choice. Thus the bowel reconstruction, usually an ileoileostomy, can remain in the pelvis away from the urinary tract reconstruction in the upper abdomen.

The senior author (JAL) prefers to locate the stoma for a transverse colon conduit in the left upper quadrant. A long midline incision is used for this procedure. The transverse colon is transilluminated, and a 15- to 20-cm segment of colon is selected based on the middle colic artery. The greater omentum is dissected from the supe-

rior surface of the transverse colon, and the colon is divided (Fig. 26-11).

The continuity of the colon is restored with a standard two-layered hand-sewn anastomosis. The butt end of the loop is closed in two layers using 2-0 chromic sutures on the mucosa and 3-0 Ti-Cron sutures on the seromuscular layer.

The peritoneum over the ureters is incised and the ureters mobilized. They are led intraperitoneally to the base of the loop where they are spatulated and anastomosed to the underside of colon in a taenia using a submucosal tunnel technique. These anastomoses are also stented in the usual fashion. When both ureters are extremely dilated, a Wallace anastomosis to the butt end is favored. When ureteral loss is extensive, the colon may be anastomosed directly to the renal pelvis for tension-free anastomoses.

Bibliography

Eyre, RC, et al. Management of urinary and bowel complications after ileal conduit diversion. J Urol 128:1177, 1982.

Hendren, WH, and Radopoulos, D. Complications of ileal loop and colon conduit urinary diversion. Urol Clin North Am 10:451, 1983.

Hensle, TW, Bredin, HC, and Dretler, SP. Diagnosis and treatment of a urinary leak after ureteroileal conduit for diversion. J Urol 116:29, 1976.

Killeen, KP, and Libertino, JA. Management of bowel and urinary tract complications after urinary diversion. Urol Clin North Am 15:183, 1988.

Libertino, JA (ed). Pediatric and Adult Reconstructive Urologic Surgery, 2d ed. Baltimore: Williams & Wilkins, 1987.

Zinman, L. The use of colon surgery in urology. In WW Bonney (ed), AUA Courses in Urology, vol 1: Bladder Cancer. Baltimore: Williams & Wilkins, 1979, pp 35–59.

Complications of Continent Urinary Diversion

AARON E. KATZ
MITCHELL C. BENSON
CARL A. OLSSON

This chapter will review the complications and reoperations associated with continent urinary diversions utilized in the adult patient population. The reader should be cautioned that all the complications may not be known, since the latency period for some may be sufficiently long and have not yet appeared (i.e., induced secondary malignancies). Also, the reader should be aware that management of the complications associated with continent diversion is not written in stone. Just as the development of these procedures remains in its early stages, the management of complications is similarly evolving.

There are in excess of 40 variants of continent urinary diversion utilized worldwide, and a complete review of all the complications unique to each form of diversion is beyond the scope of this chapter. However, many of the procedures are simple variants of parent procedures, and this chapter will address each parent operation and the possible complications expected. The very fact that there are as many continent urinary diversion procedures as described reveals an obvious corresponding fact: the "best" continent diversion has yet to be devised. In particular, controversy continues to exist as to which bowel segment should be appropriately fashioned into a urinary reservoir. Additional points of controversy relate to the many different techniques utilized for achieving urinary continence and the prevention of reflux of urine into the diverted upper urinary tract.

The principles and techniques of bowel surgery, as well as complications resulting therefrom (i.e., the management of postoperative ileus or small bowel obstruction), have been covered in detail in other texts and will not be discussed here except as they relate to continent diversion.

The numerous operative procedures that have evolved in the quest for the perfect urinary diversion attest to the higher than satisfactory complication rates and the lack of unanimity regarding which operation is "best." Although continent urinary diversion is certainly appropriate in selected patients, the procedures are technically more challenging and are potentially fraught with higher complication rates than those operations which utilize external collecting devices. Additionally, there is a recognized learning curve to continent diversion during which the complication rate is significantly higher than that encountered after standard diversion.

General Considerations

A chapter on the management of complications and the indications for reoperations following continent urinary diversion would be remiss if it did not include the techniques employed in an effort to avoid complications. The standard techniques we utilize in continent diversion are listed below.

All sutures utilized in the urinary tract should be absorbable. Individual surgeon's preference will dictate the caliber of suture material utilized, as well as whether simple chromic catgut or manmade absorbable materials (polyglycolic acid) should be used. In general, when performing surgical procedures for urinary diversions that require bowel manipulation, we prefer a stapled bowel segment division as well as stapled reconstruction of bowel continuity. It is our prejudice that this shortens operative time greatly and affords safe bowel anastomoses. Suturing techniques are not necessary except to take one or two silk Lembert sutures at the apex of side-to-side stapled bowel anastomoses. In order to avoid stone formation on the stapled butts of conduits, the ends are either oversewn with absorbable suture material, or else the single application of an absorbable staple distal to the metal stapled margin suffices.

It is our preference to utilize diverting stents that will drain urine externally, ensuring that urine is safely diverted beyond any anastomotic site during the early healing interval. These stents should be exchangeable, and therefore, any end-hole, long (90-cm), single-J ureteral diverting stent is acceptable. Ureteral stents are always sutured to the anterior abdominal wall near the edge of the stoma site, and they are directed into a urinary appliance that is applied in the operating theater.

We advocate the use of suction drain catheters in all cases of urinary diversion where anastomotic leaks may be experienced. Soft silicone rubber suction drains are preferred because they have less potential for tissue damage with migration into conduits and/or pouches. In obese patients or those with tissues of poor quality or nutritional depletion, through-and-through no. 2 nylon stay sutures are also used.

Routine Postoperative Care

Paralytic ileus can be expected after all forms of urinary diversion that involve bowel. Therefore, gastric decompression is always achieved by means of either nasogastric intubation or else the provision of a gastrostomy at the time of the operation. It is our prejudice to maintain this gastric decompression until the patient experiences the passage of flatus. Nasogastric tubes suffice in the majority of patients. However, certain patients may best be managed by formal gastrostomy decompression. These include individuals in whom multiple prior abdominal procedures have been performed and the patient with pulmonary disease, who may benefit from the improved pulmonary toilet that can be achieved in the absence of a nasogastric tube.

If the duration of paralytic ileus is projected to be in excess of 4 to 5 days, intravenous hyperalimentation is initiated on the second postoperative day. If the patient is nutritionally depleted to begin with, hyperalimentation has been suggested to be of value if initiated during the preoperative interval.

Ureteral stents are generally removed at 7 to 10 days following surgery. At the time of removal, radiologic contrast studies are first carried out to document the integrity of the reservoir. If there is any question of extravasation, the stents are left in situ, and repeat studies are carried out. Upon removal of the stents, drainage films are taken to ensure that the upper tracts are able to drain without significant dilatation.

Management of Generic Complications

Gastrointestinal Anastomosis

As many as 5 to 10 percent of individuals undergoing urinary diversion will experience bowel complications at some time in their future. These may be temporary episodes of ileus that respond to interval gastrointestinal decompression. In contrast, they may require reoperative surgery so as to repair bowel obstruction consequent to anastomotic stenosis or adhesions. It has been reported that anastomotic leakage and bowel obstruction requiring operative intervention in the postoperative period may carry a 20 percent mortality. Therefore, the surgeon is well advised to become thoroughly familiar with a technique of hand-sewn or stapling-device intestinal anastomosis that is dependable in all circumstances. In general, with normal bowel, we use a stapled anastomosis solely. If the bowel is damaged by previous irradiation, an additional layer of seromuscular silk sutures can be placed to strengthen the anastomotic site.

The preservation of a wide-based mesenteric supply to the isolated intestinal segment is usually sufficient guard against "pipestem" formation. This complication seems to be a consequence of vascular compromise. The only appropriate management for "pipestem" is replacement of the affected segment. Attempts to dilate portions of the bowel do not provide durable results but may be of some short-term benefit.

Ureteral

The incidence of ureteroileal urinary extravasation has been greatly decreased by the routine use of ureteral stents. Many operative series have been published indicating that the use of such stents reduces the incidence of urinary extravasation to 1 to 3 percent of cases. Similarly, ureteroileal stenosis, sometimes a result of anastomotic leakage, has been greatly ameliorated by the use of indwelling stents.

Ureterointestinal anastomotic stenosis may occur at any time in the patient with any urinary diversion. This should be regarded with considerable concern in

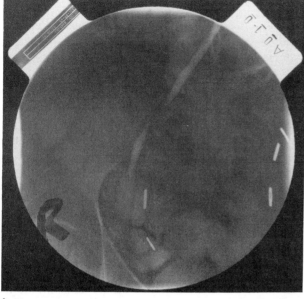

A

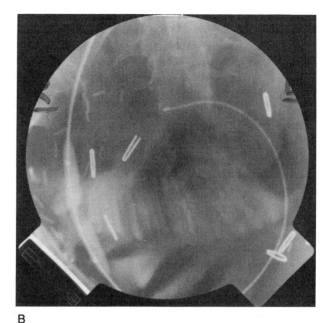

B

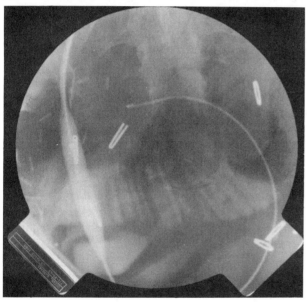

C

Figure 27-1. *A. Antegrade nephrostogram revealing a stricture of the distal right ureter. B. A double-pigtail catheter has been placed distal to the strictured segment. Under fluoroscopic guidance, a balloon is placed at the level of the stricture. C. Complete distension of the balloon with disappearance of the "waist" of the balloon.*

the individual who has undergone cystectomy for uroepithelial malignancy. One of the reasons for ureteral obstruction in this patient would be the occurrence of a primary ureteral neoplasm. Any cancer patient developing ureteral obstruction should be thoroughly investigated by means of urinary cytology, imaging, brush biopsy, and endoscopy of the bowel to rule out neoplastic causes.

Ureterointestinal anastomotic stenosis also can occur independent of recurrent uroepithelial malignancy. This is particularly true on the left side, where the need

to free a portion of ureter from its blood supply is considerably greater. Additionally, ureteroileal anastomotic failure because of angulation beneath the inferior mesenteric artery is more likely to occur in the left ureter. Lastly, antirefluxing techniques of ureterointestinal anastomosis increase the risk of ureteral stricture. When a benign ureteroileal anastomotic stenosis has been discovered, an attempt should be made to solve the problem by endoscopic technology (Fig. 27-1).

The region of the anastomotic stricture may be dilated by balloon dilation with a catheter that can be directed either from the ileal stoma or else percutaneously placed. If access is possible, a flexible sigmoidoscope will offer enhanced visualization of the bowel segment and may prove superior to a flexible cystoscope. After balloon dilation has been accomplished, ureteroileal intubation is required for a period of 6 to 8 weeks in order to ensure patency. This technique will be successful in approximately 50 percent of ureteroileal strictures, although the long-term outcome of patients managed in this fashion is not yet known. In contrast, open reoperation to revise the ureteroileal anastomosis is somewhat more dependable, although it is associated with all the complications of a major operative intervention. If ureteroileal stenosis requires long-term stenting, it should be recognized that there have been instances wherein the stent has eroded through the ureter into the

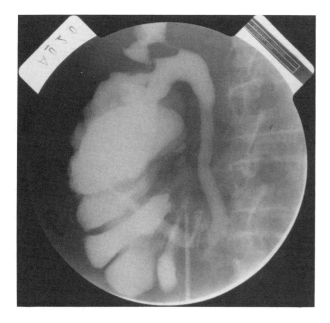

Figure 27-2. *A 60-year-old woman who previously underwent radical cystectomy with creation of an Indiana reservoir. Subsequently, she developed symptomatic pyelonephritis. Pouchogram above reveals significant right ureteral reflux. Patient required reexploration with reimplantation of right ureter.*

adjacent common iliac artery resulting in profound hemorrhage.

Ureterointestinal reflux is not uncommon despite antirefluxing anastomoses (Fig. 27-2). In patients with orthotopic voiding pouches, the presence of reflux may be of no consequence, and the isolated finding of a refluxing ureter is not an absolute indication for surgery. Rather, if the patient is maintaining sterile urine and there is no evidence of upper tract deterioration, the reflux merely should be observed.

In patients with catheterizable continent reservoirs, reflux can be more problematic. These patients may experience recurrent episodes of pyelonephritis and can become uroseptic. However, some patients tolerate low-grade reflux well and do not require reimplantation. The patient with recurrent pyelonephritis will likely require an antireflux procedure, but it is worthwhile to attempt suppression to determine if conservative measures will succeed.

Reoperations for reflux will be governed by the original operative procedure. In colonic reservoirs, a ureteral advancement procedure can be performed in a manner similar to a pediatric bladder reimplant. Alternatively, the tunnel can be lengthened from the outside if feasible. In a Kock pouch, the refluxing intussusception will have to be repaired in the same manner discussed below for incontinence.

Metabolic

It should be emphasized that all continent diversions will allow for substantial reabsorption of urinary constituents. This will necessitate increasing workload on the kidneys. No patient with substantial renal impairment should be considered for these procedures. In general, we demand that the preoperative serum creatinine level be less than 1.8 mg/dl. Surgical procedures performed in patients with renal impairment can result in severe metabolic acidosis and eventual calcium wasting and osteomalacia. This is of greater concern in the female than the male patient because of the higher incidence of baseline osteoporosis.

Even in the absence of renal impairment, metabolic acidosis can occur and should be monitored. All patients exhibiting a metabolic acidosis should be treated with alkalinization utilizing sodium or potassium citrates or sodium bicarbonate. The patient should be monitored by urinary pH both at home and in the office.

Stone Formation

Stones may form in intestinal reservoirs secondary to exposed foreign bodies (staples, sutures), urinary stasis, or mucus acting as a nidus. If stones are found at a small enough size, they usually can be managed cystoscopically by forceps extraction (along with the offending staple). If somewhat larger stones are found, electrohydraulic or ultrasound lithotripsy units may be used to fracture the stone. The remaining fragments and offending staples can be removed by a combination of forceps and irrigating techniques. We also have employed a percutaneous approach to large stones that have formed in continent reservoirs. Under CT scan guidance, we have inserted a percutaneous tube into an Indiana pouch and performed electrohydraulic lithotripsy (personal communication, Ridwan Shabsigh).

Continent Urinary Diversion

It has been suggested that continent urinary diversion should not be performed because of the higher complication rates reported with these procedures. However, an extensive review from our institution has demonstrated no statistically significant difference in reoperations, mortality, or hospital stay in patients undergoing continent diversion versus conduit diversion by the same three surgeons over a 3-year period. This review indicated that with proper patient selection, continent diversion operations can be conducted at the same cost to society and to the patient as conduit diversions.

Orthotopic Voiding Diversions

A number of operative procedures have been developed for the provision of a urinary pouch of low pressure and high capacity that will accommodate the collection of urine and allow the male patient to initiate voiding by Valsalva maneuver following cystoprostatectomy. These operations have been popularized by the singular work of Maurice Camey, whose Camey I operation was a pioneer step in this form of urinary diversion. Although these procedures vary in some aspects, many of the possible complications are shared by all.

Urethral Transitional Cell Cancer Recurrence

A feature shared by all orthotopic voiding procedures utilized for treatment of bladder cancer is the risk of urethral cancer recurrence. The incidence of anterior urethral recurrence in bladder cancer patients is approximately 4 to 5 percent overall. This is too low a percentage to warrant routine urethrectomy in all patients. However, the risk of urethral transitional cell cancer (TCC) is higher in select patient groups. Patients who have prostatic urethra transitional cell cancer are at high risk for distal urethral recurrence. Others have suggested that diffuse intravesical carcinoma in situ warrants distal urethrectomy as well. In order to ensure the proper selection of patients for this operation, our custom has been to conduct prostatic urethral biopsy in all individuals being considered.

Patients developing a urethral recurrence following cystoprostatectomy will require a total urethrectomy and mobilization of the neobladder from the pelvis. This is a technically difficult procedure and may result in vascular injury to the reservoir. If the reservoir cannot be salvaged, formation of another means of urinary diversion will be necessary. For reservoirs that can be salvaged, the options available for reconstruction will be predicated on the form of orthotopic diversion performed. One option available to all would be the placement of a Kock valve on the reservoir in a fashion similar to that described by Lieskovsky for repair of a failed valve (see Fig. 27-2). Patients who have undergone an ileal ureter neobladder as described by Studer have the advantage of the orthotopic segment that can be brought to the skin as an ileal conduit.

Enuresis

Nocturnal enuresis occurs frequently in all orthotopic voiding procedures and is the most common complica-

tion. Its true incidence is difficult to determine because there is no uniformity in reporting postoperative results. Some authors only consider nighttime incontinence a complication if it results in soilage, while others consider any void, whether in response to a planned awakening or a reflex awakening, a failure. In general, enuresis represents an expected operative risk and can be managed by planned awakenings or the use of a condom catheter.

Under normal circumstances, a spinal reflex arc ensures the continued recruitment of external sphincteric contraction during bladder filling. Since the bladder has been removed in the patient undergoing orthotopic voiding diversion, this reflex is ablated, and external sphincteric recruitment does not occur except under voluntary conscious control. However, some of our patients do describe the ability to recognize the need to void at night and have developed a "wake reflex."

Initial management of enuresis should be expectant, because reservoir pressures are higher and pouch capacities smaller in the immediate postoperative period. After 3 months, patients should be obtaining nighttime control. In general, patients are instructed to void before retiring and are advised to set an alarm clock for around 3 to 4 hours after going to bed. Others prefer the use of a nighttime condom catheter. Pharmacologic therapy is not usually of value in the treatment of enuresis, which is most related to urine production, pouch capacity, and sphincteric integrity.

Daytime Incontinence

Continence depends on preservation of the external sphincteric apparatus in the male. One of the additional benefits of the Walsh technique of nerve-sparing prostatectomy is the improved identification of the prostatic apex and resultant better preservation of the sphincteric apparatus. The preserved male sphincter results in a daytime continence rate in orthotopic voiding operations well in excess of 95 percent.

Prolonged daytime incontinence is rare in patients undergoing neobladder reconstruction and should be considered a major complication. Daytime incontinence occurring in the immediate postoperative period should be managed expectantly, since it may be secondary to high pressure and low capacity. Daytime incontinence lasting beyond 6 months is cause for concern. Potential treatments include pelvic floor exercises, gastrointestinal antispasmodics and antidiarrheals (i.e., Donnetal or Lomotil), and alpha agonists. If conservative measures fail, options include penile clamps, condom catheters, and anti-incontinence surgical procedures. Whether periurethral injections of substances such as collagen or Teflon would be of value remains to be determined. There is insufficient literature available to know what techniques will work best.

Urinary Retention

The mechanism of voiding following neobladder reconstruction is pelvic floor relaxation and Valsalva. Patients who have a difficult time mastering this procedure can be aided by sitting to void. This allows the patient to fully relax the sphincter while not fearing fecal incontinence. However, all patients should be advised of the occasional need for clean intermittent catheterization. A rare patient will be unable to void by Valsalva maneuver and pelvic floor relaxation. Such patients will necessarily be assigned to permanent intermittent catheterization in order to achieve urinary emptying.

A patient developing urinary retention as a late sequelae should be evaluated for possible tumor recurrence. Recurrent tumor can cause retention secondary to external pelvic compression or intrinsic urethral obstruction. These patients should be evaluated with pelvic imaging, voided cytologies, and urethroscopy.

Procedure-Specific Complications

Orthotopic Hemi-Kock Pouch

This operation was designed by Ghoneim and Kock to accommodate the male patient facing cystectomy. In this instance, prevention against reflux depends on the construction of a nipple valve. Nipple valve construction requires the use of staples to stabilize the intussusception of the bowel. Thus this form of voiding pouch will have a higher potential for the development of urinary calculi within the pouch, a feature not shared by the other orthotopic voiding operations.

The complication that is not shared by any other neobladder is ureteral reflux secondary to a failed proximal intussusception. The incidence of failure has been reduced dramatically by the numerous advances in nipple valve construction described by Skinner and associates. Nevertheless, nipple valve failure can be anticipated in 10 to 15 percent of cases despite the very best of operative techniques. Failed nipples can be repaired by repeat intussusception and refastening of the bowel to the wall of the reservoir. Occasionally, a new nipple must be fashioned.

Detubularized Right Colon Pouch

Right colon reservoirs have been criticized because of the loss of the ileocecal valve. While this does result in frequent bowel movements in a number of patients, at least in the short term, the majority of patients will experience bowel regularity with the use of simple pharmacologic therapy. However, it should be noted that some patients have developed rather striking diarrhea following loss of the ileocecal valve. This may be particularly true in the pediatric patient in whom there is neurogenic bowel dysfunction (i.e., myelomeningocele patient).

Sigmoid Pouch

Use of the sigmoid colon as a continent voiding pouch offers a few potential advantages as well as disadvantages. With regard to the latter, the sigmoid colon is often affected by diverticulosis and/or malignancy. For this reason, it might not be a suitable bowel segment to use for longer-term urinary diversion. However, the facility with which the sigmoid colon can be brought to the membranous urethral region and the simplicity with which it can be reconfigured in a cup cystoplasty fashion afford distinct advantages over other bowel segments. Furthermore, in contrast to other operations, the loss of the sigmoid colon has little, if any, impact on the nutritional status or bowel habits of the patient.

Continent Catheterizing Pouches

Numerous operative techniques have been developed in recent years for the continent diversion of urine wherein urine is emptied at intervals by patient self-catheterization. For these operations to be successful, certain criteria must be adhered to. First, it is mandatory that patients undergoing these procedures have sufficient hand-eye coordination to perform clean intermittent catheterization. Quadriplegic patients and some individuals with multiple sclerosis may not be candidates for this operation. Furthermore, patients with any degree of dementia that would interfere with their understanding of the catheterizing process would not be appropriate candidates.

Incontinence

There are numerous methods for creating a continence mechanism in catheterizable reservoirs. Each mechanism has its advantages and disadvantages, and each may fail with time. The construction of a continence mechanism using an intussuscepted nipple valve is certainly the most technologically demanding of all the continence mechanisms. In order that the surgeon achieve a degree of dependability in his or her own clinical results with intussuscepted valves, a significant learning curve must be overcome initially. For this reason, nipple valve construction probably should not be chosen by the surgeon carrying out occasional construction of continent pouches. It should be noted that the past decade has seen the introduction of many modifications of the original technique of Kock for construction of a stable nipple valve. The single reason for all these modifications is the rather disappointing long-term stability of nipple valve in some patients.

One of the major advances in nipple valve construction has been the removal of mesenteric attachments from the middle 6 to 8 cm of bowel to be utilized for nipple valve construction. A second major advance has been the attachment of the nipple valve to the reservoir wall itself. Nevertheless, nipple valve failure can be anticipated in 10 to 15 percent of cases despite the very best of operative techniques.

There are three general reasons for nipple valve failure: pinhole fistulas, nipple valve prolapse, and nipple valve shortening or effacement. Pinhole fistulas at the base of the nipple are a consequence of setting the aligning pin of the staple instrument. Such fistulas simply can be oversewn during formal reexploration. Nipple valve prolapse may occur, in which case bowel can be intussuscepted once more, restapled, and fixed to the reservoir wall with suture or stapling techniques. Shortening of the nipple length beneath the 2.5 to 3 cm necessary for urinary continence probably occurs as a consequence of ischemia.

A failed nipple valve must be repaired or refashioned, and this can only be performed with an open reoperation. In the case of nipple effacement, it may be possible to restaple the valve to the wall. If the nipple valve appears unrepairable secondary to either insufficient length or ischemia, a new segment of bowel can be isolated, intussuscepted, and patched to the reservoir (Fig. 27-3).

During reconstruction of the continence mechanism, intraoperative testing for pouch integrity is always performed. The continence mechanism is tested for ease of catheterization as well as continence after the pouch repair has been completed. The pouch is filled with saline, the continence mechanism catheter is removed, and the pouch can be compressed slightly to look for points of leakage as well as to test the continence mechanism for its ability to contain urine. Thereafter, the continence mechanism is catheterized to ensure ease of catheter passage.

Stone Formation

A final feature of stapled nipple valves is the potential for stone formation on exposed staples. While this has been

Figure 27-3. *Technique of efferent limb construction for failed valve mechanism. A. Intussusception of ileum. B. Placement of three lines of staples. C. Completed construction and anastomosis of new efferent limb onto original pouch. (From G Lieskovsky, S Boyd, and DJ Skinner, Management of late complications of the Kock pouch form of urinary diversion. J. Urol 137:1146, 1987.)*

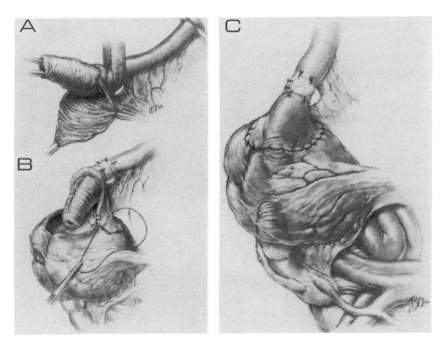

greatly lessened by the omission of staples at the tip of the nipple valve, as suggested by Skinner et al., occasionally, more proximal staples erode into the pouch and serve as a nidus for stone formation. These stones are usually able to be managed endoscopically with forceps extraction of the stone and staple or else electrohydraulic or ultrasonic disintegration of the stone with subsequent forceps staple extraction.

Urinary Tract Infection

Since all patients with catheterized pouches will have chronic bacteriuria, the problem of antibiotic management should be discussed. Most authors would suggest that bacteriuria in the absence of symptomatology does not warrant antibiotic treatment. The construction of an effective reflux mechanism in these pouches usually ensures against clinical episodes of pyelonephritis. Obviously, if pyelonephritis does occur, antibiotic treatment should be instituted. Antibiotics also should be administered for a condition manifested by pain in the region of the pouch along with increased pouch contractility ("pouchitis"). This latter condition, while infrequent, may result in temporary failure of the continence mechanism because of the hypercontractility of the bowel segment employed for construction of the pouch. The patient typically presents with a history of sudden explosive discharge of urine through the continence mechanism (rather than dribbling incontinence), along with discomfort in the region of the pouch.

If treatment of a pouch infection is necessary, a course of at least 10 days is warranted. Shorter courses of therapy may be unsuccessful secondary to retained mucous debris, bacterial penetration within intestinal crypts, and incomplete emptying.

Urinary Retention

Urinary retention is an infrequent occurrence in catheterizable pouches. It is seen most commonly with pouches whose continence mechanism consists of a nipple valve. In these circumstances, if the chimney of the nipple valve is not near the abdominal surface, the catheter can be directed into folds of bowel rather than into the nipple valve proper such that urinary retention results. This complication presents a true emergency, and the patient must seek immediate attention so that catheterization can be achieved promptly. If traditional maneuvers such as the use of Coude tip catheters are unsuccessful, a flexible cystoscope and wire can be of

great value in identifying the lumen to the reservoir. A Council tip catheter can then be advanced over the wire. After the immediate problem has been resolved by emptying the pouch, the patient should be kept under observation for the ability to successfully catheterize on a number of occasions.

Intraperitoneal Rupture

Intraperitoneal rupture of catheterizable pouches has been reported (Fig. 27-4). In general, these episodes are more common in the neurologic patient, in whom sensation of pouch fullness may be less distinct. Often there is associated mild abdominal trauma, such as a fall, that is antecedent to the rupture. In general, these patients require immediate pouch decompression and abdominal exploration with drainage of infected urine. If the amount of urinary extravasation is small and the patient does not have a surgical abdomen, occasionally catheter drainage and antibiotic administration suffice in treating intraperitoneal rupture of a pouch. We have employed this nonoperative approach successfully in one patient with a right colon pouch.

Figure 27-4. *Radiograph reveals extravasation of contrast medium from Indiana pouch. Patient required exploration and repair of rupture.*

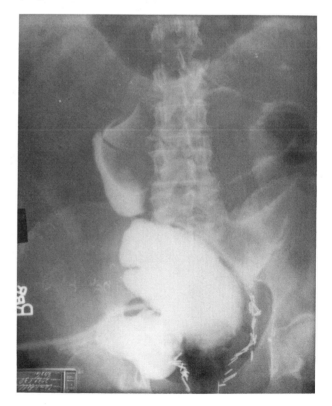

Summary

The patient facing cystectomy now has the opportunity to select various forms of urinary diversion. Although not all the newer techniques have stood the test of time, preliminary results indicate that newer forms of continent diversion should be considered safe and effective. With experience, these procedures can be performed with morbidity rates very similar to those encountered with conduit diversion. As with any procedure, however, appropriate patient selection and surgical training are imperative.

The complications that can arise following continent urinary diversion can truly test the surgeon's creativity and abilities. To manage these potential complications, one must be well versed in all procedures that are utilized in constructing continent diversions. The solution to a given complication may lie in techniques that may have nothing to do with the original operation.

Bibliography

Askanazi, J, et al. Effect of immediate postoperative nutritional support on length of hospitalization. J Urol 134:1032, 1985.

Beddoe, AM, et al. Stented versus nonstented transverse colon conduits: A comparative report. Gynecol Oncol 27:305, 1987.

Benson, MC, et al. Analysis of continent versus standard urinary diversion. Br J Urol 69(2):156, 1992.

Camey, M, and LeDuc, X. L'enetrocystoplastie avec cystoprostatectomie totale pour cancer de la vessie. Ann Urol 13:114, 1979.

Cordonnier, JJ, and Spjut, HJ. Urethral occurrence of bladder carcinoma following cystectomy. Trans Am Assoc Genitourinary Surg 53:13, 1961.

Ghoneim, MA, et al. An appliance-free, sphincter-controlled bladder substitute: The urethral Kock pouch. J Urol 138:1150, 1987.

Jakobsen, H, et al. Pathogenesis of nocturnal urinary incontinence after ileocaecal bladder replacement: Continuous measurement of urethral closure pressure during sleep. Br J Urol 59:148, 1987.

Knapp, PM, Jr, et al. Urodynamic evaluation of ileal conduit function. J Urol 137:929, 1987.

Kramolowsky, EV, Clayman, RV, and Weyman, PJ. Endourological management of ureteroileal anastomotic strictures: Is it effective? J Urol 137:390, 1987.

Kramolowsky, EV, Clayman, RV, and Weyman, PJ. Management of ureterointestinal anastomotic strictures: comparison of open surgical and endourological repair. J Urol 139:1195, 1988.

Lieskovsky, G, Boyd, SD, and Skinner, DG. Management of late complications of the Kock pouch form of urinary diversion. J Urol 137:1146, 1987.

Regan, JB, and Barrett, DM. Stented versus nonstented ureteroileal anastomoses: Is there a different with regard to leak and stricture? J Urol 134:1101, 1985.

Schellhammer, PF, and Whitmore, WF, Jr. Transitional cell carcinoma of the urethra in men having cystectomy for bladder cancer. J Urol 115:56, 1976.

Skinner, DG, Boyd, S, and Lieskovsky, G. Clinical experience with the Kock continent ileal reservoir for urinary diversion. J Urol 132:1101, 1984.

Sullivan, JW, Grabstald, H, and Whitmore, WF, Jr. Complications of ureteroileal conduit with radical cystectomy: Review of 336 cases. J Urol 124:797, 1980.

Walsh, PC, Lepor, H, and Eggleston, O. Radical prostatectomy with preservation of sexual function: anatomical and pathological considerations. Prostate 4:473, 1983.

Complications of Ureterosigmoidostomy

MARK C. ADAMS
ALAN B. RETIK

Ureterosigmoidostomy was the earliest form of urinary diversion, the first being performed by Simon in 1851. Initial experience with the procedure was complicated by leakage, peritonitis, pyelonephritis, obstruction, and significant mortality. The characteristic electrolyte disturbance of hypokalemic, hyperchloremic acidosis was recognized and well described by Ferris and Odel in 1950. Development of a direct mucosal ureterointestinal anastomosis and an antirefluxing intestinal anastomosis led to a significant decrease in the incidence of early complications after ureterosigmoidostomy.

Late complications, however, still occur in a significant number of patients after ureterosigmoidostomy. Many of these complications may necessitate reoperation. In several series, up to half of patients have suffered complications requiring secondary surgery after ureterosigmoidostomy. Some patients will have recurrent episodes of pyelonephritis, and these patients, even in the absence of obstruction or reflux, should be considered as candidates for conversion to some other diversion. Radiographic upper urinary tract deterioration is also not uncommon following ureterosigmoidostomy and may be due to infection, obstruction, reflux, or stone disease. Such deterioration is unacceptable in a patient with a long life expectancy and should be considered an indication for reoperation. Late ureteral obstruction occurs in up to 30 percent of these cases and requires reoperation, as does coloureteral reflux. Renal calculi have been reported in up to 18 percent of cases, and recurrent stone disease following ureterosigmoidostomy probably should be considered an indication for reoperation for conversion.

After ureterosigmoidostomy, urine is exposed to a large absorptive surface. Most patients with such diversion will develop hyperchloremia, with or without frank acidosis. The majority of such patients may be adequately maintained on medical therapy; however, significant metabolic derangements are an indication for conversion to a different type of urinary diversion.

The admixture of urine and feces is particularly foul smelling, and anal incontinence is unacceptable for patients with ureterosigmoidostomy. Even these patients who do well during the day may have soilage at night that eventually becomes intolerable.

Perhaps the most distressing complication of ureterosigmoidostomy is colonic neoplasia. Tumors at or near the ureterocolonic anastomosis were initially recognized in 1948. With longer follow-up, it appears that approximately 5 percent of patients with ureterosigmoidostomy have developed malignancies to date. Historically, many of these malignancies have been metastatic at the time of presentation and fatal. With better awareness of this potential and close follow-up of patients, it may be possible to detect these tumors at an early stage. The presence of such a tumor is obviously an indication for colectomy and an alternate form of urinary diversion.

With the success of primary urinary tract reconstruction and the development of effective forms of continent urinary diversion, we rarely, if ever, use ureterosigmoidostomy in children at this time. We feel that the long-term risk of upper urinary tract deterioration, metabolic acidosis, and tumor development is prohibitive. Because of those long-term risks, it is reasonable to consider elective urinary undiversion or conversion to a continent urinary reservoir even in a patient who has done well with ureterosigmoidostomy. Certainly, when complications of ureterosigmoidostomy do occur that require reoperation, consideration should be given to elective abandonment of ureterosigmoidostomy. This is particularly true when there is recurrent pyelonephritis, upper tract deterioration, or recurrent renal calculi without correctable obstruction or reflux. Significant metabolic or electrolyte abnormalities are also indications for conversion. Patients with good rectal continence are sometimes very happy with and adjusted to ureterosigmoidostomy, and reoperation for revision of the ureterocolonic anastomosis occasionally may be indicated for obstruction and/or reflux. Again, our preference in these patients would be for conversion to an alternate form of urinary diversion and resection of the old anastomotic sites due to the potential for tumor development. Certainly, however, it is the patient's decision when there is a correctable local problem.

Revision

When revision of ureterosigmoidostomy is planned, the patient should have a preoperative mechanical bowel preparation and receive perioperative intravenous antibiotics. Any patient with ureteral obstruction should have colonoscopy preoperatively to rule out a malignancy at the anastomotic site. A large rectal tube with multiple holes is inserted and anchored immediately prior to surgery. The ureter is identified and approached by incising the overlying peritoneum. The distal-most ureter is mobilized at the muscular hiatus of the taenia, taking care to preserve all the ureteral adventitia and longitudinal blood supply. When revision is necessary for obstruction or high-grade reflux, the ureterocolonic anastomosis to be revised is taken down by incising the taenia longitudinally over the underlying ureter. The distal ureter with a small rim of colonic mucosa is then removed from the tunnel, and the distal-most ureter along with any strictured ureter is excised for histologic examination. We then generally use a new site for the revised ureterocolonic anastomosis, and this is determined on the basis of ureteral length and colonic course and mobility.

The new anastomosis is made as low as possible on the colon; however, it is critical not to angulate the ureter at the muscular hiatus of the new tunnel. Once a new site is determined, we incise the taenia for a length of approximately 5 cm in a longitudinal fashion toward the antimesenteric margin of the taenia. The muscle and submucosa are then freed away from the underlying mucosa. This dissection can be facilitated by injecting

sterile saline submucosally prior to the incision. A small incision is then made through the colonic mucosa at the distal end of the new tunnel. The ureter is brought into the tunnel. A stent passed up the ureter facilitates manipulation of the ureter with a strict no-touch technique and avoids injury to the longitudinal blood supply. The distal end of the ureter is spatulated slightly, and the full thickness of ureter is approximated to the colonic mucosa circumferentially using interrupted fine chronic catgut suture. The taenia is then reapproximated over the distal ureter using interrupted nonabsorbable suture. Use of a nonabsorbable suture aids in identification of the ureteral tunnel at future operation, if necessary. The muscular hiatus is left wide to avoid compromise of the ureter at that point, and angulation of the ureter must be avoided. The edge of incised peritoneum is then approximated to the colon wall with absorbable suture to stabilize the anastomosis and place it in the retroperitoneum. We prefer to leave a small pediatric feeding tube across the anastomosis as a ureteral stent. This can be passed up the ureter and brought into the colonic lumen prior to the mucosal anastomosis. The distal end of the stent can be approximated to the end of the rectal tube. At the end of the case, the rectal tube can be withdrawn slowly, bringing the stent out transanally. The rectal tube should then be replaced and the tube and ureteral stents carefully anchored.

If revision of a ureterocolonic anastomosis is performed for low-grade reflux, it may occasionally be possible to lengthen the tunnel from outside the colon. The ureter at the muscular hiatus in such a case is mobilized. The taenia is then incised back from the old hiatus, mobilized off the mucosa, and closed over the ureter to achieve a longer appropriate tunnel length (Fig. 28-1). The ureter is often fixed in position after the previous reimplant, and angulation at the new hiatus must be avoided. It may at times be necessary to carefully mobilize the ureter with its adventitia to avoid angulation. In such a reoperative case, it is essential that a good ureterocolonic anastomosis be achieved. The surgeon should be prepared to completely revise the anastomosis if a perfect anastomosis cannot be achieved in such a manner from outside the colon (Fig. 28-2).

If both ureteral anastomoses require revision, it is preferable to reimplant both ureters separately. If one ureter is particularly dilated, shortened, or scarred, we at times use transureteroureterostomy and a single reimplant unless there is a contraindication such as prior stone disease. Good drainage and successful prevention of reflux generally can be achieved in this manner by reimplanting the better ureter rather than trying to sep-

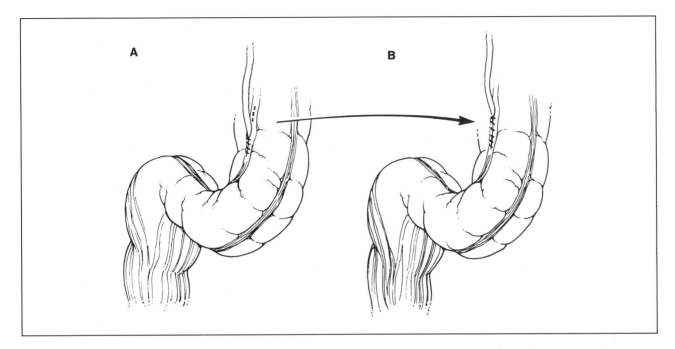

Figure 28-1. *Revision of ureterocolonic anastomosis for mild to moderate reflux. A. Taenia is incised back from muscular hiatus and mobilized. B. Taenia is closed over the ureter to lengthen tunnel. Angulation must be avoided.*

Figure 28-2. *Revision of ureterocolonic anastomosis. Ureter is mobilized and old anastomotic site closed. New anastomosis is performed lower on sigmoid.*

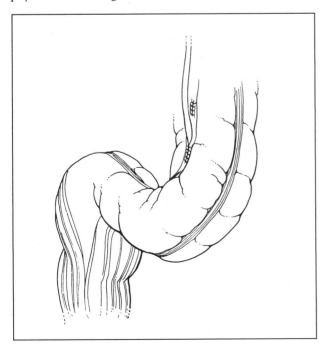

arately reimplant a compromised ureter. In such a case, the ureteroureteral anastomosis should be performed as high as possible above the ureterocolonic anastomosis. The crossing ureter should take a nice, smooth course beneath the colonic mesentery to meet the recipient ureter, and again, angulation should be avoided at this anastomosis. We leave a ureteral stent with multiple perforations across the transureteroureterostomy in this setting. When one ureterocolonic anastomosis has failed and the other is functioning well, transureteroureterostomy of the failed side into the functioning side is an alternative to revision of the ureterocolonic anastomosis.

If revision of ureterosigmoidostomy is undertaken and adequate ureteral length for conversional anastomosis is not present due to high division of the ureter at the primary diversion or loss of significant ureteral length due to stricture, a roux-en-Y limb of colon can be brought up to meet the ureter or ureters. The colon is divided, the distal colon is brought up to the ureters, and the proximal colon is then reanastomosed to the distal colon beneath the ureterocolonic anastomoses (Fig. 28-3). An alternative approach is to use an isolated ileocecal segment interposed between ureter and colon. The il-

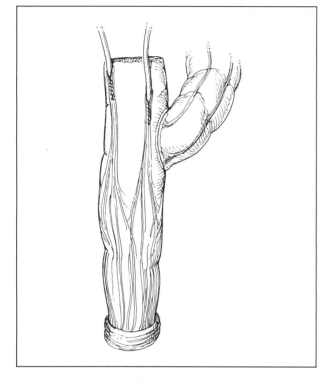

Figure 28-3. *Roux-en-Y limb of colon brought up to meet short ureters.*

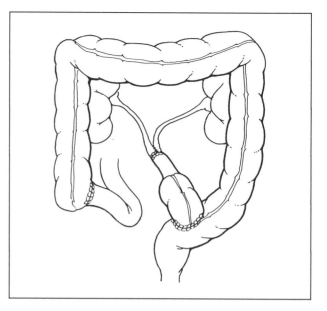

Figure 28-4. *Ureteroileocecal sigmoidostomy. Intussusception of ileocecal valve provides an antireflux mechanism. The cecum is anastomosed to the sigmoid colon in an end-to-side fashion.*

eocecal valve can be intussuscepted to provide an antireflux mechanism. A very dilated ureter, unsuitable for submucosal tunneling without tapering, can be anastomosed to the iuelum in an end-to-end fashion. This technique (Fig. 28-4) has the significant theoretical advantage of a ureteroileal anastomosis that does not appear to be at the same risk for malignant development as ureterocolonic anastomoses in animal models. Although clinical experience is not adequate to yet determine if this advantage is real in the clinical setting, ureteroileocecal sigmoidostomy may provide a means for avoiding what is essentially an iatrogenic tumor in patients who desire this type of diversion.

Conversion

When conversion from ureterosigmoidostomy to an alternate form of diversion is contemplated, the choice of diversion will depend on the patient. Most of these patients, who have had at least some continence previously, will desire continent diversion over a conduit and ostomy.

If the lower urinary tract is present and reconstruct-

able, we prefer undiversion to continent urinary diversion. In its absence, the choice of an appropriate continent urinary reservoir is a personal one based on the experience and expertise of the surgeon. Good results have been achieved using the Koch pouch or continent ileocecal (Indiana) pouch, with our preference being the latter. If the patient has a suitable appendix or ureter, a continent reservoir based on the Mitrofanoff principle can be constructed. Figure 28-5 illustrates such a case. This was a 10-year-old girl born with classic bladder exstrophy. After initial closure and failed reconstruction, she had undergone a cystectomy and diversion with ureterosigmoidostomy. She had been troubled with soilage at night and several episodes of pyelonephritis. During reconstruction, a limited colectomy was performed including the previous anastomotic sites. The descending colon immediately adjacent to that segment was isolated and reconfigured as a reservoir. An isolated segment of distal ureter left on its pelvic vasculature was tunneled submucosally into the reservoir and brought out of the abdomen as a continent, catheterizable stoma. This technique, whether using appendix or ureter, is highly continent and should provide easy catheterization as long as the catheterizable limb is made short and straight. The technique, in this setting, allows for colectomy and isolation of an adjacent segment of bowel for use as a reservoir with a single bowel anastomosis. It also allows for preservation of the ileoce-

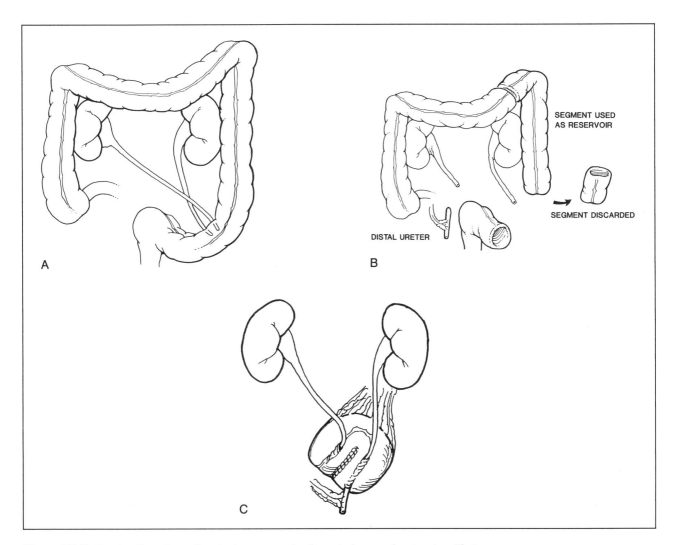

Figure 28-5. *Construction of a continent urinary reservoir after cystectomy and ureterosigmoidostomy. A. Ureterosigmoidostomy. B. Colon containing anastomotic sites is resected, and adjacent descending colon is reconfigured as a reservoir. C. Isolated segment of distal ureter, based on blood supply from iliac vessels, is used as continent stoma.*

cal valve and terminal ileum in the gastrointestinal tract.

Significant impairment in renal function may be considered a relative contraindication to continent diversion because the storage of urine within absorptive bowel for long periods of time is more likely to cause hyperchloremia and acidosis in patients with such impairment. The same problem, however, can occur with conduit diversion, particularly if drainage is poor. If a conduit is to be performed, we prefer a nonrefluxing colon conduit to an ileal conduit in children.

When conversion to another form of urinary diversion is performed, we feel strongly that a colectomy that includes the ureterocolonic anastomotic sites be performed. Those sites with approximately a 5-cm proximal and distal margin should be resected to remove that area of colon at greatest risk for tumor development. These anastomotic sites, once exposed to the admixture of urine and feces, remain at long-term risk for tumor development even with urinary diversion. A lifetime of close follow-up is otherwise imperative if these sites are not removed.

Bibliography

Allen, TD, Roehrborn, CG, and Peters, PC. Long-term follow-up of patients after cystectomy and urinary diversion via ileal loop versus ureterosigmoidostomy for bladder cancer. Presented at the American Urological Association Meeting, Dallas, Texas, May 1989.

Bennett, AH. Exstrophy of bladder treated by ureterosigmoidostomies. Urology 2:165, 1973.

Coffey, RC. Transplantation of the ureters into the large intestine in the absence of a functioning urinary bladder. Surg Gynecol Obstet 32:383, 1921.

Cordonnier, JJ. Ureterosigmoid anastomosis. Surg Gynecol Obstet 88:441, 1949.

Dixon, CF, and Weismann, RE. Polyps of the sigmoid occurring thirty years after bilateral ureterosigmoidostomy for exstrophy of the bladder. Surgery 24:1026, 1948.

Ferris, DO, and Odel, HM. Electrolyte pattern of the blood after bilateral ureterosigmoidostomy. JAMA 142:634, 1950.

Goodwin, WE, et al. Open transcolonic ureterointestinal anastomosis. Surg Gynecol Obstet 97:295, 1953.

Hendren, WH. Ureterocolic diversion of urine: Management of some difficult problems. J Urol 120:719, 1983.

Leadbetter, GW, Jr, Zickerman, P, and Pierce, E. Ureterosigmoidostomy and carcinoma of the colon. J Urol 121:732, 1979.

Leadbetter, WF, and Clarke, BG. Five years' experience with ureteroenterostomy by the "combined" technique. J Urol 73:67, 1954.

Nesbit, RM. Ureterosigmoid anastomosis by direct elliptical connection: A preliminary report. J Urol 61:728, 1949.

Rink, RC, and Retik, AB. Ureteroileocecalsigmoidostomy and avoidance carcinoma of the colon. In LR King (ed), Bladder Reconstruction and Continent Urinary Diversion. Chicago: Year Book Medical Publishers, 1987.

Spence, HM, Hoffman, WW, and Pate, VA. Exstrophy of the bladder: Long-term results in a series of 37 cases treated by ureterosigmoidostomy. J Urol 114:133, 1975.

Wear, JB, and Barquin, OP. Ureterosigmoidostomy: Long-term results. Urology 1:192, 1973.

Vesicostomy, Ureterostomy, and Pyelostomy

EDMOND T. GONZALES, JR.

Nonintubated, cutaneous urinary diversion (cutaneous ureterostomy, pyelostomy, and vesicostomy) is a time-honored management approach for many urologic disorders that result from ureteral or bladder obstruction or dysfunction. The growth of pediatric urology during the decade of the 1960s was closely tied to the development of improved techniques of nonintubated, temporizing, ureteral diversion. For the first time, the liberal use of these techniques allowed sick neonates with severe urologic obstructions to maintain stable renal function and to avoid recurring and destructive urinary tract infection. After these procedures were done, infants were generally able to maintain growth to a sufficient size and maturity to allow for a planned, elective, and technically easier reconstruction. The first group of patients to obviously benefit from these procedures were those with posterior urethral valves, although infants with ureterovesical junction obstruction, ureteroceles, prune belly anomaly, severe vesicoureteral reflux, and neurogenic vesical dysfunction were commonly managed in this fashion also. An additional indication for temporizing cutaneous urinary diversion in the past was to treat a child with severe urologic sepsis associated with obstruction and pyonephrosis that was not responding to available chemotherapy.

While the use of cutaneous vesicostomy proved particularly unacceptable in adults because of problems with poor vesical drainage, stone formation along hair growth at the stoma site, and the inability to satisfactorily fit a urine-collecting appliance to the stoma, cutaneous vesicostomy was shown to be very successful in preserving the upper tracts in infants with severe vesical dysfunction—particularly when associated with posterior urethral valves or neurogenic bladder dysfunction. When permanent urinary diversion was considered in a child who had large, thick-walled, dilated ureters, permanent end cutaneous ureterostomy seemed to offer fewer overall complications than did ileal or colon segments interposed between ureter and skin.

The current indications for cutaneous urinary diversion, whether temporary or permanent, are extremely limited. Today, the technique of clean intermittent catheterization as a means of managing disorders of the bladder is accepted worldwide. Even in the newborn and very young infant, in both males and females, properly performed clean intermittent catheterization has proven to be safe and effective. Current indications for choosing a vesicostomy in an infant with neuropathic bladder might include (1) the inability or unwillingness of the primary caretaker to perform intermittent catheterization or (2) a high-pressure, small-capacity, noncompliant bladder in a child in whom it is felt that it is inappropriate to proceed with definitive reconstructive procedures (vesical augmentation) at this time. It is also prudent to consider a vesicostomy in children with urethral obstruction (most often posterior urethral valves) when the urethra is very small and unable to safely accept the available endoscopes that have a working channel. However, modern pediatric cystoscopes with a working channel are as small as no. 7.8 French, small enough to safely negotiate the urethra of very tiny infants. In addition, endourologic techniques have been described that access the bladder percutaneously, allowing the valve to be destroyed in an antegrade fashion. Whitaker also has developed a tiny electrocautery hook that can be positioned accurately with fluoroscopy to safely incise urethral valves in the smallest premature infants.

The indications for ureterocutaneous diversion likewise have undergone careful reevaluation and are very limited today. If temporary upper tract drainage is felt to be indicated, current instrumentation and physician skills in placement of percutaneous nephrostomy tubes allow this technique to be done safely even in the newborn. It is also less likely, today, with the availability of modern antibiotics, to have to resort to open drainage to control severe urosepsis associated with obstruction. However, even if mechanical drainage is felt to be necessary in such a situation, placement of a percutaneous nephrostomy tube usually will provide satisfactory drainage, avoiding the need for open surgical diversion. Percutaneous nephrostomy drainage also can be used over an extended period of time to allow for assessment of the potential for recoverability of renal function in very young infants with congenital ureteral obstruction.

Perhaps the most controversial area today regarding the indications for high ureteral diversion involves the young infant with posterior urethral valves and severe renal insufficiency at presentation. It has been suggested by some that these infants develop better ultimate renal function after high-loop ureterostomy than do similar cases followed after endoscopic destruction of valves alone. There is evidence to suggest that during the first few months after birth the kidney is still able to develop new renal tissue. It is proposed by those who feel that high ureteral diversion is preferable to primary valve ablation that this potential is maximized when intraureteral pressures are brought to as low a level as possible. They suggest that a period of temporizing ureteral diversion offers the best chance to maximize this growth of new renal tissue and therefore provides for better glomerular filtration in the long term. The answer to this dilemma remains elusive.

Current techniques for bladder refunctionalization (enterocystoplasty), bladder replacement (continent diversion), and newer reconstructive techniques to secure continence at the bladder neck have all played a role in decreasing the need for permanent ureterocutaneous diversion. In fact, much effort has been spent over the last two decades in undiverting individuals who underwent planned "permanent" diversion during the 1960s and 1970s.

Despite these considerations and the obvious wane in enthusiasm for any sort of ureterocutaneous or vesicocutaneous diversion (temporary or permanent), there are still occasional indications for using these procedures. All cutaneous diversions are performed to provide improved drainage of urine. Most complica-

tions associated with cutaneous diversions will be related to obstruction to urinary flow. Less often, prolapse of the diverted organ may be the problem. These complications and their management will be discussed for the three separate techniques individually.

Additional problems associated with cutaneous urinary diversion also include peristomal dermatitis, poor stomal site for an appliance (with leakage), and chronic bacilluria. These particular complications are not likely to need surgical reconstruction and will not be discussed in more detail here.

Vesicostomy

Of all the cutaneous diversions that have been described, vesicostomy is the one most likely to be used today, and the only real indication for performing a vesicostomy today is as a temporary diversion in an infant with bladder dysfunction that is causing damage to the upper tracts and who cannot be managed by clean intermittent catheterization because of either medical or social reasons. Most often this will be for neurogenic disease (myelomeningocele) or severe urethral obstruction (posterior urethral valves). Although several techniques for vesicostomy have been described in the young infant, the Blocksom technique has proved to be eminently successful and is the procedure most often performed.

When fashioning the vesicostomy, it is important that an adequate stoma be placed sufficiently high in the bladder so that the more mobile, intraabdominal, peritonealized portion of the bladder is not able to prolapse through the stoma site (Figs. 29-1 and 29-2). Preferably, the stoma will be positioned posterior and cephalad to the location of the urachus. It is also important that the stoma site be adequately wide to allow for free urinary flow. I have personally found it helpful to incise the external oblique fascia and the external oblique muscle laterally on either side of the stoma site to help in preventing stenosis due to circumferential fibrosis.

If the stoma has been placed sufficiently high in the bladder but stenosis occurs, it can be managed very easily in most cases by incising the fibrous band on the inferior margin of the stoma and then advancing a small triangular flap of abdominal wall skin based inferiorly at this location in order to interpose healthy cutaneous tissue between the cut edges of the fibrous ring. I have not found it necessary in most cases to formally take down and then redo a stenotic vesicostomy stoma. In some situations, daily dilation of the stoma site may be all that is necessary to stabilize the situation temporarily

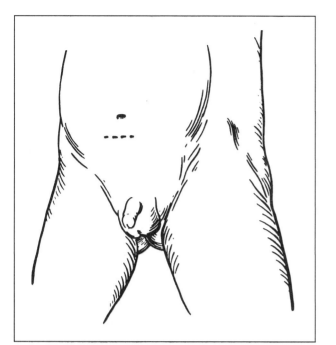

Figure 29-1. *Vesicostomy. Site of proper stoma placement. A transverse skin incision is made midway between the symphysis pubis and umbilicus. (Illustration courtesy of R. Dixon Walker, III, M.D.)*

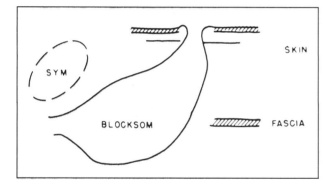

Figure 29-2. *Vesicostomy. Schematic illustrating the components of a properly prepared vesicostomy using the Blocksom technique. The stoma is placed midway between the umbilicus and symphysis pubis (sym) utilizing a well-mobilized, tension-free bladder dome. (Illustration courtesy of R. Dixon Walker, III, M.D.)*

until formal closure of the vesicostomy and refunctionalization of the bladder can be performed.

Prolapse of the bladder through the stoma, though, is a different matter. Prolapse occurs when there is too much mobile peritonealized bladder wall pushing up against the stoma site. While making this stoma somewhat narrower might reduce the tendency for prolapse, the primary problem is that the position of the stoma site on the bladder is too close to the bladder neck. It has

been my experience that the most successful means to manage prolapse is to take down the existing stoma, close the bladder at this location, and, if the vesicostomy is to be maintained, move to a more superior position on the bladder dome. In effect, this means redoing the vesicostomy.

Cutaneous Ureterostomy

Cutaneous ureterostomy can be divided into two separate procedures—end cutaneous ureterostomy and loop cutaneous ureterostomy. If a more permanent diversion is considered and the ureters are dilated and thickened, end cutaneous ureterostomy is a reasonable choice (Fig. 29-3). Several years ago it was popular to perform a transureteroureterostomy with a single abdominal stoma or to bring both ureters together at the umbilicus so as to fashion only one stoma site. If end cutaneous ureterostomy is used as a temporizing diversion with

Figure 29-3. *End cutaneous ureterostomy. This form of urinary diversion is associated with high rates of stomal stenosis. (Illustration courtesy of R. Dixon Walker, III, M.D.)*

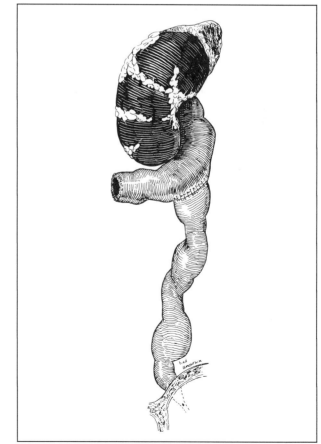

planned later ureteral reimplantation, the diversion it-self may scar the distal ureter such that reimplantation is ultimately made more difficult and the procedure is more likely to fail. As noted in the introduction, the indications for permanent end cutaneous ureterostomy today would be extremely limited.

The primary complication of end cutaneous ure-terostomy is ureteral obstruction. If an end ureteros-tomy becomes obstructed, it is likely to do so at one of three locations: as the ureter turns under the perito-neum to move anteriorly to the stoma site, at the level of the musculofascial layer of the abdominal wall, or at the skin edge itself. The incidence of ureteral stomal steno-sis is fairly common (as high as 70 percent in some series) and seems related primarily to prediversion ure-teral caliber. Excessive dissection of the ureter at the time of mobilization (devascularization) and tension on the stoma anastomosis are contributing factors. Some surgeons encourage that the ureterocutaneous meatus be made more capacious by interposing a small skin flap into the ureteral stoma.

If the obstruction appears to be intraabdominal, of course, an abdominal exploration with appropriate lysis of bands or resection of ischemic sections of ureter with reanastomosis would be necessary. If the obstruction is distal and at the margin of the fascia or skin, the stenosis often can be corrected in a fashion similar to what was described for the vesicostomy. A flap of skin is elevated from one margin of the stoma and the ureter incised proximally through the fibrous ring until an adequate lumen is encountered. The skin flap is then laid into this incised margin of the ureter. If the obstruction is rela-tively deep, special consideration must be given to the incision around the stoma to allow elevation of a larger skin flap without extending cutaneous scars too far out from the stoma site. Pitting and contracture from these scars can make it very difficult to achieve a satisfactory seal of the collection device around the stoma. This procedure, though, is only useful if the obstruction is within a centimeter or so of the skin edge. If the level of the obstruction is somewhat more proximal than that—due either to the presence of a very obese abdomen or because the obstruction is at the level of the parietal peritoneum—formal mobilization of the stoma and dis-tal ureter probably will be necessary to satisfactorily relieve the obstruction. On occasion, it may be neces-sary to interpose a small segment of bowel between ureter and skin in severe, recurrent stomal stenosis.

Another option available today would be balloon dilation of these obstructions if a balloon catheter can be passed safely beyond the obstruction. However, since these are mature, fibrous scars, it is unlikely that this technique will provide a permanent resolution to the problem.

Several techniques have been described for higher ureteral diversions. The technique used most often is the single-loop ureterostomy (Fig. 29-4). When chosen as a form of diversion, the loop ureterostomy is almost always done in a newborn or very young infant. The technique is inconvenient in older children because placement of the stoma is such that it is nearly im-possible to maintain a dependable collection device in position. In the very young infant, on the other hand, satisfactory urinary collection is achieved by using dia-pers overlying the stoma site. Obstruction is uncommon if the loop is placed through the small flank incision without interposing muscle or fascia between the limbs of the ureterostomy. When this principle is adhered to, in my experience, stenosis of a loop ureterostomy al-most never occurs.

Figure 29-4. *Loop cutaneous ureterostomy. Medial dissection and sutures as illustrated may result in a greater incidence of stenosis by compromising the ureteral blood supply. (Illustration courtesy of R. Dixon Walker, III, M.D.)*

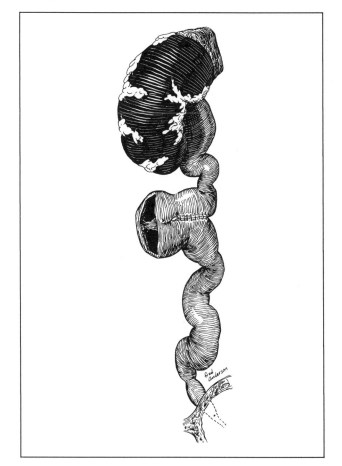

The important concept in performing a loop ureterostomy is in preparing for ultimate reconstruction of the urinary tract. When the loop of ureter is being brought to the skin, every effort is made not to disrupt the medially based blood supply to the ureter. Clamps and tapes are not passed around the ureter. All ureteral manipulation is done with delicate traction sutures placed along the lateral margin of the ureter. At the time of take-down of the ureter, the segment that traverses the abdominal wall is dissected free, and the ureter is transected at that location in the midpoint of the stoma. The blood supply then is carefully dissected proximally and distally so that the blood supply to the remaining ureteral limbs is not disrupted. This surgical principle provides for a well-vascularized anastomotic site and in itself will reduce the risk of ureteral stricture after take-down.

Pyelostomy

If a large and redundant renal pelvis is present in a child in whom temporizing cutaneous diversion is thought to be appropriate, pyelostomy has one inherent advantage over loop ureterostomy—that is, at the time of reconstruction, a formal ureteroureterostomy will not be necessary. Presumably, pyelostomy would be considered in a child with a lower ureteral or infravesical problem in whom the renal pelvis is large and pliable. After the primary pathology is corrected, the pyelostomy stoma simply can be ellipsed and closed primarily, and the child does not incur the risk of an anastomotic stricture that might occur with the ureteroureterostomy necessary at take-down of a loop ureterostomy.

Stomal stenosis of the pyelostomy can occur as it does with any cutaneous anastomosis. Revision of the stoma may then become necessary, although I would suggest that if revision is necessary, one might consider proceeding with primary total reconstruction of the infant at that time. Another problem that occasionally can occur with pyelostomy is prolapse through the pyelostomy stoma. With a very large and floppy renal pelvis, especially if the kidney is thinned and very mobile, prolapse of the entire pelvis and part of the kidney can occur if the stoma is made too large.

Summary

In summary, cutaneous diversions, whether they be vesicostomy, ureterostomy, or pyelostomy, are circumferential openings that are at risk of undergoing cicatri-

cial stenosis. Most often, this will be found either at the level of the external oblique fascia or at the level of the skin. If the stenosis is superficial, an inlay of a small skin flap is all that is usually necessary. If it is deeper, a formal revision of the stoma may be indicated. Since the bladder and the renal pelvis are partially peritonealized, cutaneous openings of either of these structures also may allow prolapse to occur. In the bladder in particular, prolapse is best avoided by proper placement of the vesicostomy stoma. For pyelostomy, the size of the stoma seems to be the best way to avoid troublesome prolapse. However, indications for performing these procedures today are very limited.

A well-functioning temporary diversion is generally taken down electively and when the overall medical situation seems ideal. However, should a complication occur in an existing diversion, it is appropriate today, considering the major advances in primary total reconstruction of the urinary tract, to proceed to definitive repair rather than to correct the complication of the cutaneous diversion.

Bibliography

Blocksom, BH. Bladder pouch for prolonged tubeless cystotomy. J Urol 78:398, 1957.

Bruce, R, and Gonzales, ET. Cutaneous vesicostomy: A useful form of temporary diversion in children. J Urol 123:927, 1980.

Burstein, JD, and Firlit, CF. Complications of cutaneous ureterostomy and other cutaneous diversion. Urol Clin North Am 10:433, 1983.

Deane, AM, Whitaker, RH, and Sherwood, T. Diathermy hook ablations of posterior urethral valves in neonates and infants. Br J Urol 62:593, 1988.

Decter, RM, and Gonzales, ET. Bladder augmentation in the pediatric age group. J Urol 94:91, 1988.

Duckett, JW. Cutaneous vesicostomy in childhood: The Blocksom technique. Urol Clin North Am 1:485, 1974.

Dykes, EH, Duffy, PG, and Ransley, PG. The use of the Mitrofanoff principle in achieving clean intermittent catheterization and urinary continence in children. J Pediatr Surg 26:535, 1991.

Hurwitz, RS, and Ehrlich, RM. Complications of cutaneous vesicostomy in children. Urol Clin North Am 10:503, 1983.

Johnston, JH. Temporary cutaneous ureterostomy in the management of advanced congenital urinary obstruction. Arch Dis Child 38:161, 1963.

Kogan, BA, and Gohary, MA. Cutaneous ureterostomy as a permanent external urinary diversion in children. J Urol 132:729, 1984.

Kropp, KA, and Angwafo, FF. Urethral lengthening and reimplantation for neurogenic incontinence in children. J Urol 135:533, 1986.

Krueger, RP, Hardy, BE, and Churchill, BM. Growth in boys with posterior urethral valves. Urol Clin North Am 7:265, 1980.

Lapides, J, et al. Further observations on self-catheterization. J Urol 116:169, 1976.

MacGregor, PS, Kay, R, and Straffon, RA. Cutaneous ureterostomy in children—long term follow-up. J Urol 134:518, 1985.

Perlmutter, AD. Temporary urinary diversion in the management of the chronically dilated urinary tract in childhood. In JH Johnston and WE Goodwin (eds), Reviews in Pediatric Urology. Amsterdam: Excerpta Medica, 1974, p 447.

Sober, I. Pelvioureterostomy-en-Y. Urology 107:473, 1972.

Williams, DJ, and Cromie, WJ. Ring ureterostomy. Br J Urol 47:789, 1975.

Zaontz, MR, and Firlit, CF. Percutaneous antegrade ablation of posterior urethral valves in premature or underweight term neonates: an alternative to primary vesicostomy. J Urol 134:139, 1985.

Index